Magic
Foods

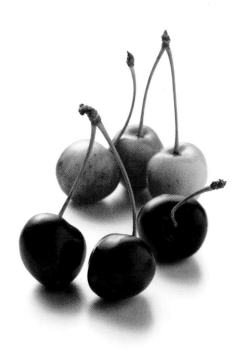

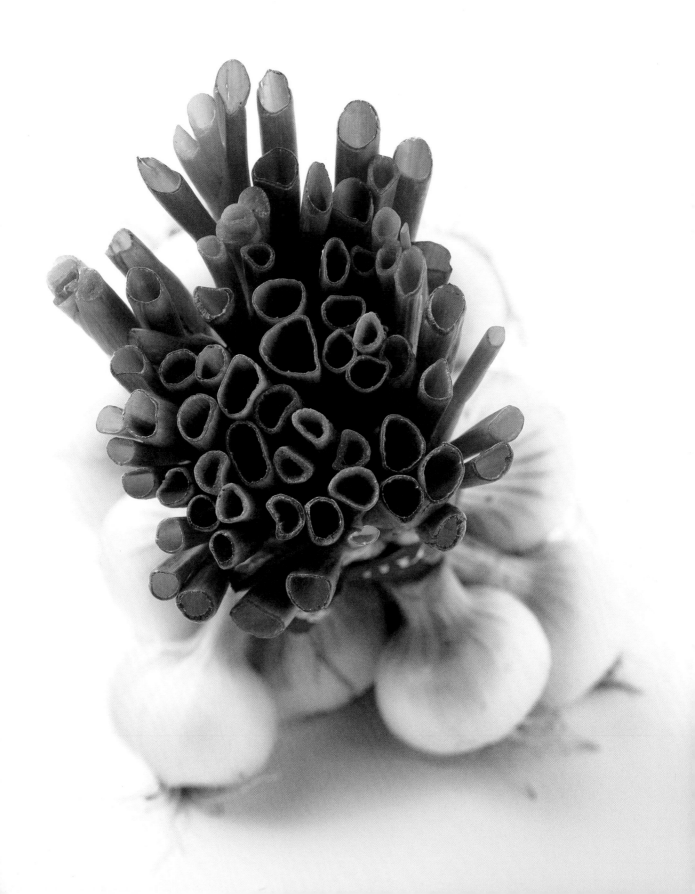

Magic Foods

Live Longer,
Supercharge Your Energy, Lose Weight,
and Stop Cravings

Reader's Digest

The Reader's Digest Association, Inc.
Pleasantville, New York | Montreal

First printing in paperback 2008

Copyright ©2007 by The Reader's Digest Association, Inc.

First published as *Magic Foods for Better Blood Sugar* in 2007

Library of Congress Cataloging-in-Publication Data
Magic foods for better blood sugar / [editor, Marianne Wait].
       p. cm.
Includes index.

ISBN 978-0-7621-0755-1 (hardcover)
ISBN 978-0-7621-0895-4 (paperback)

1. Nutrition—Popular works. 2. Food—Composition—Popular works.
3. Blood sugar—Popular works. I. Wait, Marianne, 1967-

RA784.M285 2006

613.2—dc22

2006026505

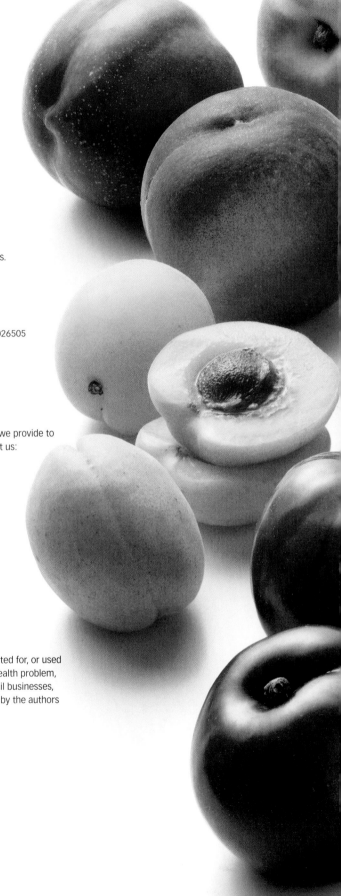

Photography: Elizabeth Watt *(Food Stylist: Anne Disrude);*
D. A. Croll; Food Collection; Getty Images:Digital Vision, PhotoAlto,
Photodisc, Stockbyte

We are committed to both the quality of our products and the service we provide to our customers. We value your comments, so please feel free to contact us:

The Reader's Digest Association, Inc.
Editor-in-Chief, Reader's Digest Books
Reader's Digest Road
Pleasantville, NY 10570-7000

For more Reader's Digest products and information, visit our website:
www.rd.com (in the United States)
www.readersdigest.ca (in Canada)

Printed in the United States

10   (hardcover)
5 7 9 10 8 6 4   (paperback)

Note to Readers: The information in this book should not be substituted for, or used to alter, medical therapy without your doctor's advice. For a specific health problem, consult your physician for guidance. The mention of any products, retail businesses, or websites in this book does not imply or constitute an endorsement by the authors or by the Reader's Digest Association, Inc.

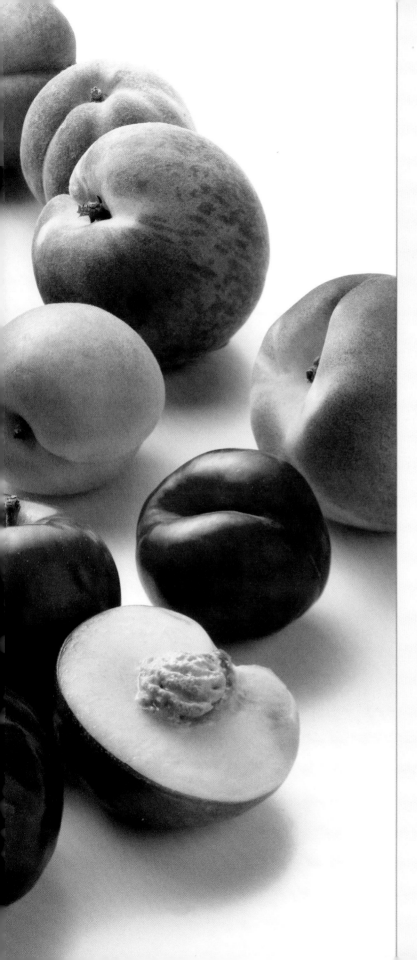

Project Staff

Editor
Marianne Wait

Senior Art Director
Elizabeth Tunnicliffe

Cover Design
Michele Laseau

Cover Photography
Elizabeth Watt

Contributing Editors
Pamela Johnson
Robert Ronald

Writers
Robert A. Barnett
Densie Webb, Ph.D., R.D.

Production Associate
Erick Swindell

Copy Editors
Jane Sherman
Marcia Mangum Cronin

Indexer
Nanette Bendyna

Consultants

Chief Nutrition Advisor
Christine L. Pelkman, Ph.D.
Assistant Professor of Nutrition
State University of New York at Buffalo

Nutrition Advisor
Brandia Joy Freiman, M.S., R.D.
Clinical Nutrition Instructor
State University of New York at Buffalo

Recipe Developer
Patsy Jamieson

Reader's Digest Home & Health Books

President, Home & Garden and Health & Wellness
Alyce Alston

Editor in Chief
Neil Wertheimer

Creative Director
Michele Laseau

Executive Managing Editor
Donna Ruvituso

Associate Director, North America Prepress
Douglas A. Croll

Manufacturing Manager
John L. Cassidy

Marketing Director
Dawn Nelson

Reader's Digest Association, Inc.

President and Chief Executive Officer
Mary Berner

President, Consumer Marketing
Dawn Zier

Reader's Digest Association (Canada) Ltd.

Vice President, Book Editorial
Robert Goyette

contents

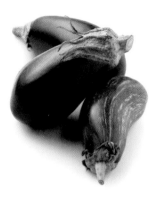 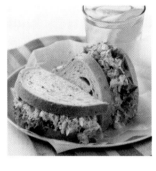 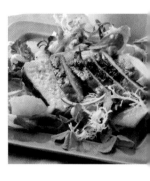 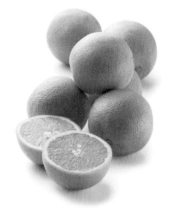

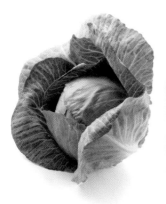
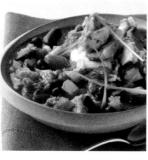
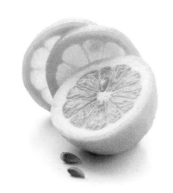
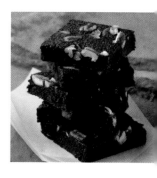

A major health crisis is emerging, one that most doctors are just beginning to recognize. You may never have heard of it, but it could very well be affecting how you feel right this minute. It's not heart disease, diabetes, or obesity, although it's linked to all three. It's out-of-control blood sugar, and you may have it without even knowing it.

Chalk it up to our modern-day diets, which are loaded with foods that send blood sugar soaring, only to crash in short order. When the crash comes, you may feel listless, irritable, headachy— and ravenously, must-eat-something-sugary-this-minute hungry. Riding this blood sugar rollercoaster is a sure way to send your hunger up, your energy down, and your waistline *out*.

introduction Magic Foods

Our love affair with sugar-raising foods, especially "white" foods such as white bread, white rice, French fries, and sugary baked goods, has led to an outbreak of insulin resistance—essentially, what happens when the body's system for handling blood sugar spikes gets worn out from overwork. Insulin resistance is linked to serious problems ranging from heart disease and memory loss to—you guessed it—diabetes. About 25 percent of adults have it. If you're overweight and over 45, the chances that you have it are nearly one in two.

Fortunately, insulin resistance is reversible. If eating the wrong foods can cause it, eating the right ones can cure it. And it's not that hard to do. We designed this book to help you get off the blood sugar rollercoaster—without turning your diet upside down.

In *Magic Foods for Better Blood Sugar,* you won't find strict eating regimens or crazy rules about carbohydrates. What you will find are 57 foods that can help you nudge your diet into sugar-friendly territory. Add just one to your plate (for instance, try barley instead of white rice), and you could see results right away. Add a few more (like avocados, which contain fats that actually improve insulin sensitivity), and you'll really be on the road to feeling better and staving off killer diseases.

Even if you already have diabetes, these strategies can help make your cells more sensitive to insulin and keep blood sugar swings in check.

You can still eat steak, if you keep it lean, as well as pasta and other carbohydrate foods if you choose the right ones (whole grains actually reduce your diabetes risk). We'll also show you how adding a few "secret ingredients" like cinnamon and vinegar to your dishes can yield amazing results.

Magic Foods is based on the latest nutrition science, but it's designed for regular folks like you who just want to know what to eat. For instance, you won't have to look up numbers before you choose a food. Our recipes, meal makeovers, meal plans, and cooks tips make it incredibly simple to get more of the 57 Magic foods onto your plate. Your meals will still taste delicious—and they'll leave you more satisfied, so you won't be hunting around for something else to eat.

At Reader's Digest, we take your health to heart. Here's something you can do to rein in insulin resistance, offload dangerous belly fat, guard yourself from diabetes (or help reverse it), and feel more fully charged and ready to embrace life every day. Don't wait for your doctor to say you have a problem. Turn the page now and start discovering the good foods and fun tools that await you.

Marianne Wait
Senior Health Editor
Reader's Digest Books

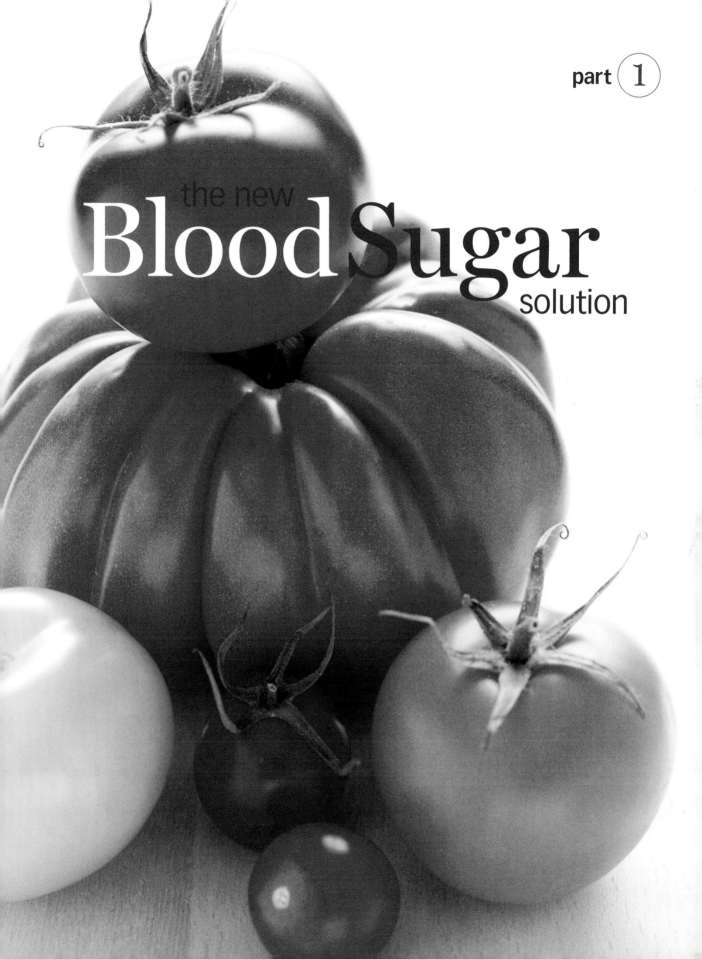

the new
Blood Sugar
solution

chapter 1

THE NATION'S SECRET
✳healthCRISIS

If you're like most people, you've probably never given your blood sugar a second thought unless you have diabetes. But doctors and researchers have recently discovered a shocking truth: If your blood sugar levels regularly soar and crash like a radio-controlled airplane, your body may sustain damage, just as the model plane does over time. Of course, in your case, the damage will occur on the inside, where you can't see it. The consequences, like low energy or weight gain, can be bothersome—or they can be deadly.

It's no longer just certain people who need to worry about their **blood sugar.** It's pretty much everyone.

Whether or not you have diabetes, a diet loaded with foods that send blood sugar up high and down low can jack up your risk of heart disease by damaging your blood vessels and raising your cholesterol. It may even chip away at your memory and increase the risk of certain cancers. You may not notice a problem, but that doesn't mean it's not there. You may have started on a path that can shave years off your life.

This realization is nothing short of a revolution in the way we understand diet and health. Fortunately, none of the damage happens overnight, and even modest changes in the foods you eat every day can start you on a healthier path and make you feel more alert, alive, and energized right away.

The Lure of "Fast-Acting" Foods

When you need a quick pick-me-up, what do you reach for? Maybe a candy bar, a handful of crackers or pretzels, or a box of raisins. It makes sense. These "fast-acting" foods take no time at all to dissolve in your stomach. Quick as light, they race into your bloodstream, flooding your body with blood sugar (glucose), and you're raring to go! The trouble is, the surge doesn't last long. In fact, it's over just as quickly as it started, leaving you feeling worse off than before—and hungry again well before your next mealtime.

Without knowing it, you may even be starting your day with foods that fizzle out in a hurry, leaving you in a slump. Think back to the last time you ate a bagel for breakfast, or a bowl of cornflakes, frozen waffles with syrup, or white toast with jam. You probably felt fine at first, but later in the morning, you may have noticed your energy level beginning to sink. Maybe you started to get irritable. Once your energy hit bottom, you may have found yourself hungry again—no, starving! So naturally, you ate a big lunch and probably a fast-acting one to boot: maybe a sandwich on a white roll the size of a softball, with a few handfuls of pretzels, a large soda or fruity drink to wash them down, and a cookie (or two) for dessert. And the cycle started over again.

Unfortunately, our diets are chock-full of foods that send us for a wild ride on the blood sugar rollercoaster. It's no wonder most of us have less energy than we'd like and feel listless too often.

It's also no wonder most of us weigh more than we want to. Yes, eating too much and exercising too little get the lion's share of the blame, but the blood sugar rollercoaster contributes by setting in motion a chain of events that eventually sends you shopping for "fat jeans."

Sound bad? Low energy and weight gain are only the tip of the iceberg in terms of what happens when your blood sugar swings high and low.

High blood sugar after meals can, over time, **damage** the body, even if it **NEVER** causes diabetes.

Why Blood Sugar Matters

For most of us, even when blood sugar skyrockets after a big meal, our bodies can bring it back to normal in a few hours with no problem. Only people with untreated diabetes have blood sugar levels that stay quite high most of the time. Thus, for a long time, doctors thought that only those people needed to be concerned about the effect of food on blood sugar.

Now we know that even in healthy people, high blood sugar after meals can, over time, damage the body, *even if it never causes diabetes*.

In short, it's no longer just certain people who need to worry about their blood sugar; it's pretty much everyone. It should concern you even if you're thin and healthy, and especially if you don't get much exercise (does that describe you? It describes most people) or you carry extra weight around your middle.

By now you're wondering, "How can I get off the rollercoaster?" Take heart: It's not that difficult—and the book you're holding will show you how. Later, we'll get into much more detail about how our diets contribute to unstable blood sugar (hint: foods like white bread, white rice, potatoes, and sugary drinks are major culprits)

Health Effects of Fast-Acting Foods

Diets full of fast-acting carbs like these send blood sugar on a wild ride, which wreaks havoc on the body.

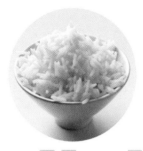
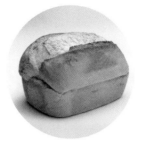
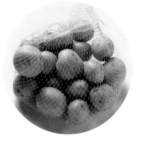

diabetes memory loss

low energy

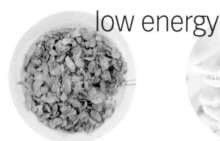
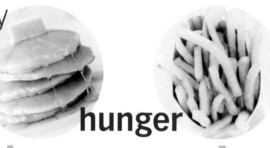

hunger

weight gain

fatigue

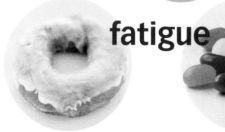
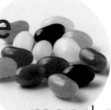
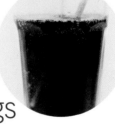

mood swings

heart attacks

and which foods can help solve the problem. But for now, let's take a deeper look at why you should care and how you stand to benefit from this book.

Energy and Weight Gain

Eating makes you feel full, right? Well, actually, that depends.

When you eat a big meal, especially one with a lot of starchy or sugary foods, the food makes its way through your stomach and intestines and then is converted into glucose, the main fuel for your muscles and even your brain. Voilá, instant energy!

But a big starchy meal can give the body more glucose than it needs. In fact, it can raise blood sugar levels twice as much as another, healthier meal would.

Most people's bodies can bring blood sugar down fairly quickly, within an hour or two of eating. The body does this by releasing insulin, a hormone produced by beta cells in the pancreas. Insulin signals the body to let that blood sugar into cells to use as fuel and to store the rest in the muscles.

But if you eat a huge pile of French fries or a big piece of bread, your body has to deal with a serious flood of blood sugar, so it overreacts, pumping out too much insulin. If you're overweight, it may pump out even more. All that extra insulin brings blood sugar down—too far. And it hangs around a long time, keeping your blood sugar low for hours. As a result, you can fall into a semi-starved state. Indeed, your blood sugar may be even lower than it was before you ate! Now you're really dragging. Your energy is low. You may get a headache.

Your body recognizes that your blood sugar is too low, so it reverses course, spewing out hormones that raise blood levels of sugars and fats (the kind that could trigger a heart attack). Your brain also sets in motion signals that tell you that you're hungry. Even though you ate more

calories at lunch than you really needed, your blood sugar is so low that your body thinks it needs more food. Those doughnuts in the conference room sure look attractive right now.

MEALS THAT MAKE YOU HUNGRY

It's not just low blood sugar but also rapidly falling blood sugar that triggers a powerful hunger signal. In 16 studies, 15 of them found that meals that raise blood sugar quickly resulted in feeling hungrier before the next meal. For example, in a study of 65 women, those whose meals were designed to keep blood sugar stable reported feeling less intense hunger and less desire to eat, especially during the afternoon.

These kinds of meals increase levels of leptin, a hormone that decreases hunger (and boosts fat burning) and lowers levels of ghrelin, a hormone that increases hunger. The women who ate blood sugar–boosting meals reported that they felt hungrier sooner.

In many studies, people who ate such meals also ate more at the next meal. In a study of overweight teenage boys, the boys ate 500 more calories within 5 hours after eating blood sugar–boosting breakfasts and lunches than they did when they ate meals that were kinder to their blood sugar. In other studies, the differences were more modest, about 150 calories. Still, eating even 100 extra calories a day may mean the difference between losing weight and gaining it.

Now, you can lose weight on any diet that cuts calories. But losing is only half the battle—and often, it's the easiest part. Sticking to a healthy eating plan that lets you keep the weight off is the hard part. Eating plenty of Magic foods is a key solution.

A MOMENT ON THE LIPS …

When you eat a meal that really bumps up your blood sugar, your body pumps out lots of insulin to bring it down, as you've just learned. But it also stops burning fat for fuel so it can use up the blood sugar instead. Your belly (or butt or thighs) pays the price. People whose diets boost blood sugar the most tend to have more body fat, especially around the abdomen, the most dangerous place for it to accumulate.

Getting off the blood sugar rollercoaster can make losing that spare tire a lot easier. In studies involving everyone from obese men to pregnant women to children, a blood sugar–stabilizing diet led to more body fat loss (or, in the case of the pregnant women, less body fat gain during the pregnancy).

> People whose diets boost blood sugar the most tend to have more **body fat,** especially around the **ABDOMEN.**

In a cruel twist of fate, a diet that causes your blood sugar to spike and dive may even slow your metabolism. Compared to a diet that keeps blood sugar levels stable, it reduces the rate at which you burn calories when you're sitting still. In a study of 39 over-weight men and women, the difference worked out to about 80 extra calories burned each day. That's an extra pound (0.5 kg) lost about every six weeks, or more than 8 pounds (3.5 kg) a year. The more overweight you are, the greater the difference may be.

A Threat to Your Heart

It's fairly easy to imagine how a diet that's rough on your blood sugar can contribute to weight gain. It's a little harder to understand how it can also contribute to a heart attack—yet it can. It can lead to clogged arteries and higher blood pressure, and it can raise the level of inflammation in the body, which doctors now know is intimately connected with heart attack risk.

High blood sugar produces unstable forms of oxygen called free radicals. These nasty molecules damage the arteries, making it harder for blood vessels to do their job of keeping blood pressure normal and making cholesterol more likely to stick like glue to artery walls.

The high levels of insulin that your body needs to tame all this blood sugar are pretty nasty, too.

BLOOD SUGAR UPS AND DOWNS

All carbs raise blood sugar. But some carb foods, like white potatoes and white rice, raise it higher and faster than others, like sweet potatoes and barley. Higher peaks mean steeper drops—your blood sugar may sink lower than before you ate— and that's when energy stalls and hunger strikes anew.

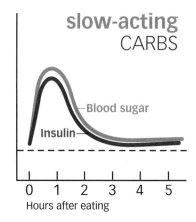

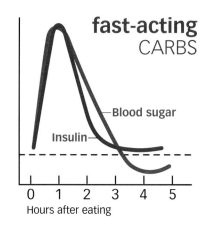

They can set in motion changes that raise blood pressure, make blood more likely to form heart-threatening clots, and increase inflammation—all of which raise your heart disease risk.

Over time, meals that cause blood sugar to spike also tend to lower "good" HDL cholesterol and raise triglycerides, fats that are toxic to cells, increasing the risk of heart disease—and of sudden cardiac arrest.

Big major studies have shown how powerful these damaging effects can be to the heart. In a study of more than 43,000 men age 40 and older, those whose diets boosted blood sugar the most were 37 percent more likely to develop heart disease in the following 6 years. In the Nurses' Health Study of more than 75,000 middle-aged women, those whose diets boosted blood sugar the most were twice as likely to develop heart disease over 10 years. For overweight women, such a diet was even more threatening. For instance, their triglycerides were 144 percent higher than those of women who ate a healthier diet, compared to 40 percent higher for women who weren't overweight.

Fortunately, the phenomenon works in reverse, too: The kinder your meals are to your blood sugar, the kinder they'll be to your heart. Several studies have found that people who ate the fewest blood sugar–boosting foods had higher levels of HDL cholesterol, lower triglycerides, and fewer heart attacks.

The Cancer Connection

It's even harder to imagine how seesawing blood sugar levels could possibly lead to cancer, but high insulin levels seem to promote an environment that makes it easier for certain tumors to grow. Research is still ongoing, and, unlike with heart disease and diabetes, it's too early to make strong statements about the connection between blood sugar levels and cancer. But there is cause for concern with the following cancers.

Colon and rectal cancer. In the Health Professionals Follow-up Study conducted by the Harvard School of Public Health and involving more than 50,000 middle-aged men, those whose diets were most likely to raise blood sugar fast and high were 32 percent more likely to develop colon or rectal cancer over 20 years. The heavier the men, the stronger the effect. In the Women's Health Study, funded in part by the U.S. National Cancer Institute, the rise in cancer risk was an astounding 185 percent higher over 8 years.

Breast cancer. In the Women's Health Study, sedentary women who followed a blood sugar–boosting diet were 135 percent more likely to develop breast cancer over seven years than women whose diets were more blood sugar friendly. These women had not yet entered menopause. On the other hand, a Canadian study of nearly 50,000 women found no link to breast cancer before premenopause, but among postmenopausal women, there was an 87 percent increase in breast cancer risk—and it was even higher if the women did little or no vigorous exercise. A Mexican study comparing women who got breast cancer with those who didn't found the risk was 62 percent greater with blood sugar–boosting diets. A similar Italian study found an 18 percent increase.

Endometrial cancer. In the Iowa Women's Health Study, which involved more than 23,000 postmenopausal women, those who didn't have diabetes and followed blood sugar–spiking diets were 46 percent more likely to get this cancer over 15 years. An Italian study that compared women who developed endometrial cancer with a similar group of women who didn't found a 110 percent increase in risk linked to this type of diet.

Prostate cancer. An Italian study looked at men ages 46 to 74 who developed prostate cancer and compared their diets with those of a similar group of men who didn't get the cancer. Those whose diets were most likely to spike blood sugar were 57 percent more likely to have prostate cancer. A similar Canadian study found a 57 percent increase in risk.

Pancreatic cancer. Even the organ that produces insulin may be more prone to cancer if it's constantly bathed in that hormone. A study using data from the Nurses' Health Study over 18 years found that women whose diets raised blood sugar the most were 53 percent more likely to develop pancreatic cancer than women whose diets raised it the least. Women in the first group who were overweight and physically inactive were 157 percent more likely to get the cancer than similar women in the second.

The Mood and Memory Connection

We began this chapter by showing how a meal that raises blood sugar fast and furiously can leave you dragging like a willow in a windstorm. Not surprisingly, it doesn't do much for your mood, either.

Our moods are intimately affected by the levels of hormones in our systems, including the hormone insulin. These hormones in turn affect neurotransmitters, chemical messengers in the brain. The different types of nutrients we eat, including carbohydrate and protein, affect these transmitters differently, triggering drowsiness or alertness. But the brain may be most sensitive to one simple compound: blood sugar.

Unlike muscles, the brain can't store sugar. It needs just the right amount of it at all times to function best, so it's not surprising that it's very sensitive to even very small differences in the amount of blood sugar available. A steady supply—which the foods in this book will help you achieve—is by far the best.

Both low and high levels of blood sugar can cause trouble when it comes to your mood and memory. People report feeling more symptoms of depression when their blood sugar is low. Memory is affected, too. In one study, people with diabetes had more trouble processing information, remembering things, and paying attention—besides being in a bad mood—when their blood sugar was low. In people with type 2 diabetes, blood sugar swings are linked not only with poor memory but also, over time, with cognitive decline and dementia.

High blood sugar levels spell trouble, too. Long before they cause diabetes, they can impair the brain, shrinking a part that stores memories and increasing the risk of Alzheimer's disease. In one study at New York University, researchers found that in people who tended to have high blood sugar levels after meals, a part of the brain called the hippocampus, which is most associated with long-term memory, was smaller than in people whose postmeal blood sugar levels were lower.

On the positive side, keeping your blood sugar on an even keel can help you feel better and stay mentally sharp. People with diabetes who control their blood sugar well report better moods, less depression, and less fatigue than those who don't. Careful studies have found that the better they control their blood sugar, the better they are able to recall a paragraph after reading it and to remember words from a list.

In general, eating a good breakfast is the best way for anyone to improve mental functioning later in the day. Studies regularly show that eating breakfast improves mood, mental alertness, concentration, and memory. Eating the *right* breakfast, one that keeps blood sugar on an even keel until lunch, is likely to work even better.

The Road to Diabetes

Perhaps the worst thing about eating meals heavy on fast-acting foods is that over time, they can greatly increase your risk of type 2 diabetes, the kind that's related to lifestyle. In type 2 diabetes—which we'll just call diabetes from now on—your body can't make enough insulin to keep your blood sugar levels under control.

In major long-term studies, eating fast-acting meals increased the risk of diabetes by 40 percent in middle-aged men and by a whopping 50 percent in middle-aged women. Fortunately, it doesn't happen overnight. It's not as if you eat a jelly doughnut on Tuesday and wake up with diabetes on Wednesday. It takes years, even decades, for your body to get to the point where it can't keep blood sugar under control on its own.

Most of us, though, are headed in the wrong direction.

The good news is that the slow journey toward diabetes can be redirected *at any point along the path*. The earlier you start, of course, the easier and more effectively you can change direction. Eating meals that are gentler to your blood sugar is key.

Insulin Resistance: A Growing Epidemic

Ever strip a screw when you're in the midst of a do-it-yourself project? Suddenly, you need to use real elbow grease to turn it just a little bit. And the more it gets stripped, the harder it is to turn.

Your body can be a little like that. The more foods you eat that spike your blood sugar, the more insulin your body has to pump out to handle the load. Over time, repeated surges of insulin can strip your cells' insulin receptors, figuratively speaking, so they don't work as well, and the insulin can't be used as efficiently. When that happens, your body has to pump out more insulin to do the same job. This condition is called insulin resistance.

In the West, where the mega-meal and the electric recliner are all too pervasive, insulin resistance is increasingly common. About 25 percent of adults have it. And if you're overweight and over 45, the chances that you have it are nearly one in two. You're much more likely to develop insulin resistance if you're overweight and sedentary.

fighting
INSULIN RESISTANCE

Eating foods that keep blood sugar levels stable is key to preventing or reversing insulin resistance. To further help your cause, take these steps.

exercise Even if you don't lose weight, exercising reduces insulin resistance. In one study, spending 30 minutes on a stationary bike three or four times a week cut insulin levels by 20 percent while lowering blood sugar levels by 13 percent—enough to take someone from "prediabetes" to "normal."

cut calories Simply eating less, even before you lose any weight, can improve insulin sensitivity and reduce levels of circulating insulin (your body needs less insulin if it's more sensitive to it). In one study of sedentary men and women, eating 25 percent fewer calories than they were used to over six months resulted in significantly lower fasting insulin levels. Other studies have found that cutting calories improves insulin sensitivity.

get enough sleep Missing out on a full night's sleep increases insulin resistance, possibly by disturbing hormone balance. Doing so for years may increase the risk of developing diabetes. In a recent study of men, those who slept less than 6 hours a night were twice as likely to develop diabetes over the following 15 years compared to men who got about 7 hours a night. (Those who got more than 8 hours a night were also at higher risk.)

do you have metabolic syndrome?

quiz

Metabolic syndrome is a cluster of risk factors that often occur together and increase your risk of diabetes and heart disease. The U.S. National Institute of Health's National Cholesterol Education Program defines it by looking at five measurements, four of which any doctor can test you to determine (the first one, waist size, you can find yourself).

Once you know your numbers, take this test.

○ **Waist size.** Check this box if yours is more than 40 inches (102 cm) for men or more than 35 inches (88 cm) for women.

○ **Triglycerides.** A normal level is below 150 mg/dL (1.70 mmol/L)*. Check this box if yours is 150 mg/dL (1.70 mmol/L) or higher.

○ **HDL cholesterol.** This is the "good" cholesterol, so a higher number is better. Check this box if yours is lower than 40 mg/dL (1.00 mmol/L) for men or 50 mg/dL (1.30 mmol/L) for women.

○ **Blood pressure.** A normal level is less than 120/80 mm/Hg. Check this box if yours is 130/85 mm/Hg or higher.

○ **Fasting blood glucose.** This is the level of blood sugar after you haven't eaten for 6 hours. A normal level is 70 to 100 mg/dL (4.0 to 5.5 mmol/L). Check this box if yours is 110 mg/dL (6.0 mmol/L) or higher.

your score
Total **how many boxes** you checked, then find your results here.

0 Congratulations; you have no signs of metabolic syndrome. Keep up the good work.

1 You don't have metabolic syndrome, but each of these is an independent risk factor for heart disease, so you should still take action.

2 You don't have metabolic syndrome, but these risk factors intensify each other, so work with your doctor to remedy them.

3 You have metabolic syndrome. You are at increased risk of developing diabetes and heart disease in the years ahead, but you can reverse the trend by losing weight, getting more exercise, and eating better. Talk with your doctor about ways to reduce your risk factors. The dietary approach outlined in this book is particularly important to you.

4 You have metabolic syndrome and then some—the more risk factors you have, the greater your overall risk. Get medical help and follow the dietary approach in this book.

5 You have metabolic syndrome and are at very high risk of developing diabetes and heart disease. Talk to your doctor and follow the recommendations in this book.

Canada measures blood glucose, blood cholesterol, and triglycerides by millimole per liter (mmol/L). The milligram per deciliter (mg/dL) method is the U.S. standard.

If you have insulin resistance, your blood sugar levels may still be normal, although they may be on the high side after meals. You don't have diabetes—yet. But you are going in a direction that's putting a lot of stress on your blood sugar control system, and you're doing some damage along the way.

The extra insulin your body has to churn out can raise blood pressure, cause cholesterol problems, and even make it easier for certain cancers to grow. It also paves the way for weight gain. And here's a real scare: There's growing evidence that the brain itself can become insulin resistant, which impairs the function of nerves and leads to the buildup of toxic deposits, increasing the risk of dementia, including Alzheimer's disease.

And of course, insulin resistance increases the risk of diabetes. High blood sugar and extra insulin can damage the beta cells in the pancreas—the ones that make insulin—so they become fatigued or die off. When that happens, you have diabetes.

Insulin resistance starts slowly, furtively, silently. It has no symptoms. But once you develop it, it's easier to become even *more* insulin resistant. In a vicious cycle, the more insulin your body has to produce to keep blood sugar down, the more insulin resistant you become—unless you do something to reverse the trend. Fortunately, changing your eating style to include more of the slow-acting foods in this book is one of the biggest keys to preventing or reversing the condition. (For other ways, see "Fighting Insulin Resistance" on page 17.)

Metabolic Syndrome: The Kitchen Sink of Conditions

Insulin resistance on its own can be dangerous, as you've just discovered. But there's worse news: If you have it, you may also have a host of related problems that tend to cluster together like birds on a telephone wire. Each of these problems on its own raises your risk of heart disease, but if you have three or more of them, your risk is double what it would be if you had only one. You're practically a heart attack waiting to happen, *even if your levels of "bad" LDL cholesterol are normal.*

This cluster of problems is known as metabolic syndrome. If you have this condition, you're also an excellent candidate for diabetes, even if your blood sugar levels aren't high yet. Indeed, 85 percent of people with type 2 diabetes have metabolic syndrome.

If you have **metabolic syndrome,** you're an excellent candidate for **DIABETES,** even if your blood sugar levels aren't high yet.

Metabolic syndrome is incredibly common here, affecting about one in four adults. Anyone can develop it, but you're much more likely to get it as you get older. In one large study of men and women age 50 and older, 44 percent had it. If you're carrying extra pounds, you're even more likely to have it.

Getting older, gaining weight, and being sedentary all contribute to the syndrome, but in many ways, this is a condition that you eat your way into. Diets low in fiber, high in calories, full of saturated fat, and loaded with foods that boost blood sugar quickly all contribute. In the Framingham Heart Study, one of the longest and largest studies of diet and disease, people whose diets tended to send blood sugar the highest after meals were 40 percent more likely to have metabolic syndrome than those who usually ate foods like the ones in this book.

According to the U.S. National Institute of Health's National Cholesterol Education Program, you have the syndrome if you have three or more of these problems.

Belly fat. A big belly isn't just somewhere you've put on extra weight. From your body's standpoint, fat around the middle is a very different kind of fat than, say, fat on your thighs. It's easier for this kind of fat to get into the bloodstream, where it can wreak havoc and increase the risk of heart disease. Indeed, researchers now suspect a large waist may be a better marker for heart disease risk than being overweight or obese in general.

High triglyceride levels. These fats are stored in the blood, ready to be broken down for energy. Even a mild elevation can increase your risk of heart disease.

Low HDL cholesterol levels. You've probably heard a lot of talk about "good" HDL cholesterol. It's the kind your body uses to pull "bad" LDL cholesterol out of the blood and transport it back to the liver, where it's broken down. Levels of HDL are often low in people with metabolic syndrome.

High blood pressure. Blood pressure is also often elevated in metabolic syndrome. It may not be high enough for your doctor to diagnose you as having high blood pressure, but along with the other factors, it's bad for your heart.

do you have prediabetes?

quiz

Only a blood glucose test can tell for sure. If your fasting blood glucose level is between 100 and 125 mg/dL (5.5 and 7.0 mmol/L), you have prediabetes. (Some doctors prefer a different test, given after you've had a sugar-rich drink.)

Should you ask your doctor to test you?
Here's how to decide.

◯ If you're **45 or older,** consider being tested.

◯ If you're **45 or older and overweight,** it's strongly recommended that you be tested.

◯ If you're **younger than 45 and overweight,** consider being tested if you also have one or more of these risk factors.

● You have a parent, brother, or sister with diabetes.

● Your ancestry is African, Asian, Native American, Native Canadian, Pacific Island, or Spanish.

● You're a mom who has had at least one baby weighing 9 pounds (4 kg) or more at birth, or you had gestational diabetes when you were pregnant.

● Your blood pressure is 140/90 mm/Hg or higher, or you've been told you have high blood pressure.

● Your cholesterol levels aren't normal: Your HDL cholesterol is 35 mg/dL (0.90 mmol/L) or lower, or your triglycerides are 250 mg/dL (2.80 mmol/L) or higher.

● You are fairly inactive, or you exercise less than three times a week.

Some of these numbers, such as those for blood pressure and HDL, are different from those in the quiz for metabolic syndrome. One reason is that borderline risk factors become more significant when they're combined, as they are in metabolic syndrome.

High fasting glucose levels. Your blood sugar may not be high enough to qualify you as having diabetes, but it still increases your risk of developing both diabetes and heart disease. The cause is insulin resistance.

Prediabetes

Even if you have insulin resistance and metabolic syndrome, a test of your blood sugar in a doctor's office may show perfectly normal levels. For a while—for years, really—your body may be able to cope with too much blood sugar after meals by pumping out extra insulin.

In some people, though, the insulin-producing beta cells in the pancreas just can't keep up. They become less effective (*exhausted* is the word doctors use), and some of them die. Then your body just can't make enough insulin to keep blood sugar levels under control.

Your blood sugar may be a little high when you wake up in the morning. A normal level after a fast, that is, after 6 hours of not eating anything, is between 70 and 100 milligrams (mg)

do you have diabetes?

quiz

If your blood sugar level after not eating for 6 hours (fasting blood glucose level) is 126 mg/dL (7.0 mmol/L) or higher, you have diabetes. Ideally, you would have been tested when you showed any of the risk factors for prediabetes (see "Do You Have Prediabetes?" on the preceding page), but many people don't find out they have diabetes until they start to have symptoms. That's unfortunate, because even though diabetes may cause no symptoms for years, it's increasing your risk of heart disease, blindness, and nerve problems. The sooner you get your blood sugar levels under control, the better your chances of avoiding these complications.

See your doctor at once if you have any of these symptoms.

○ Increased thirst

○ Increased hunger

○ Fatigue

○ Increased urination, especially at night

○ Weight loss without dieting

○ Blurred vision

○ Sores that don't heal

of glucose for every 10th of a liter (dL) of blood/ 4.0 to 5.5 millimoles (mmol) of glucose for every liter (L) of blood. If yours is between 100 and 125 mg/dL (5.5 and 7.0 mmol/L), you have prediabetes. You don't have full-blown diabetes yet, but you're on the train that takes you there.

Your chances of developing diabetes are very high over the next few years—but you can still get off the train. That was proven in a major study, called the Diabetes Prevention Program, of more than 3,000 men and women in 27 U.S. medical centers. Their ages ranged from 25 to 85, with an average of 51. All were obese. All had prediabetes. About 11 percent of those in the study who did nothing to change their lifestyles went on to develop diabetes in *each year* of the three-year study. That is, about a third got diabetes.

Those who switched to healthier diets and lost weight, however, didn't suffer the same fate. Over three years, they started walking about 30 minutes a day, ate healthier meals, and lost about 15 pounds (7 kg) each. Although some did develop diabetes, there was a 58 percent reduction in the overall incidence of the disease.

Diabetes

If insulin resistance has damaged your pancreas so much that you have prediabetes, and you do nothing to change your lifestyle, it's almost inevitable that you will develop diabetes. Your beta cells are exhausted and just can't produce nearly enough insulin to do their job. Your blood sugar levels are above 125 mg/dL (7.0 mmol/L) even when you wake up in the morning.

The train may have left the station, but you can still get off at the next stop. Your diet is an essential part of your treatment plan. You'll work with your doctor to take the right medication to improve your insulin sensitivity and insulin production. Losing weight, exercising, and choosing foods that are gentle to your blood sugar levels are key to the effectiveness of those medications.

Take this book to your doctor or nutritionist and discuss how to work our recommendations into your lifestyle plan. Working with your doctor, you may be able to reduce the medications you take. In some cases, under medical supervision, you may be able to stop taking them entirely.

The Magic Foods Solution

The nation's secret health crisis—insulin resistance and the closely related threats of diabetes, heart disease, and other health problems—is a secret no more. The way we've been eating affects our moods, our appetite, our weight, and, in the end, our longevity. But once you know what to do, you can make changes without a lot of fuss that will help you feel better and be healthier in the next 20 minutes and the next 20 years.

Magic Foods for Better Blood Sugar isn't a radical diet. It doesn't turn basic nutrition upside down. You'll find many of the same building blocks of a healthy diet here that you've heard about for decades: whole grains, fruits and vegetables, nuts, seeds, beans, eggs, lean meats and poultry, seafood, and low-fat dairy products. But we've improved this time-honored advice to help you keep your blood sugar in balance before, during, and after each meal. And you'll do it with the Magic foods you'll discover in Part 2, the meal makeovers you'll discover in Part 3, and the recipes and meal plans you'll find in Part 4.

The differences between the Magic Foods approach and a basic healthy diet are subtle but powerful. Whether you're young or not so young, thin or not so thin, with normal blood sugar levels or high ones; whether you are insulin resistant or not; and indeed, whether you have diabetes or not, this way of eating can make all the difference in the world to your health. Read on to learn more.

chapter 2

THE hidden EFFECTS OF food

The **glycemic load** is a more powerful factor in keeping you healthy than the amount of carbohydrate—or fat—you eat.

Now you're in on the secret: Most of us are damaging our health by eating too many foods that send our blood sugar soaring. Besides contributing to diabetes and other serious illnesses over the long haul, meals loaded with these foods also leave you tired, grumpy, and hungry again in no time after you eat them. Other foods barely move the blood sugar needle or move it gradually, keeping you feeling full and energized.

Unfortunately, foods don't come with labels explaining which is which. After reading this chapter, though, you'll know how to tell the difference.

In the end, it's as simple as choosing pasta over rice, baked beans instead of mashed potatoes, oil-and-vinegar dressing instead of Thousand Island, and other easy fixes. Read on to discover what makes these foods Magic.

First, we'll talk about the three so-called macronutrients in food—carbohydrate, fat, and protein—from which we get almost all of our calories, and we'll tell you how they affect your blood sugar. Then we'll talk about two "magic" food components you can use for amazingly effective blood sugar control: soluble fiber and acetic acid, found in sour foods.

Carbohydrate

We'll reveal the main plot twist right now: Carbohydrates are the foods that raise blood sugar. Plain and simple, right? The trouble is, not all carb foods are created equal.

Carbohydrates are actually found in most foods except fats and oils, meats, poultry, and fish. But of course, some foods contain more carbs than others. Beans are about one-fourth protein and three-fourths carbohydrate. Rice, on the other hand, is more than 90 percent carbohydrate. Whole milk contains all three macronutrients: fat, protein, and carbohydrate.

It's the quantity of carbohydrate in foods (and of course, how much of the food you eat) that primarily affects blood sugar, but the type of carbohydrate also has an effect.

Introducing the Glycemic Index and Glycemic Load

To figure out which carbs are best and worst for blood sugar, scientists had to do some serious detective work. First, they needed to come up with a way to measure a food's effect on blood sugar.

Nutrition scientist David Jenkins, M.D., Ph.D., developed a system called the glycemic index (GI) back in 1981 (the prefix *glyc-* means "sugar"). He had volunteers eat different foods, all containing 50 grams of carbohydrate. Then he measured the volunteers' blood sugar over the following 2 hours to see how high it went.

As a control he used pure glucose, the form of sugar that's identical to blood sugar—your body converts glucose very quickly to blood sugar—and assigned it the number 100 on his new index.

The glycemic index opened a lot of eyes. Almost everyone had assumed that table sugar would be the worst offender, much worse than the "complex carbohydrates" found in starchy staples such as rice and bread. But this didn't always prove true. Some starchy foods, like potatoes and cornflakes, ranked very high on the index, raising blood sugar nearly as much as pure glucose. That's why you won't see these foods in our list of Magic foods.

The higher the **glycemic load** in the diet, the greater the incidence of obesity, diabetes, heart disease, and cancer.

WHERE THE GLYCEMIC INDEX FELL SHORT

Something was wrong, however. Some of the results pointed fingers at healthy foods, such as carrots and strawberries. Watermelon was just about off the top of the GI chart. But no one ever gained weight from eating carrots, nor do carrots, in the real world, raise blood sugar. What was the GI missing?

The GI measured the effects of a standard amount of carbohydrate: 50 grams, or about 1 1/2 ounces. But you'd be awfully hard-pressed to eat enough carrots—seven or eight large ones—to get 50 grams of carbohydrate. The same holds true for most other vegetables and fruits. They're full of water, so there's not much room in them for carbohydrate. Bread, on the other hand, is crammed with carbohydrate. You get 50 grams by eating just one slice.

To solve the problem, scientists came up with a different measurement: the glycemic load (GL). It takes into account not only the *type* of carbohydrate in the food but also the *amount* of carbohydrate you would eat in a standard serving. (To get a bit technical, a food's GL is the GI multiplied by the amount of carbohydrate in one serving.)

This made more sense. By this criterion, carrots, strawberries, and other low-calorie foods are clearly good to eat—they all have low GL values, since the amount of carbohydrate they contain is low.

The GL has turned out to be a powerful way to think about not just individual foods but also whole meals and even entire diets. When scientists looked at the GL of typical diets in different populations, they found that the higher the GL, the greater the incidence of obesity, diabetes, heart disease, and cancer. You may remember a study we mentioned in Chapter 1 in which men who ate the most sugar-boosting foods were 40 percent more likely to get diabetes. That's GL we were talking about. We also talked about the Nurses' Health Study finding that women were twice as likely to develop heart disease over 10 years if they ate more sugar-boosting foods. Again, the GL. The converse is also true: The lower the GL of your diet, the more likely you are to keep your weight under control and stay free of chronic disease.

When it comes to eating right, controlling weight, and preventing disease, the GL is a heavy hitter. It's a more powerful factor in keeping you healthy than the amount of carbohydrate—or fat—you eat.

What Makes Some Carbs Better than Others

Why would one high-carb food have a different GL than another? Why does white rice, for instance, have a higher GL than, say, honey? It has to do with the way nature constructed them.

Carbohydrates consist of starches and sugars. Starch—think of starchy foods like beans and potatoes—is made up of sugar molecules bound together in long chains. When you eat a carbohydrate-rich food, your body converts those starches and sugars into glucose, or blood sugar. Some starches, like those in white rice, are extremely easy for the body to convert, and therefore blood sugar levels rise like a hot temper after you eat them. Others, like those in beans, take a lot more work to break down, so blood sugar levels simmer rather than explode.

Four factors determine how fast the body breaks down carbohydrate.

CARB DENSITY COUNTS

The glycemic load takes into account how much carbohydrate a serving of food contains. The amount in one bagel equals the amount in five helpings of watermelon.

55 grams of carbohydrate

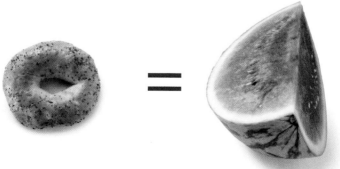

1 bagel   5 cups watermelon

THE TYPE OF STARCH—OR WHY TO AVOID STICKY RICE

Remember, starches are made of sugar molecules chained together. Some chains have straight edges, while others are branched. The straight-edged type, called amylose, is harder for your body to break down and turn into blood sugar. The branched type, called amylopectin, is much easier to break down because there are so many places for the enzymes that break down starch to get at it. Think of a tree with lots of branches—there are a lot more spots for birds to land on it compared to a simple post.

White potatoes are very high in amylopectin, the branched kind of sugar chain, which is why they raise your blood sugar in a jiffy. Peas and lentils are high in amylose, the straight kind, so they're converted to blood sugar at a snail's pace.

The more amylose a food contains, the slower it will be digested and converted into blood sugar. Take rice, for instance. Some types contain more amylose than others. In general, the softer and stickier the rice is after cooking, the lower its amylose content; this is why "sticky rice" is dastardly to your blood sugar. The firmer the rice, the higher the amylose and the harder it is for your body to turn into blood sugar quickly—making brown rice a better choice. Some genetic variants of rice—such as some

sold in Australia, for example—are particularly high in amylose (as much as 25 percent), but unfortunately, most of the rice we eat is low in amylose and thus has a high GL.

THE TYPE OF SUGAR—OR WHY FRUIT IS A-OKAY

Sugar is the molecule that makes up carbohydrates, but there is more than one kind. There's table sugar (sucrose) as well as the kind found in fruits and grains (fructose), the kind in milk (lactose), and the kind in malted barley (maltose). The sugar in milk and fruit tends to be absorbed more slowly than other sugars since it needs to be converted into glucose by the liver first, which is why these foods are gentle to your blood sugar.

Ironically, table sugar, which is half fructose and half glucose, is turned into blood sugar more slowly than some starches, like bread or potatoes. That doesn't make sugar good for you, of course. One reason is that fructose, especially in the amounts contained in packaged foods loaded with high-fructose corn syrup, raise triglycerides, blood fats that increase the risk of heart attack. (Fruit, by contrast, contains a little fructose plus plenty of water, fiber, and nutrients.) The other reason is that sugar packs a lot of carbohydrate calories in a small package.

NOT ALL STARCHES ARE EQUAL

Potatoes raise blood sugar fast because the type of starch they contain is easily broken down. Peas contain a type of starch that's broken down much more slowly.

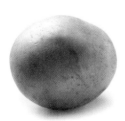

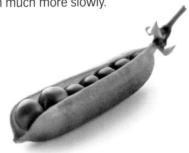

potato (amylopectin)   peas (amylose)

That's why one 32-ounce (1-liter) cola drink contains a whopping 400 calories—and will send your blood sugar soaring.

HEAT—OR WHY NOT TO OVERCOOK RICE OR PASTA

All starch, whether it's made of straight or branched chains, is composed of crystals, which don't dissolve in cold water. Think of a grain of rice or a piece of raw potato—put it in water and it stays the same. But heat breaks down those crystals so the starch can dissolve in water—a little like a snowflake that comes in from the cold. When you cook a starchy food, it absorbs water and becomes easier to digest.

The more overcooked rice or pasta is, the faster it makes your blood sugar rise. When starch is heated and then cooled, it can return, in part, to its crystal form; that's why hot potatoes have a high GL, while potato salad's is slightly lower. Just make it with olive oil instead of mayo to keep it healthier.

PROCESSING—OR WHY TO AVOID WHITE FLOUR

Have you ever noticed that some wheat breads are as smooth as white bread, while others have crunchy kernels in them? Those kernels take a long time for your body to break down. So do any whole, intact grains, such as wheatberries (small kernels of wheat, delicious in salads).

Modern commercial flour, on the other hand—especially white flour—is extremely easy for the body to turn into blood sugar, which is why we suggest throughout this book that you choose whole grains that are still intact and foods such as beans, lentils, and wheatberries instead of those made from white flour. (Unfortunately, we're surrounded by white-flour foods. You'll need to make a conscious effort to cut back.)

Until the 19th century, the main way to turn grain into flour was to grind it between stones, sometimes powered by a water wheel. Making very fine flour took a lot of work, and it was

pasta
GETS A PASSING GRADE

Bread, even many whole wheat breads, can raise your blood sugar pretty quickly. Yet pasta, even if it's made from white flour, has a much lower GL. How can that be?

Imagine putting cooked pasta and a piece of bread in a bowl of water. The bread will fall apart, but the pasta won't. That's because in pasta dough, the starch granules get trapped in a network of protein molecules, so it takes more work—and more time—to get at them. That's why **pasta releases its carbs much more slowly than potatoes** or most breads do, especially if it's served al dente (slightly undercooked). Similarly, gnocchi, a pasta-like product made from durum wheat and potato flour, has a lower GL than potatoes. You'll find pastas, especially whole wheat pastas and protein-enriched pastas, on our list of Magic foods in Part 2.

Pasta is particularly good for you if you eat it as the southern Italians do: **cooked al dente,** prepared with olive oil and beans or vegetables, served in modest portions, and followed by a piece of fish or lean meat and perhaps a side of garlicky greens and fruit for dessert. A huge bowl of overcooked pasta with a butter or cream sauce is not what the doctor ordered.

available only in small amounts to the rich. Then high-speed, high-heat steel rollers, which make very fine flour quickly and inexpensively, were invented, almost instantly transforming our diets into blood sugar nightmares.

In a study, folks who ate a **high-protein** diet consumed 25 percent **FEWER** calories than those in the high-carb group.

Modern manufacturing also allows grains to be turned into highly processed forms such as cornflakes or puffed corn snacks, which tend to have higher GLs than grains left intact, like popcorn, or those milled in an old-fashioned manner, like coarse, stone-ground whole wheat flour used in stone-ground wheat bread.

Protein

Unlike carbohydrate, protein doesn't raise blood sugar. Your body breaks it down into amino acids, which it uses as building blocks for muscles as well as many compounds such as neurotransmitters, the brain's chemical messengers. Unless you're on a diet that has no carbs, your body won't even try to convert protein into blood sugar.

That's why you'll find protein foods such as fish, chicken, beef, pork, soy, milk, eggs, and cheese on our list of Magic foods. If you substitute calories from one of these foods for some of your carbohydrate calories, your blood sugar will thank you. For instance, if you add shrimp to a rice dish, you'll eat less rice, and the meal will have less impact on your blood sugar.

While we're fans of protein, we're not suggesting a diet of fatty bacon, greasy burgers, and the like. These are packed with saturated fat, and as you'll read a bit later, saturated fat increases insulin resistance, which is bad for your blood sugar. Lean protein foods, like fat-free milk and

chicken breast without the skin, are far better choices because they contain fewer calories and less saturated fat. Fish and shellfish are definitely on the menu because they're not only low in saturated fat but also high in heart-healthy omega-3 fatty acids. Beans, peas, and lentils, all high in protein, have the added plus of being rich in fiber.

We're also not suggesting an extremely high protein, low carb diet. You'll find out why in the next chapter.

More Pluses for Protein

There are also other benefits to protein. Some of the compounds our bodies make from protein's amino acids help regulate blood sugar, so including protein in a meal means your body will handle the carbohydrates in that meal more efficiently. That's one reason we want you to include a source of protein with every meal. Another reason: Your body takes a while to break down the protein in the foods you eat, and this slows the digestion of the whole meal, including the carbs it contains, making for a slower rise in blood sugar.

In one recent study, healthy volunteers ate a starchy breakfast (white bread) followed by a starchy lunch (mashed potatoes and meatballs). On some days, however, they got extra protein in the form of whey (dairy protein). On days when they ate more protein, their blood sugar levels were more than 50 percent lower in the following 2 hours than on days when they ate mostly carbs. Another study, of people with diabetes, found that adding whey reduced their blood sugar response by 21 percent over the following 2 hours.

Protein, especially the kind found in milk, also stimulates the pancreas to produce insulin. That may not sound like a good idea since having high levels of insulin over long periods of time is unhealthy. But the earlier your body makes insulin in response to a rise in blood sugar, the less insulin it may need to make—and the less likely you are to become insulin resistant.

Protein and Weight Loss

Eating more protein-rich foods should even help you lose weight. Protein puts a damper on hunger, expanding the time between when you eat and when your stomach starts rumbling again. Research proves it. In a six-day study, one group of volunteers went on a low-GI, high-protein diet. The other group followed a low-protein, high-carb diet. Both groups were allowed to eat as much as they wanted—and the folks who ate the high-protein diet consumed 25 percent fewer calories than those in the high-carb group. In a longer study, lasting six months, high-protein dieters lost more weight than high-carb dieters. They ate less because they felt fuller.

Getting enough protein can also help keep your metabolism running at full speed. Usually, when you really cut back on calories—especially if you go on a very low carb diet—your body resorts to breaking down muscle tissue for energy. But muscle tissue burns up a lot of calories even when you're not flexing a thing, so breaking it down slows your metabolism. Eating plenty of protein helps your body keep its muscle tissue.

In diet studies, people on moderately high protein diets lost more body fat and less muscle. A moderately high protein diet might get as much as 30 percent of its calories from protein, rather than the 15 to 20 percent most people get. Twenty to 30 percent is the protein intake we recommend.

Fat

Fat has gotten a bad rap, to the point where most people think the less fat you eat, the better. Research is proving that this just isn't true.

During the height of the low-fat craze, people loaded up on carbohydrates like fat-free chips and low-fat cookies—foods laden with fast-acting carbohydrates—thinking they were doing themselves good. What a mistake! They were actually wreaking havoc on their blood sugar and eating just as many calories in the bargain.

The fact is, fat's no demon. Some fats are positively good for you and your blood sugar, and they absolutely belong in your diet.

Like protein, fat doesn't raise blood sugar, so swapping carb-rich foods such as pretzels for fat-rich foods such as nuts can be an excellent trade.

Also like protein, fat takes a while to digest. Because it slows the rate at which food leaves

THE POWER OF PROTEIN

Adding protein to a carbohydrate dish lowers the glycemic load of the dish—assuming you eat the same amount—because you end up eating less carbohydrate. Protein itself also helps steady blood sugar.

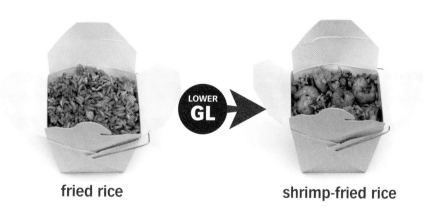

fried rice   shrimp-fried rice

your stomach, it can blunt the blood sugar effect of a whole meal, even if that meal includes carbs. Tossing your salad with olive oil or drizzling some on your pasta, adding some nuts to your rice, broiling fatty fish for dinner, or using slices of ripe avocado in your sandwich won't magically lower your blood sugar, but it will help.

Good Fat, Bad Fat

Notice that we've talked about nuts, oils, and fish instead of other fat sources such as burgers or butter. It's true that adding fat lowers the GL of a starchy food, but adding butter or sour cream to a heap of mashed potatoes doesn't make it healthy. Quite the contrary.

Butter, which comes from cow's milk, is an animal food, and as with many animal foods, most of the fat it contains is saturated. That's the kind that clogs arteries. It's also bad for blood sugar. In both animal and human studies, a diet high in saturated fat has been shown to trigger insulin resistance, which it does in many ways. Saturated fat increases inflammation, which is toxic to cells, including those that handle glucose. It also makes cell membranes less fluid, so the insulin receptors there are less responsive to insulin; the hormone bounces off them like water off a drum rather than sticking to them.

> A moderate-fat **diet** can be every bit as effective as a low-fat diet in helping you **LOSE** weight.

It's clear that people who eat the most saturated fat are at the highest risk of developing insulin resistance and metabolic syndrome. And as you read in Chapter 1, these conditions increase your risk of heart disease and diabetes.

The trick, then, is to avoid the worst of the "bad" fat foods, like marbled steak, high-fat lunchmeats, butter, whole milk, full-fat cheeses, and ice cream, and choose instead lean cuts of meat and poultry, fat-free or 1% milk, low-fat cheese, and lean lunchmeats such as turkey, chicken, and extra-lean roast beef.

Even better, embrace unsaturated fats, which can actually *improve* insulin sensitivity, thus benefiting your blood sugar. These fats come mainly from plants—think avocados, nuts and seeds, olives, and olive and canola oil—and fish and seafood. The Mediterranean diet, one of the healthiest diets in the world, gets a moderately high 30 to 35 percent of its calories from fat, mostly the unsaturated kind. This is the fat ceiling we recommend.

Protecting Your Heart

"Good" fats are also good for your heart. Swapping that cheeseburger for seafood or that butter for peanut butter (a good source of unsaturated fat) lowers your "bad" LDL cholesterol while leaving "good" HDL cholesterol alone. In fact, eating just a handful of nuts a few times a week can slash your risk of getting heart disease by 25 percent.

So can eating fish a few times a week. Seafood contains omega-3 fatty acids, which do a world of good for your heart by lowering triglycerides, helping prevent blood clots, reducing inflammation, and promoting normal heart rhythm. Eating just two servings of fish—especially fatty fish such as salmon or mackerel—a week can reduce your risk of heart disease by a third or more.

Losing Weight

You'd think that if you want to lose weight, you should cut way back on fat, which is high in calories. Pretty obvious, right? Surprisingly, recent research has shown it's not necessarily true. A moderate-fat diet can be every bit as effective as a low-fat diet in helping you lose weight—if you choose mostly beneficial fats.

A bit of fat also makes meals more satisfying, which can make it easier to stick to a healthy eating plan over the long haul. Try to go too low fat, and you'll most likely throw in the towel at some point, probably sooner rather than later. In one study of overweight men and women, those on a moderate-fat diet lost about 9 pounds (4 kg) over 18 months, while those on a low-fat diet actually wound up *gaining* more than 6 pounds (3 kg). One key reason was dieting fatigue: Only 20 percent of those on the low-fat diet were still actively participating by the end of the study, while 54 percent of those on the moderate-fat diet were still at it.

Lower Blood Sugar with Soluble Fiber

Carbs, protein, and fat are all macronutrients—nutrients that provide the vast majority of our calories. Fiber doesn't count because it isn't digested by the body, so it provides not a single calorie. Nevertheless, it's an extremely important element in a Magic diet.

There are two types of fiber: soluble and insoluble. Soluble fiber is the kind that dissolves in water. It's found in oats, barley, beans, and some fruits and vegetables. Insoluble fiber is found mostly in whole wheat and some fruits and vegetables. Both types are very good for you, but only soluble fiber will help lower your blood sugar—in a big way.

How big? Researchers at a USDA Diet and Human Performance Laboratory tested oatmeal and barley (which is even richer in soluble fiber than oatmeal) on overweight middle-aged women. On days when the women ate oatmeal for breakfast, their blood sugar levels over the following 3 hours were about 30 percent lower than when they ate a sugar-laden pudding. On days when they ate barley cereal, it was about 60 percent lower.

BEST FOODS FOR SOLUBLE

fiber

Here you'll find the amount of soluble fiber per serving of various foods. Remember, you're aiming for about 10 grams a day.

grains (1/2 cup cooked)

Barley	1 g
Oats	1 g

beans and peas (1/2 cup cooked)

Black beans	2 g
Great Northern beans	1.5 g
Kidney beans	3 g
Lima beans	3.5 g
Navy beans	2 g
Pinto beans	2 g
Black-eyed peas	1 g
Chickpeas	1 g

vegetables (1/2 cup cooked)

Broccoli	1 g
Brussels sprouts	3 g
Carrots	1 g

fruit (1 medium fruit, except where noted)

Apple	1 g
Blackberries (1/2 cup)	1 g
Grapefruit	2 g
Orange	2 g
Pear	2 g
Prunes (1/4 cup)	1.5 g

How does soluble fiber work its magic? When it mixes with water, it forms a gum. Think of oatmeal; you can pick out the grains or flakes when it's dry, but once you cook it, it's one big mush. This gooey gum forms a barrier between the digestive enzymes in your stomach and the starch molecules in food— not just in the oatmeal but also in the toast you ate with it. Thus, it takes longer for your body to convert the whole meal into blood sugar.

> Eating more foods rich in soluble **fiber** is a key strategy for lowering your blood sugar after meals.

Eating more foods rich in soluble fiber is a key strategy for lowering your blood sugar after meals. It will also improve your health in other ways. Oatmeal is famous by now for lowering cholesterol, but it may lower high levels of triglycerides and reduce blood pressure as well. There's even a health claim allowed on oatmeal packaging: "Eating 3 grams of soluble fiber from oatmeal in a diet low in saturated fat and cholesterol may reduce the risk of heart disease." (About 1 1/2 cups of cooked oatmeal supplies 3 grams.) Lots of other foods are also rich in soluble fiber (see "Best Foods for Soluble Fiber" on page 31).

Nutrition experts tell us to aim for at least 20 grams of total fiber a day, both insoluble and soluble. A good goal for soluble fiber is 10 grams. Sound like a hard goal to reach? Here are some foods you might eat in a typical day that would add up to more than 10 grams.

Breakfast: A cup of cooked oatmeal with a chopped medium apple; soluble fiber: 3 grams.

Lunch: Add a side dish of black beans (1/2 cup); soluble fiber: 2 grams.

Dinner: Add a side dish of roasted Brussels sprouts (about 1 cup); soluble fiber: 6 grams.

In case you're counting, that's 11 grams. Not surprisingly, many of these fiber-rich foods also have low GLs, so they can help lower the GL of a meal if you use them to replace other carbs. For instance, if you ate a combination of 1/2 cup of rice and 1/2 cup of beans instead of 1 cup of rice, you'd drop the GL by almost half.

Pucker Power

Wouldn't it be terrific if there were a simple ingredient you could add to your meals that would act like an anchor, keeping blood sugar from rising too high? As it turns out, there is. It's acetic acid, the sour-tasting compound that gives that characteristic tang to vinegar, pickles, and sourdough bread.

The effect can be quite dramatic. In one small study, people who ate a buttered 3-ounce (85-g) bagel and orange juice—a high-GL breakfast— saw their blood sugar shoot up in the next hour. But when they also drank about a tablespoon of apple cider vinegar (with artificial sweetener added to improve the taste), their blood sugar levels after the meal were 50 percent lower! A similar 50 percent reduction in blood sugar happened when they had the vinegar along with a chicken-and-rice meal.

How does acetic acid make it happen? Scientists aren't sure, but they do know that it interferes with the enzymes that break apart the chemical bonds in starches and the kinds of sugars found in table sugar and milk. This means it takes your body longer to break down those foods into blood sugar. Other researchers believe acetic acid keeps foods in the stomach longer so they aren't digested as quickly. Acetic acid may also speed up the rate at which glucose is moved out of the bloodstream and into muscle cells for storage.

No matter how it works, it does, and taking advantage of it is as easy as adding vinegar to salads and other foods and having a pickle with your sandwich at lunchtime. Lemon juice also has "pucker power" and seems to help control blood sugar. You'll read more about vinegar, lemon juice, and sourdough bread in Part 2.

The Secrets of a Magic Diet

Now you understand why rice raises blood sugar fast while oatmeal raises it more slowly and chicken doesn't raise it at all. And why the soluble fiber in beans and the acetic acid in vinegar help keep your blood sugar steady. If you don't feel like remembering the details, don't. You don't need to. In Chapter 4, we'll reveal the Seven Secrets of Magic Eating, and if you follow these rules, you'll be eating for better blood sugar.

You don't even need to bother with the exact GL numbers of the foods you eat (although we do supply them for some common foods on pages 55-58). In this book, we've simply classified foods according to very low, low, medium, high, and very high GL. The foods you'll read about in Part 2 have very low, low, or medium GLs—part of what makes them Magic.

It's important to note that you don't always have to choose foods in the "low" category. Eating just one low-GL food in a meal in place of a high-GL food is enough to tame your blood sugar response to the whole meal. Also remember that a food's GL is based on a moderate portion; if you eat twice as much, the effect on your blood sugar will be twice as great. Of course, the converse is also true: If you eat 50 percent less of a starchy food, your blood sugar response will be 50 percent lower. In each Magic food entry in Part 2, you'll find out the size of an appropriate serving of that food. Keeping your portions under control is of course the best way to lose weight, whether or not you choose low-GL foods.

You'll learn much more about how to focus on Magic foods later in the book. First, in case you're tempted after reading this chapter to switch to a very low carb diet, let us explain why that's a bad idea.

WHAT ABOUT wine?

Alcohol, in the right amounts, can benefit blood sugar. Moderate drinking—from one drink a few times a week up to one a day for women or two a day for men—is associated with lower fasting insulin levels, higher levels of "good" HDL cholesterol, smaller waist circumference, and lower triglycerides … in other words, a lower risk of metabolic syndrome (see page 19).

It also **lowers the risk of developing diabetes** by between 33 and 56 percent, according to a comprehensive review of more than 30 studies. And if you have diabetes, it reduces your risk of developing heart disease by 34 to 55 percent.

Wine, especially red wine, may have extra benefits. It contains antioxidants that, in animal studies, help prevent insulin resistance. Wine is also acidic, so in theory, it should reduce the blood sugar effect of foods you eat. But beer is fine, too; despite what you may have heard, even regular beer is fairly low in carbohydrates.

The main benefits come from the alcohol itself, but **don't forget the moderation part.** People who have three or more drinks a day have a much higher risk of diabetes and heart disease. A drink is defined as a 12-ounce (341 ml) beer, 5 ounces (150 ml) of wine, or a 1.5-ounce (45 ml) shot of distilled spirits, such as vodka.

If you have diabetes, ask your doctor about drinking. Because alcohol lowers blood sugar, it could cause hypoglycemia.

chapter 3

WHY low-CARB
DIETS AREN'T THE ANSWER

What raises blood sugar? The simple answer is carbohydrates. So why not just yank them out of your diet like weeds in your garden? Why not quash blood sugar by swearing off bread, pasta, rice, and cereal? Been there, done that. The low-carb craze is on the downswing, and that's a good thing because over the long haul, very low carb diets simply aren't good for you, as you'll discover in this chapter. That doesn't mean it's not smart to cut back on carbs—but don't go crazy.

When low-carb diets first became popular, they seemed to be a breath of fresh air after the low-fat (and high-carb) diets that preceded them. Remember low-fat cookies, low-fat snack cakes, and low-fat everything else? With low-carb diets, suddenly people could load up on bacon and still lose weight as long as they were willing to eat hamburgers without buns and pretty much give up sandwiches and spaghetti. People were amazed at how effective these diets could be. Weight loss could happen

Many **low-carb** diets have turned out to be less effective, and less healthy, than originally claimed.

very quickly, sometimes within days. And amazingly, it often seemed to come with added health benefits, including lower cholesterol, blood pressure, and triglycerides (blood fats linked to heart attacks.)

The most extreme kind of low-carb diet was pioneered by the late Robert Atkins, M.D., whose first book, *Dr. Atkins' Diet Revolution*, came out in 1972. It promised quick and long-lasting weight loss and prevention of chronic disease, all while allowing high-fat steak and ice cream. Since then, other, more moderate low-carb diets have allowed small amounts of carbohydrate-rich foods, but they still cut out most grains as well as starchy vegetables and even fruit.

The Downsides of These Diets

The Atkins diet and the many other low-carb diets that followed in its footsteps have turned out to be less effective, and less healthy, than originally claimed. Often, the weight returned, and as it did, problems such as high cholesterol and high blood pressure came back, too. Also, in the end, many people decided they didn't want to go through life without ever eating pasta again.

Let's look at what would happen if you followed one of the more extreme low-carb diets.

You'll Feel Terrible

Low-carb diets usually begin with an "induction" phase that eliminates nearly every source of carbohydrate. Often, you'll consume as few as 20 grams of carbohydrate a day. That's less than 100 calories' worth—about what's in a small dinner roll. On a 1,200-calorie diet, that's only about 8 percent of your daily calories. By contrast, health experts recommend that we get between 45 and 65 percent of our calories from carbs.

When carbohydrate consumption falls below 100 grams, the body usually responds by burning

muscle tissue for the glycogen (stored glucose) it contains. When those glycogen stores start to run out, the body resorts to burning body fat. But that's a very inefficient, complicated way to produce blood sugar. The body tries to do it only when it absolutely has to (such as when it's starving)—and for good reason. Turning fat into blood sugar comes at a price in the form of by-products called ketones. They make your breath smell funny. They can also make you tired, lightheaded, headachy, and nauseated. Feeling lousy is certainly one way to dampen the appetite, but not one that most people would choose.

> Burning fat for blood sugar produces **ketones,** which can make you tired, lightheaded, headachy, and nauseated.

With virtually no carbs in your system, you may even have trouble concentrating. According to the Institute of Medicine of the National Academy of Sciences, the human brain requires the equivalent of 130 grams of carbohydrate a day to function optimally—and that's a minimum.

Your Health May Suffer

If you're overweight or obese, and you have insulin resistance—and especially if you have prediabetes or diabetes—cutting way back on carbohydrates can have immediate health benefits. Your blood sugar and insulin levels will go down, your triglycerides and blood pressure may fall, and your levels of "good" HDL cholesterol may rise.

But the low-carb diet will also wreak some havoc. When your body breaks down lean body mass—muscle—for energy, your metabolism slows because muscle tissue burns up a lot of calories. This may be one reason that the weight often comes back after you've been shunning carbs for a while.

The effects on your heart are also questionable. Especially if you switch to a high-saturated-fat diet, as people do when they start eating their fill of steak and bacon, your "bad" LDL cholesterol will go up. Levels of homocysteine, an amino acid that increases the risk of heart disease, may also rise if you eat a lot of meat and too few vegetables. And to get rid of the ketones produced when your body burns fat for energy, your kidneys need to work overtime, which raises your risk of kidney stones.

Ironically, low-carb diets may even interfere with insulin sensitivity; a certain amount of carbohydrate in your diet may be needed in order for the pancreas, which produces the insulin that keeps blood sugar in check, to work well.

You'll Miss Out

It's not just that you'll feel deprived because you've had to give up bread, fruit, and all the rest. Your body will also be deprived of foods and nutrients that are essential for good health, including the following.

Whole grains. These protect against metabolic syndrome, diabetes, heart disease, stroke, and cancer.

Fruits and vegetables. Produce helps prevent heart disease, stroke, and some cancers. Most fruits and vegetables are very filling while providing few calories, so they can help you cut calories without deprivation. Indeed, the more fruits and vegetables people eat, studies show, the thinner they tend to be.

Beans. Rich in protein, complex carbohydrates, and B vitamins, beans have no saturated fat and lots of soluble fiber. They also contain plant chemicals that protect against heart disease and cancer.

Low-fat dairy foods. Sure, you can have butter and cream on a carb-restricted diet, but you won't get much calcium or protein from them. Fat-free and low-fat versions of milk and yogurt are excellent sources of those nutrients.

Fiber. Getting fiber from these foods (except dairy) helps reduce the risk of heart disease and diabetes. Beans and many fruits and vegetables are particularly rich in soluble fiber, which helps lower blood sugar, curbs hunger, and lowers LDL cholesterol.

Vitamins, minerals, and health-protective plant chemicals. Whole grains, for example, are rich in components such as lignans, which may protect against diabetes independently of their effects on blood sugar. And without fruits and vegetables, you'd be awfully hard-pressed to get enough vitamin C or other disease-fighting antioxidants.

You'll Eat Too Much "Bad" Fat

The original Atkins diet became popular largely because it allowed people to eat foods forbidden on most other diets, such as cheeseburgers (without buns). More recently, the diet has been revised to include sources of healthier fats, such as fish and olive oil, and other low-carb diets have shied away from saturated fats as well. But in practice, once you stop eating bread, fruit, and beans, it's all too easy to eat too many fatty animal foods. After all, how many foods can you take out of your diet?

If you load up on saturated fats—the original Atkins diet got as much as 26 percent of its calories from saturated fat versus the 10 percent or less that experts recommend—it's bad for your health. Saturated fats are still the major culprits behind elevated LDL cholesterol. The latest revisions to the diet, to be fair, do emphasize lean poultry and seafood, but in practice, many people are attracted to this diet for the bacon and butter.

What's more, saturated fats also directly impair the body's ability to react to insulin, so following a low-carb, high-saturated-fat diet may help you lose weight in the short term, but it may also speed the development of insulin resistance. Eventually, that can lead to metabolic syndrome, diabetes, and heart disease.

The Weight Will Come Back

Two major studies of low-carb diets, published in the *New England Journal of Medicine*, looked at obese men and women who stuck with either a low-carb, high-fat diet or a low-fat, high-carb diet. Both diets were low in calories.

In one study, which lasted six months, the low-carb diet seemed to win hands down. The people on it lost nearly 13 pounds (6 kg); the low-fat dieters shed just 4 pounds (2 kg). But the second study lasted six months longer, revealing a truth about low-carb diets: The results don't last. This study too found that the low-carb dieters lost more weight in the first six months, but in the second half of the year, the weight came roaring back. By the end of a year, there was no significant difference in weight loss between the two groups. This weight "snap-back" may be one reason that extremely low carb diets have fallen out of favor.

Take the Good, Leave the Bad

The good news? Many of the weight-loss advantages of low-carb diets may have nothing at all to do with restricting carbohydrates. The main benefit may be due to the extra protein—and you can add protein to your diet even if you don't drastically cut carbs. As you discovered in Chapter 2, protein-rich foods can really help with weight control. One reason may be that protein stimulates the body to burn slightly more calories than carbohydrates or fats do.

The main reason, though, is that protein foods curb hunger better. When people eat protein-rich foods, they feel fuller longer, and when they diet, they consume fewer calories and lose more weight when they eat a lot of protein.

One recent study puts it in perspective. Researchers at the University of Washington School of Medicine in Seattle gave volunteers a diet that got 50 percent of its calories from carbohydrates. That's certainly not a low-carb diet, though it's not a high-carb diet either. It's actually a good goal, on par with what we suggest in this book.

To start, the volunteers got only 15 percent of their calories from protein and 35 percent from fat. That's about what most people get. Then they switched: Carbs stayed the same, but fat was decreased to 20 percent of calories, and protein was doubled to 30 percent. The participants were allowed to eat as much as they wanted—but they ate less. Over 14 weeks, they lost an average of 11 pounds (5 kg), including 8 pounds (3.5 kg) of body fat, thanks to the extra protein.

> The main **BENEFIT** of low-carb diets may be due to the extra **protein** in them.

More Protein, and Carbohydrates in Moderation

No matter how you slice it, we eat too many carbohydrates. We consume many more calories than we used to, and most of those extra calories come from extra carbs (so many chips and cookies!). Thus, it makes sense to cut back some on carbs. It also makes sense to choose lower-GL carbohydrate foods instead of "fast-acting" carbs that send your blood sugar soaring. These strategies are a big part of the Magic Foods approach to eating.

That approach, which we spell out in the next chapter, provides the benefits of a drastically low carb diet with none of the hazards. You'll get the blood sugar advantages, including lower insulin levels. By eating plenty of lean protein, you'll feel satisfied and less hungry. And by choosing "good" fats and limiting "bad" ones, you'll keep LDL cholesterol from rising and protect your heart in the process. You'll also discover a way of eating that you can enjoy—rather than endure—for the rest of your life.

chapter 4

A BREAKTHROUGH eating APPROACH

This is not a "diet" in the dieting sense. It's a **delicious,** practical, long-term strategy for healthy eating.

Now that you know how important it is to eat foods that help keep your blood sugar steady, you're probably wondering, "So what's for dinner?" We've given you some heavy hints already, but it's time to spell it all out so you know exactly how to eat the *Magic Foods* way—and can start doing it today. Get ready for the ultimate sugar-busting, health-enhancing diet. You'll feel so good, you'll never look back.

In this chapter, you'll discover the Seven Secrets of Magic Eating and how to put them to practical use. The great news is that it's easier than you may think. In fact, changing just a few of the foods you eat every day can help you feel more energized and prevent the chronic diseases that slow us all down as we age.

This is not a "diet" in the dieting sense. It's a delicious, practical, long-term strategy for healthy eating, one that will not only help stabilize your blood sugar but also make it easier to leave that extra weight behind. The best part is that you can start by making as many or as few changes to your current diet as you'd like. You can decide to do only one or two new things—for instance, switching from rice to barley and snacking on hard-boiled eggs instead of pretzels—until you're ready for another change. Or you can be a bit more ambitious right from the start. Our goal is to give you the tools you need to eat for better blood sugar, to use as you wish.

With the *Magic Foods* approach to eating, you don't have to give up bread, although you will want to navigate the bread aisle carefully and eat a little less. You don't have to swear off potatoes and white rice, although you'll definitely eat them more sparingly than you do now. You can also have pasta, in moderation (we'll explain which types are best for better blood sugar). And we encourage you to pour yourself cereal for breakfast—assuming it's one of the kinds we describe in this chapter.

You'll enjoy eating more protein-rich foods to keep you full and help keep your blood sugar low and steady. And while you'll say goodbye to unhealthy fats, your diet will actually contain plenty of fat in the form of "good" fats to add appeal to meals and blunt the blood sugar effects of the carbs you eat.

Along the way, you'll learn a few clever tricks of the trade, such as how to finish your salad with a dressing that can lower the blood sugar impact of your entire meal, how to use a little-known Middle Eastern spice to pull the plug on blood sugar, which sour fruit has a sweet benefit, and which little seeds pack a powerful health kick.

We're not asking you to throw your current diet out the window—just to tweak it a bit. Magic eating is really a series of very small, simple steps, such as adding a chopped apple to oatmeal, choosing sourdough bread instead of regular white bread, and making sweet potato fries your fries of choice (try them; you'll love them). Whether you make one change a meal,

one change a day, or only one change in all, your blood sugar will benefit.

Although the changes are easy, the rewards are real: more energy, less weight, a healthier heart, lower risk of diabetes, protection against certain cancers, and greatly improved quality of life.

The Seven Secrets of Magic Eating

If you remember only one strategy from this book, remember the Seven Secrets of Magic Eating. Some of them may sound unusual, while others seem like the good old rules of healthy eating you already know about. But each one was chosen for a specific reason: to keep your blood sugar levels steady throughout the day. Here's a quick summary. You may even want to jot down the seven secrets and post them on your fridge as a daily reminder to keep you on the *Magic Foods* course. You'll read more about each of these secrets shortly.

1. Choose low-GL carbs and limit carb portions. Carbohydrate-rich foods, especially grains and starchy vegetables, are the main contributors to high blood sugar. By choosing "slow-acting" (low-GL) carbs instead of "fast-acting" (higher-GL) carbs, you can help keep blood sugar low and steady. You'll also want to limit your portions no matter what kind of carbs you choose.

2. Make three of your carb servings whole grains. You're not eating as many carbs, so make those you do eat count by choosing whole grains, which help prevent heart disease and diabetes independently of their effects on blood sugar.

3. Eat more fruits and vegetables. Aim for at least seven to nine small servings a day. Most fruits and vegetables have little carbohydrate and are packed with vitamins, fiber, and health-protective compounds, with few calories. Eating fruits or adding vegetables to carbohydrate-rich dishes helps make your diet blood sugar friendly.

4. Eat protein at every meal. Protein lowers the GL of meals and helps curb hunger, making weight loss easier.

5. Favor good fats. "Bad" saturated fats can interfere with your ability to control blood sugar, but "good" unsaturated fats help your body control it better. Good fats also lower the GL of meals.

6. Add acidic foods to your meals. It's an amazingly simple way to blunt the blood sugar effect of a meal.

7. Eat smaller portions. We're talking not about just carb-rich foods here but about all foods. Even when you eat a low-GL diet, calories count. Cutting calories can help you fight insulin resistance—and of course, along with exercise, it's still the way to lose weight.

1
SECRET

Choose Low-GL Carbs and Limit Carb Portions

Most of the carbs we eat are the kind that send blood sugar soaring. We eat lots of potatoes, mostly fried. We consume enormous quantities of bread in all forms, but mostly bread that's made with refined white flour and has little fiber. We eat a lot of rice, most of it white. We treat ourselves to muffins, cakes, and pastries made with white flour. We snack on bags of potato chips and pretzels (it's true pretzels are low in fat, but they're more or less just empty carbs). And we wash it all down with sugar-sweetened sodas and fruit drinks.

If you're going to tackle your dietary weak points, this is the place to start. The good news is that it's relatively easy to make improvements. Because we eat so many of these foods to begin with, any change is a change for the better!

"Just Say Less"

One approach is to simply eat less of these high-GL foods. In the past decade or two, we've started to eat more calories, nearly all of them from carbohydrates—and nearly all of those carbohydrates are high GL. So it's time to dial down the carbohydrate mania: Eat fewer salty snacks out of bags, fewer French fries, less bread, and fewer pastries, and drink a lot less soda and other sweetened drinks. Ask yourself, "Do I really need that sugar-coated cereal, that whole takeout container of white rice, those French fries on the 'side' (which take up half the plate), or that giant slice of leftover birthday cake?"

We're not talking about a "just say no" approach but rather a "just say less" approach.

Let's say you start your day with a great big bowl of cornflakes or Rice Krispies or Corn Chex. If you measured how much you poured, it would probably be at least twice the serving size suggested on the box. So the "just say less" approach is to pour out less cereal. Fill the rest of the bowl with berries, low-GL fruits that will bring down the overall GL of your breakfast. And like many fruits, berries are rich in fiber that can help fill you up.

Go Low GL

Even better, why not choose a lower-GL breakfast cereal? If you fill your bowl with a single serving of a medium-GL cereal—such as Grape-Nuts, Cheerios, Special K, or Life—instead of a high-GL one, your blood sugar will be lower after breakfast. And it'll be even lower if you choose a low-GL cereal, such as All-Bran, Bran Buds, or Alpen Muesli—or, if you like hot cereal, oatmeal. Keep watching portions and slicing berries or an apple into your bowl, and you'll really lower your blood sugar response to breakfast. Plus, you'll give yourself a seriously healthy start to the day.

If you like numbers, consider this: A 2-ounce (60 g) bowlful of Kellogg's Cornflakes has a GL of 48; a 1-ounce (30 g) bowlful of All-Bran cereal plus a whole medium apple has a GL of 15—more than two-thirds less. That means your blood sugar will rise two-thirds less as well.

Here's another example. At dinner, instead of a potato, you might decide to make pasta since it has a lower GL. That's a good substitution. A 5-ounce (140 g) baked potato has a GL of 26; the same size serving of pasta has a GL of 17. So the switch itself lowers the GL of that side dish by 9 points, changing it from a "high" to a "medium" GL choice. You could serve the pasta with a little olive oil, freshly ground black pepper, and a tablespoon of Parmesan cheese and never miss the potato a bit.

Now, to lower the GL of your pasta side dish even further, you could cut some red bell peppers into strips, microwave them for a minute, and toss them with the pasta, oil, pepper, and cheese. Because the vegetables add volume to the dish, if you serve yourself the same 5-ounce (140 g) portion, you'll eat half as much pasta, so the GL of the dish has been cut in half—to 4.5. This means the GL of your side dish is only 20 percent of what it would have been if you'd had the baked potato, which means it should raise your blood sugar 80 percent less!

Take a look at "The Glycemic Load of Common Foods" on page 55 and "The Magic Carb Pyramid" on page 43. Pick out a high-GL food that you eat frequently and figure out ways to eat less of it—such as substituting a low-GL or a medium-GL food for it and eating small portions. Now you're cooking.

A final note: Even if you're choosing lower-GL foods, it's still important to watch your portion sizes. That's because if you eat twice the recommended portion of the food, the GL will double. It's a simple concept, but one that many people miss. Even if you choose beans—a low-GL food—doubling the serving size will double the GL.

WHAT'S BOOSTING YOUR BLOOD SUGAR THE MOST?

The best way to lower the GL of your diet is to figure out which high-GL foods you eat the most and then eat less, either by cutting back on portions or choosing a different food in its place.

In a major study of middle-aged women, these five foods were the biggest contributors to GL in the diet. Together, they made up about 30 percent of the GL of the women's entire diets. Try the smart substitutions instead. Each of them has a GL that's at least 50 percent lower than that of the food it replaces. These are only a few examples; you'll find more throughout this book.

Food	Percent of GL in the Diet	Smart Substitution
Cooked potatoes	7.7	Pasta
Cold breakfast cereal	6.5	High-fiber cereal
White bread	5.2	Sourdough bread
Muffin	5.0	Apple
White rice	4.6	Pearled barley

For kids, studies show, the biggest contributors to a high-GL diet are often candy, soft drinks, cakes, cookies, and salty snacks. So this age group will require a different strategy. For them, encouraging fruits as snacks and low-fat milk as a beverage may be the best thing you can do.

2 | Make Three of Your Carb Servings Whole Grains

SECRET

If we are gorging ourselves on refined carbs, we're doing it largely at the expense of whole grains. And that's a shame because when it comes to preventing chronic disease, there's nothing like whole grains. There's clear, strong evidence that if you eat at least three servings of these foods a day, you'll substantially lower your risk of developing metabolic syndrome, diabetes, heart disease, and cancer. Most of us, though, have less than one serving a day. A serving is about an ounce (30 g)—one slice of 100 percent whole grain bread or 1/2 cup of cooked grains.

Eating more whole grains has been shown to cut heart disease risk by 25 percent in women and 18 percent in men and reduce diabetes risk by 35 percent in both. One key way grains may protect against these diseases is by helping to prevent a root cause: metabolic syndrome (described on page 19). In one study of more than 750 men and women over age 60, those who ate about three servings of whole grains a day were 54 percent less likely to have metabolic syndrome than people who ate less than one serving a day. Their fasting blood sugar levels were lower, and they tended to have less body fat. They also had 52 percent fewer fatal heart attacks. In fact, just six weeks on a whole grain diet can markedly improve insulin sensitivity, according to one study of overweight men and women.

Why are whole grains so good for us? They contain all the parts of the grain, not just the starchy low-fiber center (endosperm) but also the nutrient-rich germ layer and the fiber-rich bran layer on the outside. Whole grains are rich in fiber, antioxidants, vitamins, minerals, and a wide range of plant compounds that protect against chronic disease in many different ways.

Most whole grains have lower GLs than most refined grains, but there are exceptions. Finely milled 100 percent whole wheat bread, for instance, actually has a fairly high GL, while some refined foods, like pastas made from white semolina flour, have medium GLs. In general, though, you're better off with whole grains, which offer benefits to blood sugar that are totally unrelated to their GLs.

When it comes to the grain-based carbs you eat, don't be a perfectionist. As long as you get three servings of whole grains a day, there's room for some refined grain foods, especially if they're low GL. Just watch portion sizes no matter what kind you're eating.

How many carbs should you eat in total? In the *Magic Foods* approach, your goal is to get 45 to 55 percent of your calories from carbs every day. Turn to the Magic Meal Plans in Part 4 to see what this looks like in an actual menu.

WHAT COUNTS AS WHOLE GRAIN?

Bread with the word *whole* in the first ingredient (such as *whole wheat*)

Brown rice

Dehulled barley (pearled barley isn't technically a whole grain, although it is good for you)

Oats

Whole wheat pasta

Popcorn

Wheatberries

Exotic grains, including amaranth, buckwheat, and quinoa

The Magic **carb** Pyramid

choose least often

potatoes
French fries
white bread
overcooked pasta
udon noodles
white rice
sticky rice
rice-based cereal

cornflakes
millet
instant Cream of Wheat
most baked goods
nondiet soda
sweetened fruit drinks
dried dates
raisins

choose more often

converted white rice
wild rice
brown rice
wheatberries
pasta cooked al dente
whole wheat pasta
rye crispbread

chocolate milk
apple juice
pineapple juice
dried figs
bananas

sweet potatoes
black-eyed peas
whole grain cereals
low-sugar cereals
regular Cream of Wheat
whole grain and sourdough
bread

choose most often

coarse barley bread
whole-grain pumpernickel
pearled barley
oatmeal
bran cereal
muesli
lima beans
split peas

milk
soy milk
tomato juice
dried prunes
dried apricots

popcorn
yogurt
most vegetables (except potatoes)
lentils
all dried beans (except black-eyed peas)
most fresh fruits (and 100% fruit juice
if limited to 6 ounces)

3 | Eat More Fruits and Vegetables
SECRET

It's no secret that fruits and vegetables are good for you. You probably already know some of their health benefits, such as lower blood pressure and lower risk of heart disease, diabetes, stroke, and certain cancers. You may even know that eating produce can reduce your risk of losing your vision as you age. Yes, fruits and vegetables are rich in vitamins, thousands of health-protective compounds, and fiber.

But did you know that eating more of them is a key strategy in losing weight and keeping it off? With the exception of a few very starchy vegetables—like potatoes—the vast majority are very low in calories. That's largely because they're mostly water and fiber (which has no calories). Studies show that the more fruits and vegetables people eat, the less they tend to weigh.

It can be as simple as eating a salad. In one study at Pennsylvania State University, women who started a meal with a low-calorie salad and then ate a pasta dish ate about 12 percent fewer calories in total than women who skipped the salad and started in on the pasta. In another study, adding about 6 ounces (170 g) of vegetables (in this case, carrots and spinach) to dinner helped people feel fuller on fewer calories.

> Studies show that the more **FRUITS** and **VEGETABLES** people eat, the less they tend to weigh.

With a few exceptions, you can forget anything you've heard about not eating this fruit or that vegetable because it contains sugar or will raise your blood sugar. Most fruits and vegetables are actually quite low in total carbohydrates, and they have fiber—often the soluble fiber that slows blood sugar's rise—so their GLs are quite low.

Foils for High-GL Carbs

You'll lower the GL of a typical portion of any carb dish by mixing in almost any vegetable or fruit (again, potatoes don't count). If you add tomatoes, carrots, and spinach to a pasta salad, for example, you'll eat less pasta. If you add chopped broccoli to a rice side dish, you'll eat less rice; the same goes for adding strawberries to hot or cold cereal. And fewer carbs equals lower blood sugar.

Let's consider a rice side dish. A cup of cooked long-grain white rice has a GL of 23, making it a high-GL food. But a cup of green peas has a GL of only 6, so if you mix an equal amount of peas with the rice, a cup of the side dish would have a GL of only 15, changing it from a high- to a medium-GL food. Really, mixing any vegetable into your rice—chopped cooked onions or carrots or asparagus—similarly lowers its GL.

Snack Perfection

Whole fruit is almost always a good snack choice. Two ounces (60 g) of corn chips, for example, has a GL of 17—making it a medium-GL food (and that's if you buy a small snack-size bag). But a medium peach or plum has a GL of only 5, and a similar-size apple's GL is 6. Plus, you're eating twice as much food, so which do you think is likely to satisfy your hunger best? Even if you ate a plum, a peach, *and* an apple, the GL would be only 16. On the other hand, if you munched 4 ounces (125 g) of corn chips instead of 2, the GL for your snack would be a whopping 34!

Raw veggies are also Magic snacks, dipped in low-fat sour cream, low-fat dressing, or one of the bean dips on pages 204–206. Pack some carrot sticks or cherry tomatoes in a sandwich bag, and you'll have no reason to hit the vending machine—practically devoid of Magic foods—in the afternoon. Fill up on veggies of different colors, since different hues indicate different health-protective compounds. You don't want to miss out on any!

You'll find plenty of tips for adding specific fruits and vegetables to your meals in Part 2, where we introduce you to all the Magic foods. The bottom line? Load up. When it comes to these nonstarchy fruits and vegetables, the more the merrier.

A Few Exceptions

Pretty much all fruits and vegetables are good for us, but some aren't as good for our blood sugar. When we tell you to eat more fruits and veggies, we're talking about colorful veggies (not starches like potatoes) and fresh, whole fruit. Here's the scoop.

Potatoes. These are the big exception: They're dense in easily absorbed carbohydrates, so their GL is quite high. In fact, the more potatoes, including French fries, that people eat, the higher their risk of diabetes. Many nutritionists think potatoes should be classified with grains rather than with vegetables, and even there, they're at the top of the carbohydrate pyramid.

Other starchy vegetables. Sweet potatoes and winter squash are rich in carotenoids and other important nutrients as well as fiber, which is also beneficial. But they're also high in carbohydrates, although their carbs aren't as easily absorbed as those in white potatoes. That makes them a better choice than white potatoes, and we include some delicious recipes for them in Part 4. But as with other carbohydrate-rich foods, watch portions.

Dried fruits. Drying concentrates the sugars in fruit and can make for intensely caloric treats. It's fine to have some raisins, dried plums, dates, figs, and apricots, but don't overindulge in them. Consider what happens when grapes (GL 8) turn into raisins (GL 28) or plums (GL 5) turn into dried plums (GL 10). Two ounces (60 g) of dried dates has a whopping GL of 25.

WHAT ABOUT TROPICAL fruits?

Some nutritionists warn against tropical fruits, which can be starchy, but mostly, these foods are fine. It's true that bananas are starchy and are a medium-GL fruit while nearly all others are low GL, so you shouldn't overeat them, but don't ban them either. And mangoes, which are extraordinarily nutritious (and oh, so good), have gotten a bad rap, but they are low GL, so keep them on the menu. Papayas are fine, too, as are pineapple and watermelon. Coconut isn't a great choice, but it has nothing to do with GL; it's high in saturated fat, which is bad for the heart and insulin sensitivity.

Juices. You'll miss out on most of the fiber and some of the vitamins in the whole fruit, and you'll get a lot more calories—and a higher GL. If you eat 4 ounces (125 g) of fresh pineapple, for example, the GL is 6. But if you drink a small juice glass (6 ounces or 177 ml) of pineapple juice, the GL is 12. Ditto for an orange (GL 5) versus a small glass of OJ (GL 10), and for grapefruit (GL 3) versus a small glass of grapefruit juice (GL 7). And if you go for a sweetened fruit drink, all bets are off: A 12-ounce (375 ml) serving of cranberry juice cocktail—about the size of a small soda—has a GL of 36. When you drink juices, keep portions small, and make sure they're unsweetened (read labels carefully).

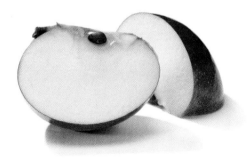

The Magic **protein** Pyramid

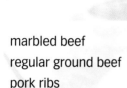

choose least often

marbled beef
regular ground beef
pork ribs
pork sausage
bacon
bologna
salami

hot dogs
chicken with skin
whole milk
butter
cream
full-fat cheese

choose more often

lean beef
extra-lean ground beef
lean pork

lean ham
lean lamb

choose most often

soy foods
fish and shellfish
poultry without skin
nuts
seeds
low-fat cheese
fat-free or 1% milk

fat-free or low-fat yogurt
eggs
split peas
lentils
green peas
All dry beans
  (except black-eyed peas)

Note: Beans are about one-third protein and two-thirds carbohydrate, so they appear in both the protein and carbohydrate pyramids. Similarly, milk and other dairy foods also contain some carbohydrate, so they also appear in both pyramids.

4 SECRET | Eat Protein at Every Meal

Want to control your blood sugar and your weight? Get enough protein.

A moderately high protein diet may get as much as 30 percent of its calories from protein, rather than the 15 to 20 percent most people get. In the *Magic Foods* approach, 20 to 30 percent of the calories you eat should come from protein.

Protein has little or no effect on your blood sugar, so any time you mix protein-rich foods with carbohydrate-rich foods, you automatically lower the GL of each portion. But protein has other benefits, as you saw in Chapters 2 and 3. It helps keep hunger at bay between meals. And if you're trying to lose weight, taking in more protein will help your body hold on to its calorie-burning muscle tissue so the weight comes off more easily.

There's no need to go overboard, though. A serving of a protein-rich food like chicken breast or sirloin steak is a mere 2 to 3 ounces (60 to 85 g), although a more typical portion is 6 ounces (170 g). The main thing to focus on is having at least a small portion of a protein-rich food at *every* meal (and as part of as many snacks as you can). It can be side dish of beans, a glass of fat-free milk, a slice or two of lean turkey, a few ounces of sirloin steak in a stir-fry, a snack of unsweetened yogurt, or a handful of nuts. Among the list of Magic foods in Part 2, you'll find these excellent protein sources.

Beans, lentils, and peas. These "vegetarian" sources of protein are excellent: They have essentially no saturated fat, and they're very low GL, in large part because they contain so much soluble fiber. And they pack a lot of minerals in small packages. Try to eat meals based on these foods at least once or twice a week.

Soy foods. Like beans, these are low-saturated-fat, low-GL, high-protein foods. Try a stir-fry with tofu; experiment with soy milk on your cereal (it tastes better than it once did, so give it

a chance); and grill some tempeh, a textured soybean product with a nutty flavor. Or stock up on frozen soy-based vegetarian burgers.

Nuts and seeds. It's hard to find a protein-rich snack, but nuts are one of the few. These little nuggets serve up not only protein but also good-for-you fats. Just stick to a palmful, since they're high in calories.

Fish and shellfish. All fish and shellfish are low in saturated fat, so they're excellent protein choices. Fatty fish are also rich in omega-3 fatty acids, which help prevent heart disease and may improve insulin sensitivity. You'll make a good choice either way: low-fat fish like cod and flounder are sources of low-saturated-fat protein, while fattier fish like wild salmon and rainbow trout provide both protein and omega-3's.

SNEAKING IN PROTEIN

It's easy to add protein to your meals and snacks.

Starting the day with **whole grain toast**? Instead of buttering it, spread it with a tablespoon of peanut butter.

When summer **berries** are in season (or frozen berries are on sale), make a quick smoothie with fat-free yogurt, a good protein source.

Making a salad? Toss in some **chickpeas** (garbanzo beans) or leftover **chicken**.

Center your lunch around **bean soup**, either vegetarian or flavored with a small amount of **pork**.

Buy single-serving packs of **nuts** to take to work for a quick snack.

Keep some hard-boiled **eggs** in your fridge as snacks or easy protein-rich additions to salads and sandwiches.

Keep **soy-based veggie burgers** in your freezer for quick dinners or high-protein, meaty boosts to pasta sauce (just crumble them into the sauce).

Look for brands of cereals and frozen waffles that contain protein sources such as **soy**.

For a healthy heart, aim for two or three servings of fish or shellfish a week.

Chicken and turkey. These are also low in saturated fat and quite low in calories if you choose white meat without the skin.

Eggs. Eggs are nutritious and versatile. A large egg has only 1.5 grams of saturated fat, and even though it's high in cholesterol, an egg a day won't raise most adults' cholesterol levels. Have eggs for breakfast or enjoy an egg salad sandwich on whole grain bread with low-fat mayo. A hard-boiled egg makes a perfect high-protein snack.

Red meat. Beef, pork, lamb, and other red meats are major contributors to saturated fat in our diets, but that doesn't mean you can't eat them. The key is to choose the leanest cuts, which have more protein—and less saturated fat. And don't eat red meat every day; leave room for meals centered on fish, beans, and so on.

Dairy foods. Fat-free or 1% milk, low-fat or fat-free yogurt, and low-fat cheeses contribute high-quality protein with very little saturated fat. Like all dairy foods, they're high in calcium, a key mineral. But full-fat cheeses, along with butter and high-fat dairy desserts like ice cream, are major contributors to saturated fat in our diets. Have milk and other dairy products every day, but go lean.

THE LEANEST MEATS

Even red meat can be a fine source of low-saturated-fat protein if you choose the right cuts.

For **beef**, choose round steaks and roasts (eye of round, top round, bottom round, round tip), top loin, top sirloin, or chuck shoulder.

When buying **ground beef**, look for extra-lean—90 percent lean or preferably 95 percent, if you can find it.

For **pork**, choose tenderloin or loin chops.

If you like **ham**, ask for extra lean.

For **lamb**, go for leg, arm, or loin.

For **lunchmeats**, check nutrition labels. Look for less than 1 gram of saturated fat per serving.

5
SECRET

Favor Good Fats

With all the emphasis on low-fat foods in recent years, you might think we'd be advocating a low-fat diet. But we're not. Instead of following a low-fat diet—which is almost by necessity a high-carbohydrate diet—you can get as much as 35 percent of your calories from fat in the *Magic Foods* approach. Check out the Magic Meal Plans in Part 4 to see what this amount looks like.

Fat, as you read in Chapter 2, isn't all bad, especially where your blood sugar is concerned. Fat doesn't raise blood sugar a bit, and it doesn't require insulin in order to be metabolized, so it doesn't raise insulin levels either. Its GL is zero. Because it slows the rate at which food leaves your stomach, it can blunt the blood sugar effect of a whole meal, even if that meal includes carbs.

Including fat-rich foods in your meals can also help your body metabolize carbohydrates better—provided they're the right fats. That means monounsaturated fat (the kind in olive oil, nuts, and avocados) and omega-3 fatty acids (found in fatty fish) instead of saturated fat (the kind in red meat and dairy foods). Good fats are remarkable because they can actually help reverse insulin resistance (turn back to page 30 if you want to refresh yourself on this). Saturated fat, on the other hand, not only raises "bad" LDL cholesterol and increases heart disease risk, but we now know that it increases insulin resistance, too.

Favoring good fats means eating fish at least once a week; adding avocado instead of full-fat cheese to your salads and sandwiches; tossing your pasta salad with, say, olive oil and toasted walnuts instead of cream sauce; and putting peanut butter instead of butter on your toast (or dipping your bread in olive oil). Adding good fats to foods means each portion will have a lower GL.

The Magic fats Pyramid

fatty red meats
butter
cream
full-fat cheese
whole milk
premium ice cream

solid shortening
solid margarine
lard
mayonnaise
partially hydrogenated
vegetable oils

**choose
least often**

corn oil
soybean oil

safflower oil
sunflower oil

**choose
more often**

olive oil
canola oil
nuts
nut oils

seeds
flaxseeds
fatty fish
avocados

**choose
most often**

fats AT A GLANCE

THE GOOD FATS

monounsaturated fats: Olive
oil, canola oil, avocados, peanuts, almonds, cashews, and most other nuts. When they replace saturated fats, they have a beneficial effect on cholesterol and help reverse insulin resistance.

omega-3 fats: Fatty fish. Related fats,
which the body can convert to a degree to the more active form found in fish, are found in flaxseed and canola oil. Omega-3 fats, especially from fish, help prevent heart disease and may improve insulin sensitivity.

polyunsaturated fats: Corn,
soybean, and safflower oils can be beneficial, but most of us already get plenty of polyunsaturated fats, so don't go out of your way to get more. You're much more likely to need more monounsaturated fat in your diet.

THE BAD FATS

saturated fats: Red meats; full-fat
dairy foods; and a few vegetable oils, such as coconut oil. These increase levels of "bad" LDL cholesterol, promote heart disease, and reduce insulin sensitivity.

trans fats: These are found in solid
margarine; vegetable shortening; partially hydrogenated vegetable oils; and many deep-fried snacks, fast foods, and commercial baked goods. They raise "bad" LDL cholesterol, lower "good" HDL cholesterol, increase heart disease risk, and may increase insulin resistance. Trans fats are now listed on nutrition labels, and manufacturers are offering new foods with "no trans fats." These are fine as long as they're also low GL, which is rarely the case!

Making the Switch

If you're used to steaks and butter, how do you make the switch to better fats? With these steps.

Cut back on the major sources of saturated fat in your diet. Start by identifying them: Look at the top tier of "The Magic Fats Pyramid" on page 49 and check out "The Top 10 Sources of Saturated Fat" on page 51. How often do you eat these foods? What single change do you think you could make in the next week—using a leaner sandwich meat at lunch, having steak instead of ribs, choosing low-fat frozen yogurt instead of ice cream? Make that one change, and when you have, start thinking about your next one. Work toward eating more foods from the bases (and middle tiers) of the fat and protein pyramids— and much fewer from the top tiers. Just cutting back on cheese, full-fat yogurt, and regular sour cream—or choosing low-fat substitutes—can substantially reduce the amount of saturated fat you eat with very little effort. So can switching from whole milk to 1% or fat free.

Eat more nonmeat protein. We're talking beans, lentils, peas, and soy foods. By swapping a few meat-based meals a week for vegetarian options, you can go a long way toward building a healthier diet. Aim for one new vegetarian meal each week for a month. Ultimately, turn it into a lifetime habit.

Eat fish or shellfish twice a week. It can be fresh, canned, or frozen (but skip the breaded fish sticks). Experiment with different cooking methods. As a start, try our recipe suggestions in Part 4.

When you eat red meat, choose lean cuts. It can make a big difference in how much saturated fat you get, and you won't need to sacrifice taste. Three ounces (85 g) of cooked regular ground beef has 6 grams of saturated fat, while the same amount of extra-lean ground beef has only 2.5 grams. Check out "The Leanest Meats" on page 48 and try to stick with these options whenever you can.

Cook and season with olive oil. Use it for sautéing, grilling, and roasting; as an ingredient in salad dressing; or drizzled over vegetables, grains, and fish. Reach for the olive oil instead of butter whenever you cook. You'll hardly notice the difference in most foods, and making this change can dramatically decrease the amount of saturated fat you add to your diet. If you simply must have the taste of butter in a dish, add a teaspoon or two to olive oil to impart that buttery flavor.

Make canola oil your second choice. Use it for a more neutral taste when sautéing and in baking. It's very versatile yet low in saturated fat.

Add more nuts, seeds, and avocado to your menus. You can add nuts to practically any main dish or baked item, and avocado is an easy addition to salads and sandwiches. Or simply carve up a few slices of avocado, drizzle with lemon juice, and enjoy as a snack. See the Nuts and Avocado entries in Part 2 for more menu suggestions.

THE TOP 10 SOURCES OF SATURATED FAT

A quick glance at this list can make it easier to target the foods that are adding the most saturated fat to your diet.

1	Cheese
2	Beef
3	Milk
4	Oils (such as palm, palm kernel, and coconut oil)
5	Ice cream/sherbet/frozen yogurt
6	Cakes/cookies/quick breads/doughnuts
7	Butter
8	Shortening, lard, other animal fats
9	Salad dressings/mayonnaise
10	Poultry with skin

Source: Dietary Guidelines for Americans 2005

6
SECRET

Add Acidic Foods to Your Meals

As you discovered in Chapter 2, even a little bit of pucker power from acidic ingredients can lower your blood sugar response to a carb-rich meal. Making foods more acidic slows the breakdown of starches into blood sugar, so your blood sugar rises more slowly.

Certain acidic foods, though, such as vinegar (acetic acid), seem to work in additional ways, making them more effective. So think vinegar! Toss out those creamy salad dressings and buy or make dressings that combine vinegar with olive oil, such as mustard vinaigrette. It takes just a tablespoon of vinegar per serving to substantially lower the GL of a meal.

Eat a small green salad drizzled with vinaigrette before lunch or dinner several times a week. You'll get some acetic acid in your meals *and* squeeze more vegetables into your diet.

But don't stop there. Soak fish in vinegar and water before cooking, suggests the Vinegar Institute; it'll be sweeter and more tender and hold its shape better. When poaching fish, toss a tablespoon of vinegar into the simmering water for the same reasons. Make a vinegar-based marinade for meat destined for the grill. Mix in a little vinegar when cooking canned soup to perk it up, and add some to the water in which you simmer vegetables. See the Vinegar entry in Part 2 for more suggestions.

If you like Japanese food, you can feel a little better about the rice if you're having sushi, since sushi rice is made with rice wine vinegar.

More Ways to Add Acids

Go beyond vinegar with these tips for adding bite to your meals.

Use mustard, which is made with vinegar, instead of mayonnaise on sandwiches, as a base to coat chicken and meats, and in bean dishes.

Eat that pickle with your sandwich. It gets its sour taste from vinegar.

Go beyond pickled cucumbers and try pickled tomatoes, carrots, celery, broccoli, cauliflower florets, and red and green bell peppers. If you're at a Japanese restaurant, ask for *oshinko* (pickled vegetables).

Don't throw out the pickle liquid! It makes an excellent marinade, especially when mixed with a little olive oil and chopped fresh herbs.

Eat sauerkraut, which is pickled cabbage. Look for low-sodium varieties.

Squeeze lemon juice, which is also acidic, over fish and seafood. Fresh lemon juice can revitalize a lackluster soup or stew, and it livens up green vegetables, rice, and chicken.

Try lime juice on fish, turkey, avocados, melon, sweet potatoes, and black beans.

Eat citrus fruit such as fresh grapefruit, which, as your tongue has already told you, is somewhat acidic.

Ask for sourdough bread. As the dough ferments, it releases lactic acid, which, like vinegar, has a beneficial effect on the food's GL

Cook with wine. It's acidic, too, and gives a tasty tang to sauces, stews, soups, and roasts. Try cooking fish in wine: Sauté garlic (and onions if you want) in olive oil, add seasoning, then pour in some wine and reduce the heat. Add the fish and cook in the simmering liquid. Squeeze in a little lemon juice at the end.

Drink wine with your dinner. It's another way to include an acidic liquid with your meal. Drinking wine (as well as other alcoholic beverages) in moderation—a glass a day for women, up to two for men—can help keep blood insulin levels low and is linked with a lower risk of developing diabetes. Moderate alcohol consumption also raises "good" HDL cholesterol levels and helps protect against heart disease. (If you have diabetes, check with your doctor first.)

7 | Eat Smaller Portions

SECRET

We've already stressed the importance of doling out smaller portions of fast-acting carb foods, such as mashed potatoes and rice, and even slower-acting foods such as whole grain cereal. But portion sizes count almost no matter what you're eating. That's because calories matter.

Eating fewer calories is one of the best ways to improve your insulin sensitivity. You'll do better if you go ahead and lower the GL of your overall diet, with the help of the Magic foods in this book, but simply eating less also helps by improving your insulin sensitivity (which ultimately lowers your blood sugar). It does this even if you don't lose weight. But of course, eating less does help you shed pounds—another key element in preventing insulin resistance, diabetes, and heart disease.

So where should you cut back on calories? Everywhere. Carbs are of course a main target, especially high-GL carbs such as rice, sodas, and sweetened drinks. But so is anything you tend to go overboard on. Yes, we want you to make protein a part of every meal, but that doesn't mean gorging on a 1-pound (450 g) porterhouse is okay. Six ounces (170 g) of a much leaner sirloin is plenty. We also recommend eating nuts, but again, the devil is in the details. An ounce (30 g) of almonds—about 25—has about 165 calories. That's fine. But if you eat a cup's worth, you're taking in more than 800 calories—more than you should get from an entire meal. Few of us have the room in our diets to eat that many extra calories without gaining weight, which increases insulin resistance. Olive oil is great for your heart and your blood sugar, but don't soak your bread in it. At 119 calories per tablespoon, you won't want to consume more than 1 or 2 tablespoons a day.

Fortunately, there's one category of food that doesn't require much portion control: nonstarchy fruits and vegetables. It's quite difficult to eat too many apples, carrots, tomatoes, salad greens, or raspberries. They'll fill you up, with few calories and a low GL, and take the place of more caloric foods.

How Much Should You Eat?

Of course, the answer to this depends on how much you currently weigh and how active you are. If you know approximately how many calories you want to aim for each day, see our Magic Meal Plans in Part 4 to get a good sense of how much food this means.

Not sure how many calories you need each day? Here's a nifty rule of thumb. If you're trying for modest weight loss, simply add a zero to your weight to get a ballpark calorie target. For instance, if you weigh 160 pounds, your target for modest weight loss would be 1,600 calories a day.

It's worth keeping a food diary for a few days to see how many calories you're really eating; the number may well be more than you think (and aren't you a little curious?). Use the nutrition labels on packaged foods to get the calories per serving (be careful; some packages contain two servings, so you'll have to double that number if you eat the whole thing). For fresh foods, use a Web site like www.calorie-count.com, www.thecaloriecounter.com, www.calorieking.com, or www.nal.usda.gov/fnic/foodcomp/search to get the calorie counts of common foods.

Another way to get a handle on portion sizes is simply to train your eye to identify what a reasonable serving looks like (see "What Does a Serving Look Like?"). Bring these images to mind when you're serving food, ordering food, and of course, eating food. The serving sizes are quite small, so don't feel bad if your portion is twice as large. A serving of pasta or rice is 1/2 cup, but most people eat a cup, so that counts as two servings. Most of us need no more than six servings of grains a day—preferably low- or medium-GL grains—so if you're eating three

or four servings at a sitting, that's too much. A single dense bagel can equal six servings of grains—an entire day's worth!

A serving of meat or chicken is about 3 ounces (85 g), but most people can eat two servings a day—the size of two decks of cards.

Cutting Back

Unfortunately, in this age of super-size servings, we've been trained to eat a lot. It's up to you to fight back.

Start by putting less food on your plate or in your bowl. Studies show that when large portions are put in front of us, most of us eat more—often

WHAT DOES A SERVING LOOK LIKE?

Here are some images to keep in mind. Each is one serving.

A 3-ounce (85 g) serving of cooked **meat** is the size of a deck of cards.

A 3-ounce (85 g) serving of **fish** is the size of a checkbook.

An ounce (30 g) of **cheese** is the size of four dice.

An ounce (30 g) of **sliced cheese** is the diameter of a CD.

A half cup of **pasta or rice** is the size of a baseball cut in half.

A cup of cold **cereal** is the size of a baseball.

A medium **baked potato** is the size of a personal-size bar of soap.

Two tablespoons of **peanut butter** is the size of a Ping-Pong ball.

Two tablespoons of **salad dressing** is the size of a shot glass.

A 6-ounce (180 ml) serving of **juice** is the size of a small yogurt container.

A medium piece of **fruit,** such as an apple, is the size of a tennis ball.

50 percent more at a single meal. Put your meals on plates in the kitchen rather than putting a big plate or bowl on the table for everyone to dig into at will. Buy small single-portion bags of snacks rather than eating out of a big bag (which always disappears). If you do buy a big bag, dole out a reasonable portion onto a small plate or a napkin, then close the bag and put it away out of sight before you sit down to munch.

When you're eating out, order smaller dishes (don't be afraid to order from the children's menu at fast-food places) or ask the server to put half the dish in a doggie bag before you start to eat. It's also a good idea to share one main dish and a separate dish of vegetables or share one main dish and fill up with a salad or broth-based soup.

In general, though, try to eat most of your meals at home. It's much easier to control your calorie intake as well as the amount of fat and number of high-GL foods that go into your meal.

Putting It All Together

Are you ready to eat the *Magic Foods* way? In the first chapter, you learned how important it is to your health and well-being to eat in ways that keep your blood sugar levels stable throughout the day. In the second chapter, you found out what makes certain foods catapult your blood sugar, while others keep it humming steadily. In the third chapter, you learned the pitfalls of a quick-fix low-carb approach. And now you've learned the Seven Secrets of Magic Eating. In the next chapter, you'll quiz yourself to see where your diet stands now, discover some fixes for your dietary downfalls, and bone up on smart strategies for eating out.

Then it's on to the real meat of the book (lean meat, of course!). In Part 2, you'll find profiles of the 57 Magic foods, from apples to yogurt. Each profile tells you how the GL of the food stacks up (either very low, low, or medium; you won't find Magic foods with a high or very high GL) plus other important health benefits it offers. You'll also learn the proper portion size—because remember, portions count—as well as menu suggestions and cooking tips.

In Part 3, the Magic Meal Makeovers show you how to make simple changes to your breakfasts, lunches, snacks, dinners, and desserts to help you make your meals more blood sugar friendly without a lot of fuss.

To really help you put Magic eating into action, in Part 4 we've supplied more than 100 Magic recipes. These make low-GL cooking come alive, incorporating the Magic foods in clever, simple, and delicious ways. Each recipe includes full nutritional information, but you don't have to worry about that if you don't want to; we've made sure the dishes are good for your blood sugar.

You'll even find meal plans that fit these recipes into a week's worth of eating based on three different calorie goals to help you manage your weight. All the tools you need are right at your fingertips!

THE GLYCEMIC LOAD OF COMMON FOODS

The GL is the best measure of a food's effect on blood sugar. Here, we've listed some common foods and grouped them into three categories: low GL (10 and under), medium GL (11 to 19), and high GL (20 and up). You want to aim for as many low-GL foods as possible and eat high-GL foods more sparingly.

Since carbohydrate foods are the ones that contribute most to the GL of your diet, we've focused on those foods here. Foods that are mostly protein or fat—such as meats, fish, and cheeses—have little or no GL, so you won't find many of

them in this list, although you will find them in the Magic foods entries in Part 2. Including protein-rich foods and "good" fats in your meals and snacks will help keep your GL score for the day moderate.

Remember that portion size makes a big difference: If you eat two servings of a medium-GL breakfast cereal, it suddenly qualifies as a high-GL food. On the other hand, if you just love a food in the high-GL category, go ahead and eat a small portion, preferably along with a small portion of a low- or medium-GL food.

LOW (GL = 10 or less)

Breads, Tortillas, Grains	Serving size	GL
Coarse barley bread (75% intact kernels)	2 slices	10
Soy and flaxseed bread	2 slices	10
Whole grain pumpernickel bread	2 slices	10
Pearled barley	1 cup	8
Popcorn	2 cups	8
Wheat tortillas	2 6" (15 cm)	6

Breakfast Cereals	Serving size	GL
Alpen Muesli	1/3 cup (1 oz [30 g])	10
Oatmeal, instant	1 cup prepared (1 oz [30 g dry])	10
All Bran	1/2 cup (1 oz [30 g])	9
Bran Buds	1/3 cup (1 oz [30 g])	7
Oatmeal made from rolled oats	1 cup prepared (1 oz [30 g dry])	7

Beans and Peas	Serving size	GL
Lima beans	1 cup	10
Pinto beans	1 cup	10
Chickpeas	1 cup	8
Baked beans	1 cup	7
Kidney beans	1 cup	7
Navy beans	1 cup	7
Butter beans	1 cup	6
Green peas	1 cup	6
Split peas, yellow	1 cup	6
Lentils, green or red	1 cup	5

LOW (GL = 10 or less)

Dairy and Soy Drinks	Serving size	GL
Low-fat yogurt with fruit and sugar	7 oz (200 ml)	9
Soy milk	1 cup (8 oz [250 ml])	7
Low-fat chocolate milk, sweetened with aspartame	8 oz (250 ml)	3
Low-fat yogurt with fruit, sweetened with aspartame	7 oz (200 ml)	2

Fruits and Vegetables	Serving size	GL
Prunes, pitted, chopped	1/3 cup (2 oz [60 g])	10
Apricots, dried, chopped	1/3 cup (2 oz [60 g])	9
Peaches, canned in light syrup	1/2 cup (4 oz [125 g])	9
Grapes, medium bunch (about 50)	4 oz (125 g)	8
Mango, sliced	2/3 cup (4 oz [125 g])	8
Pineapple, diced	2/3 cup (4 oz [125 g])	7
Apple	1 small	6
Kiwifruit, sliced	2/3 cup (4 oz [125 g])	6
Beets, sliced	1/2 cup	5
Orange	1 small	5
Peach	1 small	5
Plums	2 small	5
Pear	1 small	4
Strawberries	about 6 medium	4
Watermelon, chopped	2/3 cup (4 oz [125 g])	4
Carrots, raw	1 large	3
Cherries	about 16 (4 oz [125 g])	3
Grapefruit	1/2	3

Beverages	Serving size	GL
Orange juice, unsweetened	3/4 cup (6 oz [180 ml])	10
Grapefruit juice, unsweetened	3/4 cup (6 oz [180 ml])	7
Tomato juice	3/4 cup (6 oz [180 ml])	4

Sweets	Serving size	GL
M&Ms with peanuts	25 (1 oz [30 g])	6
Nutella (chocolate hazelnut spread)	4 Tbsp	4

Nuts	Serving size	GL
Mixed nuts, roasted	1/3 cup (1.5 oz [45 g])	4
Cashew nuts	about 13 (1.5 oz [45 g])	3
Peanuts	1/3 cup (1.5 oz [45 g])	1

Medium (GL =11–19)

Bread, Tortillas, Crackers, Chips	Serving size	GL
Coarse barley bread (50% intact kernels)	2 slices	18
High-fiber white bread	2 slices	18
Corn chips	2 oz (60 g)	17
100% whole grain bread	2 slices	14
Sourdough rye bread	2 slices	12
Stone-ground wheat thins	4	12
Corn tortillas	2 6" (15 cm)	11
Rye crispbreads	2 1/2	11

Grains	Serving size	GL
Converted long-grain white rice	2/3 cup cooked	16
Brown rice	2/3 cup cooked	18
Quinoa	2/3 cup cooked	16
Wild rice	2/3 cup cooked	18
Wheatberries	2/3 cup cooked	14
Bulgur	2/3 cup cooked	12

Pasta	Serving size	GL
Spaghetti (cooked 15 minutes)	1 cup	17
Whole wheat spaghetti	1 cup	13
High-protein spaghetti	1 cup	12

Beverages	Serving size	GL
Low-fat chocolate milk	8 oz (250 ml)	12
Pineapple juice, unsweetened	6 oz (180 ml)	12
Apple juice	8 oz (250 ml)	8

Fruits, Vegetables, Beans	Serving size	GL
Sweet corn	1 cup	18
Sweet potato	1 medium (5 oz [140 g])	17
Figs, dried, chopped	1/3 cup (2 oz [60 g])	16
Banana	1 small (4 oz [125 g])	11
Black-eyed peas	1 cup	11

Breakfast Cereals	Serving size	GL
Nabisco Cream of Wheat, regular	1 cup prepared (1 oz [30 g])	17
Post Grape-Nuts	1/2 cup (1 oz [30 g])	16
Cheerios	1 cup (1 oz [30 g])	15
Life	3/4 cup (1 oz [30 g])	15
Special K	1 cup (1 oz [30 g])	14

High (GL = 20 or higher)

Potatoes	Serving size	GL
Baked russet Burbank potato	1 medium	26
French fries	5 oz (140 g)	22

Grains	Serving size	GL
Sticky white rice	2/3 cup cooked	31
Millet	2/3 cup cooked	25
Couscous	2/3 cup cooked	23
Long-grain white rice	2/3 cup cooked	23

Pasta	Serving size	GL
Udon Japanese noodles	1 cup cooked	25
Spaghetti (cooked 20 minutes)	1 cup	22

Breads	Serving size	GL
French baguette	2 slices	30
Middle Eastern flatbread	1 large	30
Italian white bread	2 slices	22
Hamburger roll	1	21
Light rye bread	2 slices	20
Mini-bagel (Lender's)	1	20
Wonder Bread	2 slices	20

Breakfast Cereals	Serving size	GL
Kellogg's Cornflakes	1 cup (1 oz [30 g])	24
Rice Chex	1 1/4 cups (1 oz [30 g])	23
Nabisco Cream of Wheat, instant	1 cup prepared (1 oz [30 g])	22
Rice Krispies	3/4 cup (1 oz [30 g])	22
Corn Chex	1 cup (1 oz [30 g])	21

Dried Fruit	Serving size	GL
Raisins	1/3 cup	28
Dates, dried, chopped	1/3 cup	25

Beverages	Serving size	GL
Ocean Spray Cranberry Juice Cocktail	12 oz (375 ml)	36
Coca-Cola	12 oz (375 ml)	24

Sweets	Serving size	GL
Mars Bar	2 oz (60 g)	26
Jelly beans	20	22
Betty Crocker chocolate cake with chocolate icing	4 oz (125 g)	20

Source: "International Table of Glycemic Index and Glycemic Load Values 2002," Kaye Foster-Powell, Susanna H. A. Holt, and Janette C. Brand-Miller, *American Journal of Clinical Nutrition* vol. 76, no. 1 (2002), 5–56. Additional data from www.glycemicindex.com, www.mypyramid.gov, and www.ars.usda.gov.

chapter 5

THE MAGIC FOODS
approach
in ACTION

Now that you're armed with the Seven Secrets of Magic Eating, where do you go from here? Altering your diet can seem dizzyingly difficult, but it doesn't have to be, especially if you make one tiny change at a time. A good first step is to take stock of your eating habits and find out what you're doing right—and where you could stand to make some gentle adjustments.

You'll be **amazed** how the simple act of acknowledging your eating habits can make you more open to **changing** them.

In this chapter you'll:

• **Quiz yourself** to find out how Magic your diet is. You'll be amazed how the simple act of acknowledging your eating habits can make you more open to changing them.

• **Find and fix** your dietary downfalls (we all have 'em).

• **Learn the art** of eating out. Since we eat so many of our meals out of the house, learning to outsmart restaurant menus and navigate the minefield of fast-food dining is key.

In Part 2, you'll discover the 57 Magic foods and how to reap their blood sugar and weight-loss benefits. The Magic Meal Plans and Magic Recipes in Part 4 will be a great help, too, not to mention the Magic Meal Makeovers in Part 3. But before we take you there, let's get you ready to go.

quiz How Magic is your diet?

Circle the number next to your answer for each question, then add up your score.
Turn to page 62 to see how you did.

1 If you were in my kitchen in the morning, you'd see me drinking:

a. Coffee or tea, plain or with low-fat milk and/or a little sugar or sugar substitute — **1**

b. Coffee or tea with full-fat cream and/or loads of sugar — **2**

c. A soft drink — **3**

2 When I eat cereal for breakfast, I'm most likely to pick one like:

a. Cornflakes, Rice Krispies, or Corn Chex — **3**

b. Grape-Nuts or Cheerios — **2**

c. All Bran, Bran Buds, or Muesli — **1**

3 When I drink juice, it's:

a. A small glass of unsweetened juice such as orange or grapefruit — **1**

b. A large glass of unsweetened juice such as orange or grapefruit — **2**

c. A large glass of juice drink (5 to 30% juice) — **3**

4 When I drink milk (or pour it over my cereal), it's:

a. Whole — **3**

b. 2% — **2**

c. 1% or fat-free — **1**

5 The bread on my counter right now is:

a. 100% whole grain (wheat, rye, pumpernickel, sourdough) — **1**

b. Made with white flour and some whole grain flour ("wheat" bread as opposed to "whole wheat" bread) — **2**

c. White — **3**

6 Potatoes (including mashed potatoes, French fries, hash browns, etc.) are:

a. The vegetables I eat most often — **3**

b. On my plate two or three times a week — **2**

c. On my plate once a week or less — **1**

7 Spinach, broccoli, and other dark green vegetables are:

a. Strangers in my house — **3**

b. Welcome as occasional visitors, if they keep quiet — **2**

c. Practically family — **1**

8 When I make or buy a deli sandwich, I:

a. Pile on the bologna, salami, and other full-fat meats — **3**

b. Use roast beef — **2**

c. Have low-fat meats like sliced turkey breast or lean ham — **1**

9 When I'm hungry in the afternoon, I grab:

a. Some fruit, nuts, or low-fat yogurt — **1**

b. Crackers and cheese or a cereal bar — **2**

c. Chips or a candy bar — **3**

10 I eat nuts:

a. Rarely   3

b. By the bagful; can't get enough   2

c. By the small handful every day or two   1

11 I eat at fast-food places:

a. At least twice a week   3

b. Once a week or so   2

c. Less than once a week   1

12 In my refrigerator, you're most likely to find:

a. Soft drinks or sports/energy drinks   3

b. Diet soft drinks   2

c. Water or sparkling water   1

13 When I get pizza, I usually eat:

a. One or two slices with a side salad and a noncaloric drink   1

b. One or two slices, no salad, and a soft drink   2

c. Two or more slices plus a big soft drink and a side of garlic bread   3

14 My favorite salad dressing is:

a. Something creamy or cheesy   2

b. Olive oil and vinegar   1

c. Who eats salad?   3

15 When I eat pasta, I:

a. Pile it high and top it with cheese sauce or meat sauce   3

b. Have a moderate amount paired with chicken, fish, or shellfish   1

c. Enjoy it as a side dish with some olive oil and grated cheese   1

16 When I'm offered vegetarian bean chili for dinner, I think:

a. Looks good!   1

b. Okay, I guess, but I hope I'm not hungry later   2

c. Where's the beef?   3

17 When I eat beef for dinner, it's likely to be:

a. A large juicy steak, like T-bone or prime rib, or a big serving of pot roast swimming in gravy   3

b. A moderate serving of lean grilled beef, such as sirloin, with rice or potatoes   2

c. A small serving of lean beef that's grilled or mixed into a stir-fry   1

18 Fish? I'll eat it:

a. Only if it's battered and deep-fried, if ever   3

b. Baked or broiled, a couple of times a week   1

c. Baked or broiled, every couple of weeks or so   2

19 When I eat Chinese food, I eat this much rice:

a. About 1/2 cup   1

b. About 1 cup   2

c. Lots—as much as it takes to soak up all the sauce   3

20 When it comes to dessert, I:

a. Live for it—usually a big slice of pie or cake or a bowl of full-fat ice cream   3

b. Eat it once in a while when I feel like indulging   1

c. Have fruit or a small bowl of reduced-fat ice cream or sorbet   1

Your Score

30 or under You're generally eating the *Magic Foods* way—choosing low-GL carbs most of the time, keeping portions under control, limiting saturated fats, and getting some fruits and vegetables. Use the Magic food profiles, recipes, and meal plans in the rest of the book to help you further fine-tune your eating.

31 to 40 Your diet could use some improvement. Pay particular attention to answers that were "3s"—these are your dietary downfalls. You do have some good things going for you in your diet, though, so build on them. Use the rest of this book to strengthen your healthy habits and retool your least healthy ones.

41 or over No blue ribbon for you—but that means you have your pick of small improvements to make. Look back over your answers and pick out some "3s" that you think you can edge into "2s" or "1s." You'll find lots of tips, tools, suggestions, and recipes in this book to help you improve your diet.

Understanding Your Score

1 Having a little sugar in your coffee isn't a big deal, but add 3 teaspoons, and you add nearly 50 calories and 12 grams of carbohydrate. Starting the day with a soft drink—an increasingly common habit—is a dietary downfall to be sure. One 16-ounce (473 ml) bottle of cola has the equivalent of 11 or 12 teaspoons of sugar and will push up your day's GL before you even get out the door.

2 The (a.) cereal choices have the highest GLs, the (b.) choices are medium GL, and the (c.) cereals have the lowest GLs and are kindest to your blood sugar. If you like a higher-GL cereal, try mixing it with a lower-GL kind and/or pouring a smaller bowl. One cup is plenty.

3 Orange juice is a healthy beverage, but it has a fair amount of sugar and calories, so don't drink it like water. Use small juice glasses for juice and save large glasses for water and low-calorie drinks only. Juice "drinks" are mostly sugar and water, so we suggest you avoid them altogether.

4 Whole milk is a major source of saturated fat in our diets, and that's bad for your heart and insulin sensitivity. Drinking 2% milk is better, but this type still gets about a third of its calories from fat, much of it saturated. Fat-free (skim) and 1% are the best choices.

5 When choosing bread, 100 percent whole grain varieties are best (and if they're made from coarsely ground flours with kernels and seeds, so much the better). Wheat breads that have some white flour are second choices, and white bread comes in last in terms of its effect on your blood sugar.

6 Potatoes are a high-GL food; there's no getting around it. You don't need to ban them, but don't rely on them as a staple. Sweet potatoes, on the other hand, are a much better choice.

7 You're not surprised, right? These dark green veggies are incredibly nutritious and have very little carbohydrate. Adding them to any dish or meal—a side of sautéed spinach, lightly steamed broccoli florets in a pasta salad—lowers the meal's overall GL per portion. So does adding nearly any other vegetable.

8 Sandwich meats are a main source of saturated fat in our diets. Lean meats, on the other hand, provide blood sugar–friendly protein without all the fat. Roast beef is in between—better than salami and bologna but fattier than turkey breast. Ask for your roast beef on rye or sourdough, and the sandwich is a step better already. Add mustard instead of mayo for the best blood sugar–lowering effect (it contains vinegar, a Magic food).

9 You can't go wrong with low-cal, high-fiber fruit. Low-fat yogurt, with its sugar-stabilizing protein, is another good choice if it's not overly sweetened. Crackers and cheese are okay, too, especially if the crackers are whole grain (with no trans fats), and you keep your portions in check. Potato or corn chips, though, have easily digested starches, and candy bars offer nothing much but fat and sugar.

10 Nuts are a Magic food thanks to their "good" fats and blood sugar–stabilizing protein. People who eat just a handful each day tend to have healthier hearts and may even have an easier time losing weight (nuts are that filling!). But eat too many, and the benefits will vanish.

11 If you eat at fast-food places often, chances are you're eating lots of fried foods, with too much saturated fat, and high-GL carbs in the bread and fries. Have fast-food meals a few times a month (or less), not a few times a week.

12 The GL of soft drinks isn't as sky-high as you might expect, but it's easy to down huge amounts. Remember, GL is related to portion size; double the amount you drink, and the GL doubles as well. Switching to water or sparkling water can have a dramatic effect on your calorie and sugar intake—and your waistline.

13 Pizza's another food that's okay in moderation, but more than a slice can really pile on the blood sugar–raising carbs and cheesy fat. When ordering, favor thinner crust and lots of veggies on top. Don't tip the scales by adding a big soft drink; have a small one or, better still, water, seltzer, or unsweetened iced tea.

14 A green salad topped with a vinegar-based dressing is perhaps the ideal Magic side dish. The vinegar even helps lower the GL of whatever you eat with your salad. Creamy dressings don't have the same effect, and they add a lot more calories, but even a salad with a little creamy dressing is better than no salad at all; try to limit dressing to a tablespoon or less.

15 Pasta's not bad for you; in fact, it's a Magic food. For a carb food, its GL is not very high, but it's still best eaten in moderation, as a base for lean protein or vegetables. Most cheese and meat sauces, though, are anything but low fat.

16 Beans are a high-protein, low-GL food, making them ideal for anyone concerned about heart health, weight, and blood sugar. Try to have a meatless main meal a few times a week.

17 Beef is a Magic food, but only when it's lean (and eaten in moderation). Even a "lean" hamburger has more saturated fat than the same amount of sirloin or chuck steak.

18 All fish is low in saturated fat, and the high-fat varieties have omega-3 fatty acids, which are good for your heart and even your blood sugar. Try to eat a couple of fish meals a week. Eating fish or seafood deep-fried erases all the benefits.

19 Rice has a surprising number of calories (about 200 per cup), and if you're eating white rice, a high GL. Stick with brown rice and keep your serving small.

20 Everyone should indulge in dessert once in a while, because eating well is not about depriving yourself. If you eat it every day, though, you're probably getting too many calories (unless your dessert is fruit or you're extremely good at controlling your portion sizes).

Find—And Fix—Your Dietary Downfalls

All of us have dietary strengths and weaknesses, just as we have strengths and weaknesses in other areas of our lives. No one is perfect—and that's fine! But if you're like most people, there are a few things you're doing out of habit that are sabotaging your efforts to control your blood sugar and lose weight. If you change just one or two of them by setting your mind to it, you'll reap rewards in spades. First, though, you have to recognize them.

PROBLEM I like a big bowl of cereal in the morning.

solution Your first course of action is to make sure you're eating a low-GL cereal, such as Raisin Bran, All-Bran, or Bran Flakes, or at least a medium-GL type like Kellogg's Special K (see "How Cereals Rate" on page 85). If you're not used to these cereals, mix them with a bit of your usual cereal at first to make the transition easier. Second, pour less into the bowl and add something else to fill it up. You can top your cereal with fresh fruit, like chopped apples, strawberries, or blueberries. Adding a table-spoon of chopped nuts is an excellent strategy because nuts add protein and "good" fat, both of which help stabilize your blood sugar and keep you feeling full.

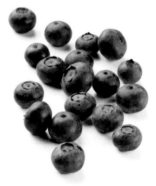

PROBLEM I don't eat breakfast until I get to work, and then there's not much to choose from except bagels or muffins.

solution Pack your breakfast in an insulated lunch bag the night before so you can grab it on the way out of the house. A fine breakfast is a piece of fruit, a plastic bag with a small handful of nuts, and 8 ounces (250 ml) of low-fat yogurt. Or make a batch of healthy bran muffins (see our recipe on page 197) over the weekend and grab one along with an orange. Another option: Keep a box of high-fiber, low-GL breakfast cereal (along with plastic spoons and bowls) at your desk, and bring the milk (in a Thermos), fruit, and nuts with you.

PROBLEM I like sweet drinks, not water.

solution That's okay. But think of these drinks, whether they're soft drinks, sweetened iced tea, or sugary fruit drinks, as a treat, like dessert. You wouldn't eat dessert more than once a day, so don't indulge in these drinks more often than that either. Wait until the afternoon and then get the smallest size you can find. In the meantime, cultivate another habit—sipping sparkling water. Some flavored varieties have few or no calories, and a good squeeze of lemon or lime juice makes plain sparkling water much more interesting and palatable. Buy seltzer or mineral water in bulk and make sure there's plenty at home and at the office. Changing this one habit can be a really effective way of improving your diet and even losing weight.

PROBLEM There's no place to get a healthy lunch near my office.

solution One strategy is to think through what changes would make it easier for you to bring lunch from home. If you're lucky, your office has a refrigerator, a microwave, or even a toaster oven. If so, get into the habit of making more of whatever you're having for dinner, then pack up the leftovers for lunch the next day. If there's no fridge, pack your lunch in a small insulated lunch bag with an ice pack. It will stay cold through lunchtime. On days when you don't pack your lunch, check out page 71 for our tips on eating better at fast-food places.

PROBLEM I like pizza. Is that so bad?

solution The devil is in the details. The thicker the crust—especially Sicilian—the higher the GL of the meal. If you add pepperoni, you really sabotage yourself with extra calories and saturated fat, which contributes to insulin resistance. So think healthier pizza: thin crust with veggies on top. Go for whole wheat crust if it's available. Stick with one or two slices. Add a salad with vinaigrette dressing so you get enough food to feel full; the vinegar in the dressing will also help lower the GL of the meal. And make the soft drink a small one or, better yet, have sparkling water.

PROBLEM When I get salad from the salad bar, I usually load it with cheese, croutons, and creamy dressing. Is it still good for me?

solution You might as well eat a hamburger with a side of lettuce. Full-fat cheeses and creamy dressings are high in saturated fat, which is bad for insulin sensitivity. They and the croutons (which are fried) are also loaded with calories. Don't abandon salads, just look for ways to keep them interesting and healthy. Add toasted sunflower seeds for crunch (and healthy fat) or a few black olives for richness (and again, "good" fat). Add hot peppers, if you like them, for kick. Throw on some chickpeas for addi-

tional texture. Top it all off with a vinegar-based dressing; experiment to find a tasty one you like, such as mustard vinaigrette for extra flavor.

PROBLEM I am starving at about 3:00 in the afternoon, and I eat whatever junk food is in sight.

solution If you eat Magic foods for breakfast and lunch, this won't happen. And that's good, because research shows that when they're really hungry, people can eat as much as twice as much food as they normally would. Snacking itself isn't bad at all, though, so keep healthy snacks on hand (think carrot sticks, apples, low-fat yogurt, a few whole grain crackers and peanut butter, or a handful of peanuts or almonds) to keep the sailing smooth between lunch and dinner.

PROBLEM I eat carbs when I'm stressed or anxious.

solution A lot of people reach for carbs when they're stressed. (The scientific jury is out as to whether carbs actually help calm you down. The effect may simply be due to a sense of comfort from a familiar food.) There's no quick solution here. The key is to figure out ways to cope other than eating. Practice deep breathing or give yourself a "timeout" by taking a 10-minute stroll, after which the craving should have passed. One of the best ways to deal with anxiety in general is to exercise; even a brisk 20-minute walk can lift your mood and calm you down. Studies show that people who exercise regularly have lower responses to stress than people who don't. You can also practice prevention at the supermarket: Avoid buying simple carbohydrates so they aren't within reach when you want them.

PROBLEM I know portion sizes are important, but it's so easy to finish what's on my plate.

solution Use a smaller plate! Really. Manufacturers are actually making many plates and bowls larger because we eat so much bigger portions than we used to. Fight the trend by serving dinner on a lunch plate. Serve juice in real juice glasses—they're much smaller than regular glasses. Instead of using a big bowl for cereal, try a smaller dessert bowl. And always spoon out your dinner onto individual plates rather than leaving bowls or platters on the table within easy reach.

PROBLEM I'd like to eat more beans, but I don't know much about cooking them.

solution You don't have to make bean dishes from scratch. Canned beans can be no-fuss additions to something you're already making. Making a salad? Rinse some canned chickpeas and toss them on top. Add canned kidney beans to nearly any vegetable soup. For a quick bean side dish, drain a can of white beans, put them into a microwavable bowl, and add some olive oil, grated Parmesan, and fresh pepper. Microwave for a minute or two, then mash for a delicious, high-protein, low-GL dish.

PROBLEM When I eat small portions at dinner, I'm still hungry.

solution First, make sure your dinner contains protein and "good fat," not just carbs. That way, it will keep you full longer (plus, you're less likely to overeat broiled chicken breast than buttery mashed potatoes). Second, try to eat a little slower so your stomach has more time to send the message to your brain that you're full. Take plenty of time between bites for conversation or sips of water. If these don't do the trick, start the meal with clear soup or a salad, both of which will occupy a lot of space in your stomach and help you put down your fork sooner. And remember: It's okay to leave the dinner table a tiny bit hungry. You'll feel fuller as your food digests.

PROBLEM I'd like to snack on fruit, but I just don't think of it.

solution Put it in front of your face, literally. Studies show that people eat more fruit when it's in a bowl on the counter rather than tucked away in the refrigerator. Lots of fruits stay fresh on the counter, 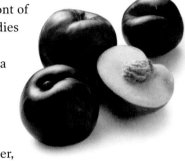 such as apples, pears, plums, nectarines, and bananas. When you buy fruit, wash it as soon as you come home, then put it in a bowl. If you keep fruit in the fridge—such as grapes, which taste great cold—make sure it's on the top shelf where it's easy to grab. Like melon? Cut it into slices or cubes and refrigerate it in an airtight container so it's ready to eat come snack time.

PROBLEM My pitfall is late-night desserts.

solution Try to have your dessert earlier. If you normally eat it at 10:00 p.m., aim for 8:30, and then brush your teeth so you're not tempted to eat again. Another strategy: Avoid bringing home the kinds of desserts that you most tend to overeat; most people won't leave the house at night just to get dessert. Finally, train yourself to enjoy healthier desserts, such as a bowl of berries with a dollop of low-fat ice cream or light whipped cream or a container of light pre-portioned pudding, and you won't have to worry as much.

The Art of Eating Out

If most restaurants offered menus full of Magic fare like lean grilled meats, whole grain side dishes, and fruit-based desserts, it would be a snap to eat out the Magic way. But they don't. Nearly all of the most common carbohydrate-rich foods on menus reflect those in the typical Western diet. In other words, they are high-GL foods. And at most restaurants, from fast-food joints to the fanciest white-tablecloth establishments, the food is floating in fat and stuffed with extra calories. Add to that the amazingly large portions that we have grown to expect for our dining dollars, and eating out seems impossible to do well.

It can be done, though, and learning to do it is a survival skill. That's because we eat out—or have takeout meals—so often now that it's a staple of our lives. Fifty years ago, about one out of four meals was prepared outside the home; today, it's closer to one in two.

The first step is to accept how commonly you eat meals you haven't made yourself, then plan to order better.

BE CAREFUL WHERE YOU EAT

Make the challenge of eating out easier by being smart about what kinds of restaurants you patronize. Avoid the temptation of all-you-can-eat places, or buffet-style restaurants, where portions are hard to control. Avoid places known for enormous portions, like most steak houses. And you probably won't find a lot of Magic foods on the menu at eateries that specialize in deep-frying an entire breaded onion. Enjoy a meal at one of these on your birthday, sure, but don't do it on a regular basis.

MAKE FRIENDS WITH THE WAITPERSON

Once you're in the right kind of restaurant, get ready to get friendly with the waitperson. Ask them to hold the breadbasket so you're not tempted to fill up on usually high-GL carbs while waiting for your meal to arrive. Inquire about how a dish you're considering is prepared (Is it swimming in butter? Are the vegetables present in only token amounts?) and find out how big the portions are.

ORDER CREATIVELY

When you order, be bold: Order soup, salad, and an appetizer (not fried) for your meal rather than an entrée. Split an entrée and share a side order of vegetables to get more veggies into your meal—and fewer calories. If a main dish comes with a potato, ask if you can get an extra vegetable instead. (Especially if you're a regular customer, you're likely to get your way.) If you plan to order dessert, plan to share it, too. The best situation is when you get to know a restaurant's regular fare, including how big the portions are, and use that knowledge to outsmart the menu.

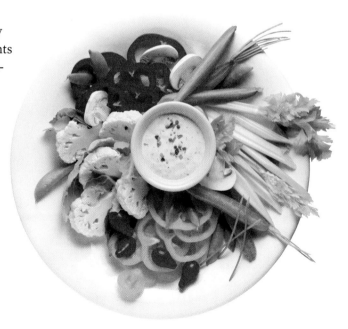

Eating Out
Chinese

The traditional Chinese diet is a healthy one, with lots of vegetables, stir-fries with small chunks of meat or fish, and soy foods. But that's not evident in the typical fare in a Chinese restaurant here, where the meal is likely to be heavy on greasy meats and swimming in sauces with lots and lots of calories. Even the vegetables are usually in a fatty sauce.

Do you have to give up Chinese takeout? Of course not; that would be almost unthinkable. But to get a Magic meal, you do have to order carefully.

YOUR GAME PLAN

1. **Ask for brown rice.** Most restaurants give you the option. Remember, white rice is a blood sugar disaster waiting to happen. And don't eat the whole bowl or container of rice. Spoon a half cup onto your plate and leave the rest. Or do as a Chinese native would: Put a small amount in a small bowl and hold the bowl up, using your chopsticks (or fork) to eat a little rice in between bites of your main dish. Or be bold and don't eat any rice at all.

2. **Start your meal with wonton, egg drop, or hot-and-sour soup.** This will take the edge off your hunger without a lot of calories (avoid soups with coconut milk). If you want a ravioli-type appetizer, order steamed vegetable dumplings, but nothing fried.

3. **When it comes to entrées, order from the "health" menu.** Here is where you'll find steamed chicken and vegetables with sauce on the side and similar low-fat choices. Another good choice is moo goo gai pan (chicken with mushrooms). If you like stir-fries, ask the waitperson to have yours prepared with less oil and more veggies, and get the sauce on the side.

4. **Make sure you order plenty of vegetables.** If you really want to make the meal healthier, order a plate of steamed vegetables and add them to other dishes. Or ask for sautéed vegetables or Szechuan-style string beans.

5. **Take advantage of the bean curd (tofu).** Include a heart-healthy, low-GL dish like bean curd with sautéed Chinese mixed vegetables (ask for sautéed bean curd, not deep-fried).

6. **Plan to take home leftovers.** Portions are often large. Think of about a cup of a dish (without rice) as a serving.

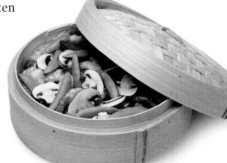

Eating Out
Italian

A single slice of pizza with vegetables is a fine choice, especially if it's made with a whole wheat and/or thin crust. A cup of pasta with marinara sauce is all right, too. The problem is, few of us stop there.

Ironically, southern Italian food, prepared the traditional way, is among the healthiest in the world. Unfortunately, Italian restaurants are often parlors for the presentation of huge mounds of overcooked pasta and pizza. And even before these arrive, you'll have ample opportunity to eat bread. So unless you want to overload on carbs and send your blood sugar for a wild post-meal ride, tread carefully.

YOUR GAME PLAN

1. **Ask the waitperson not to bring the bread-basket.** Instead, order minestrone or another broth-based soup to fill up on while you await your entrée. Pasta e fagioli, another Italian classic, is a delicious bean/pasta soup that's also a good starter.

2. **If you want pasta, order a dish from the appetizer section of the menu, or share.** That's the traditional way—a small first course of pasta followed by simple grilled meat, poultry, or fish and a side of sautéed greens. As for pasta sauces, opt for those based on tomatoes (marinara), vegetables, white wine, and garlic—not cream. Watch out: Pasta primavera is often made with lots of cream.

3. **If it's on the menu, order simple grilled beef, veal, pork, chicken, fish, or shellfish.** Add a side order of sautéed spinach or broccoli rabe (a slightly bitter Italian version of broccoli). Finish with a mixed green salad with vinaigrette dressing.

4. **For dessert, ask for fresh berries or fruit ice, if it's available, or a small plate of cookies to share.** Stay away from the custards and cheesecake, the cannoli, and the tiramisu.

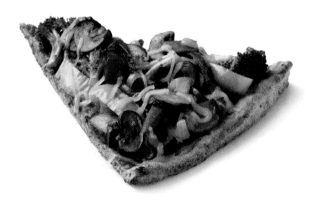

Mexican

Ordering from a fast-food Mexican place is about as big as a blood sugar challenge can get. Portions are generally huge, the tortillas used for burritos are larger than your head and filled with a cup or more of white rice (blood sugar enemy #1), and the entrées tend to be loaded with cheese—and we don't mean the Magic low-fat variety. Thread your way around these potholes, and you can arrive at a delicious, moderate-GL meal.

just say NO

Tortilla chips

Nachos

Chimichangas

Quesadillas

Enchiladas (beef, cheese, or any other kind)

Chiles rellenos

Refried beans

Anything "grande"

YOUR GAME PLAN

1. **Ask the waitperson to take away the tortilla chips.** The Mexican equivalent of a big breadbasket is either a bowl of chips with salsa or nacho chips covered with cheese. Just say no.

2. **Order a healthy starter instead.** Look for ceviches (marinated raw fish or seafood); guacamole, which is full of "good" fats (ask for soft tortillas instead of deep-fried chips to dip, and don't overeat them); gazpacho, a spicy cold vegetable soup; black bean soup; and tortilla soup (chicken in broth with vegetables and thin fried tortilla chips). Ask for extra salsa for the table and eat it with a spoon rather than on chips.

3. **For an entrée, look to fajitas.** These are made with lean beef (or chicken or shrimp) grilled with onions and peppers. Other good choices are grilled chicken or fish dishes.

4. **Order tacos or burritos without high-fat sour cream.** Ask for extra salsa instead. Hard tacos are fried, so you're better off with soft tacos; soft tortillas are even better. A small tortilla is the equivalent of a slice of bread.

If you're not eating rice, two or three soft tacos are fine, but stick to one or two if you are having rice. If you're getting a burrito, ask for no rice and more beans.

5. **As a side dish, go for rice and beans instead of Mexican rice.** Thanks to the beans, this dish has a lower GL than rice alone. But check first to be sure the beans aren't refried. Refried beans are loaded with fat.

6. **Have dessert at home.** Desserts at Mexican restaurants, such as flan and fried ice cream, are usually high in calories and fat, so skip them and eat something healthier elsewhere.

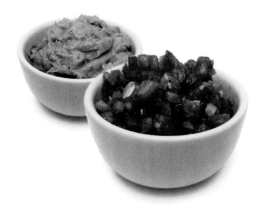

Eating Out
Fast Food

An occasional visit to a fast-food joint never killed anyone. Burgers and fries are still the staples on these menus, but the restaurants are now offering a greater selection of healthier fare. True, you'll have trouble locating a decent vegetable, but you can keep the fat and calorie damage under control by ordering grilled sandwiches, salads, and even vegetarian burgers, chili, soup, and low-fat dairy desserts. Aim to make your meals "fast" ones less than once a week.

YOUR GAME PLAN

1. **Opt for simple grilled fare,** if you can find it. If there's a grilled chicken sandwich and the chicken isn't breaded, that's a good start. Wendy's Ultimate Chicken Grill (360 calories) is a good choice, as is McDonald's Chicken McGrill.

2. **A simple hamburger isn't bad either—if you order the smallest one.** At 280 calories, Wendy's Jr. Hamburger is a low-cal burger. (By contrast, a Burger King Double Whopper with Cheese has 1,060 calories.) Another good option is a vegetarian burger. Burger King regularly offers vegetarian burgers (the BK Veggie; 380 calories), and McDonald's has them at some locations (the McVeggie; 350 calories).

3. **Order à la carte.** A meal that includes fries and a big soft drink is often cheaper, but it's no nutritional bargain. Skip the soft drink and ask for water—or orange juice, hot tea, coffee, or low-fat milk—instead. If it's a special treat, get the fries but buy the smallest size.

4. **Take advantage of the salads.** Just skip the cheese, bacon bits, and other add-ons. Ask for vinaigrette dressing. Try a salad as an entrée. Good choices include Burger King's Fire-Grilled Chicken (with vinaigrette) and Wendy's Mandarin Chicken Salad (with Oriental sesame dressing).

5. **Have yogurt.** At Wendy's, you can get fresh fruit with yogurt (220 calories); McDonald's offers Fruit 'n' Yogurt Parfait (160 calories).

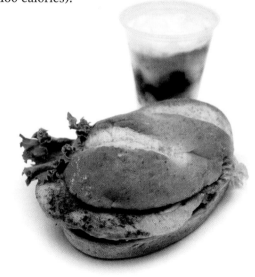

A (Scary) Trip to the Mall

Be prepared: The mall is a very dangerous place—for your nutritional safety. Before you leave, you'll get hungry, but like a fly in a spider's web, you're caught in a matrix of sticky choices that are nearly all disastrous.

If you succumb to a Classic Cinnabon, for example, you'll take in 730 calories, nearly all of them in the form of high-GL starches, sugar, and saturated fat. Go for the Cinnabon Caramel Pecanbon, and you get 1,100 calories—more than half the amount most people need in an entire day!

Or maybe Dunkin' Donuts is nearby. Grab a croissant (330 calories) and wash it down with a Coffee Coolata with cream (350), and you're up to 680 calories. And you haven't even had a meal, just a snack!

Maybe you're hungrier. If you're eyeing up Chick-fil-A, watch out: A Chicken Deluxe Sandwich with medium waffle fries and a large iced tea will cost you 950 calories.

Can you escape without catastrophe? Perhaps, if you keep your wits about you.

If there's a Subway, for instance, you can have a 6-inch (15 cm) roast beef sandwich on whole wheat bread for only 290 calories, with very little saturated fat and only a modest amount of carbohydrate (45 grams). You can get a similar low-fat, low-cal sandwich made with ham, oven-roasted chicken breast, turkey breast, or club style. Get it with minestrone soup for only 90 more calories. Wash it down with a diet soft drink or water, and you've eaten a real, satisfying meal for only 380 calories.

On the other hand, if you want only a snack, and you're smart, you'll have one with you. A handful of nuts is easy to throw into a resealable plastic bag. Baby carrots are similarly easy to bag and transport. And the old snack standby, an apple, always works well.

Now, throw away the apple core, put on your coat, get on the escalator, and walk out of the mall. No one will get hurt.

A Hidden Hazard: Coffee Drinks

It's easy to drink yourself into a bad place. And we're not talking about alcohol, just big "coffee" drinks. We're highlighting Starbucks here, but it's the same story at Dunkin' Donuts and other establishments that use coffee as a vehicle for cream, chocolate, caramel, and sugar.

Consider the Double Chocolate Chip Frappucino Blended Crème with whipped cream, Venti size (24 ounces/710 milliliters). It has 86 grams of sugar. Since 10 grams of table sugar—about 2 1/2 teaspoons—has a GL of 6, you could estimate that the sugar in this drink would provide a GL of about 52. Since any food with a GL over 20 is high GL, this is *very* high. But that sweet beverage also contributes a whopping 25 grams of fat, more than half of it saturated—the kind that not only clogs arteries but also contributes to insulin resistance. That drink has more fat and saturated fat than you'd get in a McDonald's Quarter Pounder with Cheese.

A Mocha Frappucino Blended Coffee might be a little better, but a Venti size still packs 530 calories, 18 grams of fat, and 69 grams of sugar (the equivalent of about 17 teaspoons). Consider as an alternative a cappuccino made with fat-free milk. Even a huge Venti has only 130 calories and about 16 grams of sugar (about 4 teaspoons' worth, with a GL of 10).

Of course, freshly brewed black coffee has almost no calories at all. Consider a tall black coffee from Starbucks with 2 teaspoons of sugar. It has fewer than 40 calories. You'd have to drink more than 18 of them to get the same number of calories as in the Frappucino Blended Crème. Its GL is about 5. Even if you add 2 tablespoons of 2% milk, it has only 57 calories.

If you prefer a cold drink, ask for plain iced coffee (with fat-free milk if you like) and add your own sugar.

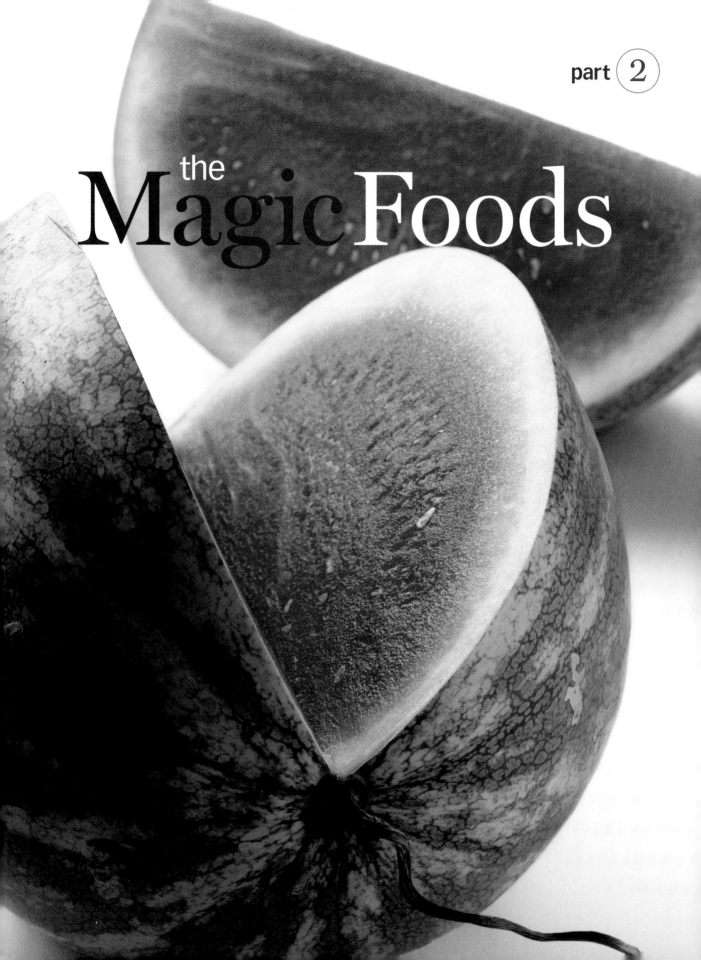

the Magic Foods

apples

GL LOW

Can eating an apple a day really help keep the doctor away? It can certainly help you control your blood sugar and gain all the benefits that come with that control. In fact, researchers have discovered that women who eat at least one apple a day are 28 percent less likely to develop type 2 diabetes than those who don't eat apples. That's probably because apples, from tart Granny Smiths to sweet, juicy Pink Ladies, are loaded with soluble fiber—number one for blunting blood sugar swings. A medium apple dishes up an impressive 4 grams of fiber, mostly pectin, which is also known for its ability to lower cholesterol.

Looking to trim your tummy? (Remember, belly fat is bad for blood sugar.) Try eating three small apples a day. A study from the State University of Rio de Janeiro found that doing so as part of a reduced-calorie diet helped women not only lose more weight but also lower their blood sugar more than women who ate another food instead of apples.

To press every bit of benefit from apples, opt for whole, unpeeled fruit. For apples with a lower GL, look for Braeburns, which have more acid and less sugar than Golden Delicious. Next on the glycemic scale is unsweetened applesauce, which offers many of the same health benefits. But steer clear of apple juice; it's not much better than apple-flavored liquid sugar.

Health Bonus

Apples aren't particularly rich in vitamins or minerals, but that doesn't mean they're not good for you. In fact, they're loaded with antioxidant compounds called flavonoids, believed to reduce the risk of cancer and heart disease. One study found that eating a small apple with the skin provided total antioxidant and anti-cancer activity equal to 1,500 milligrams of vitamin C.

PERFECT portions: 1 apple

At about 80 calories each, apples are the perfect snack size just the way nature grew them.

Menu Magic

- Snack on half an apple with a smear of peanut butter (another Magic food).

- Add thinly sliced apples to sandwiches for a bit of tang and crunch.

- Mix chopped apples with low-fat yogurt and wheat germ (two other Magic foods) for a healthy mid-morning snack.

- Doctor up jarred salsa by adding chopped apples, cucumbers, onions, jalapeño peppers, and lime juice.

- Put together an apple-cabbage skillet dinner with chopped apples, shredded cabbage, low-fat turkey sausage, chopped onions, cider vinegar, and fresh parsley.

- Make applesauce by cubing apples and simmering them in a small amount of water until desirably mushy. Add a sprinkling of cinnamon, a Magic spice.

Smart Substitutions

Instead of raisins: Try sliced apples on your oatmeal or other cereal. Unlike apples, raisins have concentrated sugars that raise blood sugar more quickly than apples do.

Instead of oil: Replace three-quarters of the butter or oil called for in cookie, cake, and brownie recipes with unsweetened applesauce.

RELATED recipes

Apple-Bran Muffins *197*
Apple-Cranberry Crumble *286*
Chicken Sauté with Apple *235*
Maple-Walnut Roasted Apples *282*
Oatmeal with Apple and Flaxseeds *193*

avocado

GL VERY LOW

Unlike virtually all other fruits (yes, avocados are fruits), these rich, creamy treats are loaded with fat—a whopping 25 to 30 grams each. Since fat has no impact on blood sugar, avocados are great additions to a low-GL diet if you eat them in moderation.

But, you may wonder, what about all that fat? There is a saving grace: Most of it is monounsaturated fat, the same heart-healthy kind found in olive oil. Research suggests that diets rich in this type of fat may help keep blood sugar in check. That's the main reason for secret number 5 of Magic eating, Favor Good Fats. Add some avocado to a sandwich or anything else with bread or carbs, and the fat will slow digestion of the meal, thus making it easier on your blood sugar.

Unlike the saturated fats in butter and meat, monounsaturated fat won't increase insulin resistance, a condition that makes blood sugar control more difficult. In fact, the good fat in avocados (as well as olive oil and nuts) may actually *reverse* insulin resistance, helping your body steady its blood sugar levels. Avocados also contain more soluble fiber (which stabilizes blood sugar and lowers cholesterol) and protein than any other fruit.

Of course, with fat come calories, so you don't want to start eating avocados with total abandon—though you probably wouldn't anyway, since a little avocado goes a long way.

Health Bonus

Avocados are rich in sterols, compounds shown to lower cholesterol. They're also packed with vitamins and minerals, including vitamin E, magnesium, vitamin C, folate, and zinc. Ounce for ounce, they provide more potassium than bananas!

Cooks Tips

To choose just the right avocado, try this: Hold the avocado in your hand and press it gently, then roll it to the other side and press again. If it gives just a

---

PERFECT portions: 1/5th avocado

Cut an avocado into five pieces and have one piece for 55 calories. If that sounds high to you, consider how it stacks up against a tablespoon of mayonnaise (100 calories), butter (also 100 calories), or salad dressing (about 75 calories). The avocado has fewer calories and offers a lot more nutrition.

---

bit but pressure doesn't leave a permanent dent (an indication that it's too ripe), it's ready to eat.

Menu Magic

- Guacamole is the classic avocado dish. Add some curry for an Indian flair; hot bean sauce or oriental chili paste for an Asian influence; or basil, sun-dried tomatoes, Parmesan cheese, and pine nuts for a taste of Italy.

- Mash some avocado and use as a spread on sandwiches (made with whole grain bread, of course), bagels, or English muffins to lower the GL of your breakfast or lunch.

- Add chunks of avocado to a side salad to lower the GL of the meal. Adding it to salads also increases your body's ability to absorb the good-for-you carotenoids, such as beta-carotene, in salad greens.

Smart Substitutions

Instead of cheese in your sandwich: Add a slice of avocado. You'll swap good fats for bad ones.

Instead of cheese as a snack: Have a slice of ripe avocado drizzled with lemon juice.

RELATED recipes

Spinach, Grapefruit and Avocado Salad
   with Poppy Seed Dressing *216*
Turkey and Bean Chili with Avocado Salsa *243*

barley

GL LOW | If you've only encountered barley in mushroom-barley soup, get ready to make friends with this underappreciated cereal grain. Whether pearled, hulled, or quick cooking, it can help transform your diet into a Magic one. In fact, think of barley as your new white rice.

Unlike white rice, which has a sky-high GL, barley's is low, thanks to its significant stash of soluble fiber. In fact, eating barley instead of white rice slashes the effect on your blood sugar by almost 70 percent. Add it to soups, use it instead of Arborio rice (the worst rice offender of all) in risotto, and serve it as a nutty, flavorful side dish. The possibilities are endless.

Because its insoluble fiber slows the rate at which food leaves the stomach, barley also helps you feel full on fewer calories.

Health Bonus

Because it contains the same kind of cholesterol-lowering fiber found in oats, barley has FDA-approved bragging rights for its ability to lower cholesterol and cut the risk of heart disease.

Menu Magic

While barley is a natural for soups, think outside the stockpot. Broaden your barley horizons and experiment.

PERFECT portion: 1/2 cup

This is a good amount for a side dish. For main dishes you can have 3/4 cup and still keep the GL in the "low" category.

- Instead of rice pilaf, make barley pilaf to serve with any main dish.
- Add barley to casseroles and use it in place of rice in rice salads.
- Serve barley and diced apples with rosemary baked chicken.
- Add cooked, chilled barley to a bean salad for a fantastic lunch.
- Try corn and barley relish. Add canned or frozen corn to cooked barley along with olive oil; wine vinegar; chopped fresh basil; salt; pepper; and chopped tomatoes, bell peppers, and onions.

RELATED recipes

Barley Risotto with Asparagus and Lemon *262*
Barley Salad with Snow Peas and Lemon Dressing *211*
Bean and Barley Soup *222*
Black Bean and Barley Salad *213*
Mushroom-Barley Pilaf *264*

BARLEY glossary

Like oats, barley comes in different varieties determined by how the grain is processed. All are beneficial to blood sugar.

Hulled barley (barley groats): Only the outer hull of the grain is removed; the bran is left intact. This is the least processed, most nutritious type.

Pot or Scotch barley: This is more processed than hulled barley but retains some of the bran layer.

Pearled barley: This is much more processed, with the outer hull and bran removed. Because the soluble fiber runs all the way through the grain, however, this type is still a smart choice.

Quick-cooking barley: Similar to pearled barley in taste and nutrition, this is presteamed, so it takes only about 10 minutes to cook compared to an hour for other types.

Barley flour: This provides more than three times the fiber of refined white flour. For baking, combine it with wheat flour; otherwise, it won't rise.

Barley flakes: Made from steam-rolled and dried barley, these are cooked for hot cereal.

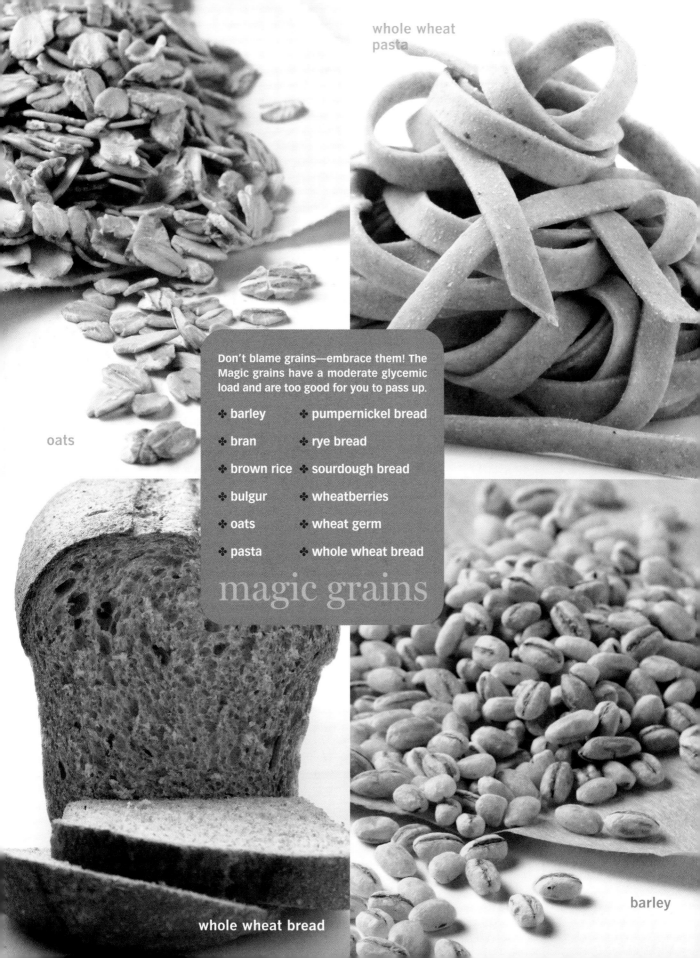

whole wheat pasta

oats

Don't blame grains—embrace them! The Magic grains have a moderate glycemic load and are too good for you to pass up.

- barley
- bran
- brown rice
- bulgur
- oats
- pasta
- pumpernickel bread
- rye bread
- sourdough bread
- wheatberries
- wheat germ
- whole wheat bread

magic grains

whole wheat bread

barley

beans

GL
LOW

Surely you remember the old childhood rhyme that begins "Beans, beans, they're good for your heart ... " Well, beans *are* good for your heart. But these slow-acting foods, rich in complex carbohydrates, are also fantastic for your blood sugar and are surely one of the foods most deserving of special attention in your Magic diet.

All beans, canned or dried, from black to white and chickpeas to cannellini, can tame both insulin and blood sugar levels thanks to their high soluble fiber content. In a recent study, men and women who ate a meal that included about 6 ounces (170 g) of chickpeas had 40 percent lower blood sugar an hour after eating than those who ate an equal amount of white bread with jam.

The soluble fiber in beans slows down digestion, leading to a slow, steady blood sugar rise rather than a spike. Beans also pack loads of protein, which doesn't raise blood sugar and actually helps your body process the carbohydrates in a meal more efficiently. Are they the perfect food for people with diabetes? Perhaps. Just stick with 1/2 cup or so per meal, since beans do contain carbohydrates.

If you're trying to lose weight, eat beans! Not only are they incredibly filling, they also pack a heap of nutrition in a relatively low-calorie package. Better still, some of the starch in beans is a type called resistant starch that the body can't even digest, so the calories don't count.

Beans are also full of folate, a B vitamin that may help reduce some of the nasty consequences of diabetes by helping to keep arteries clean.

Dietary guidelines recommend eating at least 3 cups of beans a week, but most of us lag far behind: We don't average even 1 cup a week. We would have to eat almost triple our current intake to meet the recommendation.

Health Bonus

Looking for antioxidants? Look no further. A recent study ranked beans among the top ten foods richest in these health protectors. What's more, the same soluble fiber in beans that helps stabilize blood sugar also helps lower cholesterol.

Perfect Pairings

Beans and rice is a classic dish, and for good reason, since together they make a complete protein (alone, each lacks certain amino acids, the building blocks of

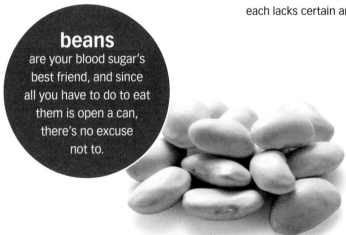

beans
are your blood sugar's best friend, and since all you have to do to eat them is open a can, there's no excuse not to.

protein). While white rice has a high GL, combining it with beans—and therefore eating less rice—makes the GL of the dish much lower. To lower the GL of a pasta meal, use less pasta and top it with beans.

Cooks Tips

The only black mark for beans is the sodium content of canned beans. Cut it in half by rinsing them in cold water before using.

Chickpeas can be ground into flour, allowing you to use less white flour and therefore lower the GL of baked goods. Bake some whole wheat bread with chickpea flour, and your blood sugar will be substantially lower a half hour after eating it than if you ate regular whole wheat bread, studies show.

Silencing the Musical Fruit

Beans have the dubious distinction of being the "musical fruit" (translation: They give you gas). That's because they're rich in a specific type of carbohydrate that you can't digest but that provides fodder for the bacteria that live in your intestinal tract. Gas is the by-product. It's a big reason why people shy away from beans, but there's no need to do without this blood sugar fixer-upper.

You can "degas" beans by soaking them. Short on time? Boil the beans in water for 2 minutes, then remove from the heat and let stand for 2 to 4 hours with the lid on. Or, if you have the luxury of planning ahead, soak them for at least 12 hours. After either method, drain, then rinse twice and cover with fresh cold water before cooking.

Another degassing option: Take Beano with meals containing beans. It's a natural food enzyme that helps digest the gas-producing compounds in beans and other foods.

PERFECT portions: 1/2 cup

This amount provides 105 to 147 calories and keeps the GL low.

Menu Magic

❂ Serve bean dip or hummus with a whole wheat pita cut into wedges.

❂ Mash beans or chickpeas to make a low-GL spread and serve on coarse-ground whole grain bread.

❂ Use drained and rinsed canned beans as the basis for easy weeknight bean soups.

❂ Add canned kidney beans (or any other kind) to green salads.

❂ Cook up a big pot of black bean chili on the weekend and freeze the leftovers.

❂ Mix mango, red pepper, onion, and black beans for a zesty summer salad. Add some cilantro if you like.

RELATED recipes

Bean and Barley Soup 222

Black Bean and Barley Salad 213

Black Bean and Sweet Potato Burritos 263

Black Bean Spread with Mexican Flavors 206

Dahl with Spinach 261

Hearty Split Pea Soup with Rye Croutons 223

Lentil and Bean Chili 262

Mediterranean Split Pea Spread 205

Tuna and Cannellini Salad with Lemon 213

Turkey and Bean Chili with Avocado Salsa 243

Warm Artichoke and Bean Dip 204

Whole Wheat Pasta with Sausage, Beans and Greens 254

beef

GL VERY LOW

Beef for dinner? You bet! Beef is an important source of protein, and as long as you choose lean cuts and eat moderate portions (no giant T-bones that give the waiter a workout), there's no reason it can't be part of a Magic diet. In fact, here's how important protein is to your blood sugar: A study at the University of Minnesota tested two different diets, one high in protein and one with only half as much. The fat content was the same in both diets. In the group that followed the high-protein diet (which was also lower in carbs), blood sugar levels were reduced by as much as if the participants had taken pills prescribed to lower blood sugar.

Your leanest choices are the "skinny six": eye of round, top round, sirloin, bottom round, top loin, and tenderloin. The not-so-skinny cuts to trim from your diet include rib eye, prime rib, T-bone, and most ground beef, which are all high in saturated fat. (To get the leanest ground beef for hamburgers or meat loaf, look for "extra lean," or 93 percent to 95 percent lean, whether it's ground beef, ground round, or ground sirloin.) Saturated fat not only clogs your arteries, it can also contribute to insulin resistance, which makes it harder for your body to use insulin to get blood sugar out of the bloodstream and into cells.

Lean beef isn't just good for your blood sugar, it's even good for your waistline. Dieters tend to lose muscle along with fat, which slows their metabolisms, since muscle tissue burns more calories than fat tissue does. Eating protein helps you hang on to that muscle mass—and keep your metabolism burning on "high."

We're not advocating a diet super-high in protein or super-low in carbs, which simply isn't healthy. (If you haven't already, read "Why Radical Low-Carb Diets Aren't the Answer," starting on page 34.) Aim to keep your protein intake at 20 to 30 percent of the calories you eat.

Health Bonus

Protein isn't the only selling point. Beef is also one of the best sources of zinc, a mineral that people often come up short on, especially if they're counting calories, and vitamin B_{12}, which you can get only from eating animal foods such as eggs, milk, and of course, beef. Another beef bonus: Its fat is rich in conjugated linoleic acid, or CLA, a fatty acid that helps lower blood sugar.

Love Me Tender

While lean cuts of beef are better for you, they're also not as tender as fattier cuts (the fat is what makes a knife cut through a prime rib like butter). But there are ways to turn up the tenderness of healthier cuts.

- Pound and flatten the meat into thinner, more tender slices.

- Use the juice from a fresh pineapple as a marinade. It contains a powerful enzyme that breaks down the meat, tenderizing it. Canned pineapple juice won't work; the enzymes are destroyed during processing.

- Use a marinade that contains vinegar, wine, or citrus juice. The acid softens the tissues of meat, making it more tender and tastier.

- Cook tenderized beef either quickly at a high temperature or for an extended period with moist heat at a low to medium temperature.

Cooks Tips

Want to beef up the health benefits of beef? If you can find it, you may want to opt for grass-fed beef, which can have as much as 60 percent more heart-healthy omega-3 fatty acids and about twice as much CLA as regular beef. But be prepared to pay: Grass-fed beef can cost at least twice as much.

Menu Magic

☢ Throw together fajitas made with flank steak, bell peppers, and onions for a quick weeknight meal.

☢ Toss hot grilled beef with cold, crisp lettuce; lime juice; and chopped onion for a refreshingly delicious Asian-inspired salad.

☢ When company comes, serve up a nice (and lean) beef tenderloin.

☢ Stir-fry strips of beef with lots of veggies for an easy way to have your beef and get your vegetables, too.

☢ Cook up three-bean chili with a small amount of extra-lean ground beef.

☢ Make Asian kebabs with beef marinated in soy sauce, sesame oil, crushed garlic, and ginger. Serve over brown rice.

☢ Create healthier meat loaf by combining finely chopped spinach and onions and grated carrots with lean ground beef. Use oats as a binder.

☢ Make any cut of beef a taste standout by marinating it in balsamic vinegar, olive oil, basil, Dijon mustard, and garlic.

RELATED recipes

Beef and Veggie Meat Loaf *230*
Flank Steak with Balsamic Sauce *228*
Greek Pasta and Beef Casserole *230*
Orange Beef Stir-Fry with Broccoli and Red Pepper *226*
Slow-Cooker Beef and Vegetable Stew *228*

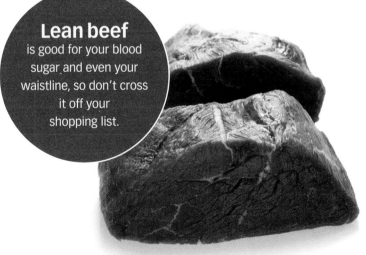

Lean beef is good for your blood sugar and even your waistline, so don't cross it off your shopping list.

berries

GL VERY LOW

Berries, from ruby red strawberries to midnight-blue blueberries, may be candy for your taste buds, but they're Magic for your blood sugar. Their sweetness is deceptive. Fructose, the natural sugar found in most fruits, is sweeter than what's in your sugar bowl (sucrose), so it takes much less (with fewer calories) to get that sweet taste. And fructose is friendlier to blood sugar, causing a much slower rise than table sugar does.

Berries are full of fiber and red-blue natural plant compounds called anthocyanins that may help keep your blood sugar in check. Scientists believe anthocyanins, also found in cherries, may help lower blood sugar by boosting insulin production.

Opt for fresh or frozen berries over berry juices. While the juices are packed with the same phytonutrients as whole berries, they are concentrated sources of carbs, and they lack an important ingredient for blood sugar control—fiber.

What about that jar of jam or jelly in your fridge? Spread lightly. Even those whose labels say they're 100 percent natural fruit spread contain either added sugar or added fruit juice and have higher GLs than whole fresh fruit. Still, a tablespoon is fine if you spread it on whole wheat toast or a whole wheat English muffin.

Health Bonus

Berries, especially blueberries, have a well-earned reputation for being especially rich in powerful disease-fighting antioxidants. Studies show that if you make berries a daily indulgence, they can help keep your eyes healthy, reduce your risk of heart disease and cancer, and work to keep your brain and memory in tiptop shape.

Strawberries are a surprisingly good source of heart-healthy vitamin C, giving even oranges a run for their money; a cup of strawberry halves provides as much C as a cup of orange sections. And studies show that people who eat a serving of strawberries a day tend to have lower blood pressure and higher blood levels of the B vitamin folate, important for keeping arteries clear.

Eating cranberries can help fend off urinary tract infections. Experts say that about 1 1/2 ounces (45 g) of dried cranberries a day could do the trick. Researchers have discovered that blueberries contain some of the same infection-fighting compounds as cranberries.

Cooks Tips

Berries are nutrition powerhouses, but they're also fragile fruits. Choose berries that are plump and free of bruises or mold. The skin of blueberries should be smooth and not shriveled. The hazy white coating you see on blueberries is a natural protective coating, so don't try to wash it off. Look for blackberries and raspberries that aren't leaking (if the small bumps that make up a berry burst, the juice inside leaks out, causing quicker spoilage).

Store berries in the fridge and rinse them just before serving; otherwise, they'll go bad faster.

Since strawberries have been named by the Environmental Working Group as one of the "dirty dozen" fruits and vegetables most likely to contain pesticide residues, buy organic when you can.

To get berry benefits year round, buy berries when they're in season and freeze them. Here are a few pointers.

- Blueberries and strawberries freeze the best. Raspberries and blackberries are more delicate, and freezing can change their texture.

- Wash the berries in cold water and let them dry completely on a paper towel or in a colander.

- Spread the dry berries out on a sheet of wax paper on a baking sheet and place in the freezer.

- Once they are completely frozen, pack them in a tightly sealed freezer container and put them back in the freezer right away.

Menu Magic

Berries can complement countless dishes, adding eye appeal as well as sweetness and flavor.

- Top your waffles, pancakes, and cereal with berries.

- Add berries to muffin batter.

- Stir fresh or frozen blueberries into plain yogurt for a satisfying snack.

- Be adventurous and make wild blueberry salsa (wild blueberries are smaller, so they work better) with diced onion, jalapeño pepper, red bell pepper, cilantro, and lemon juice.

- Use whole strawberries as edible garnishes at breakfast, lunch, or dinner.

- Drizzle a tablespoon of chocolate syrup over fresh strawberries for a decadent but healthy dessert.

- Spoon a generous amount of fresh berries over a smallish serving of frozen yogurt or ice cream.

- Sprinkle fresh berries over tossed green salads.

- Add dried cranberries to green salads or grain side dishes.

- Make a very berry smoothie with yogurt, mixed berries (fresh or frozen), vanilla extract, and orange juice.

PERFECT portions: 1/2 cup

A handful of berries makes a perfect low-calorie snack.

RELATED recipes

Berry-Flaxseed Smoothie *208*

Blueberry-Oatmeal Muffins *198*

Cantaloupe and Blueberry Compote with Green Tea and Lime *276*

Cherry-Raspberry Crumble *287*

Chocolate-Raspberry Cheesecake *284*

Instant Strawberry Frozen Yogurt *277*

Lemony Blueberry Cheesecake Bars *279*

Mixed Berry-Almond Gratin *288*

Mixed Berry and Stone Fruit Soup *276*

Multi-Grain Pancakes or Waffles *192*

Peach-Raspberry Crumble *287*

Pear-Berry Clafouti *283*

Rhubarb-Blackberry Crumble *286*

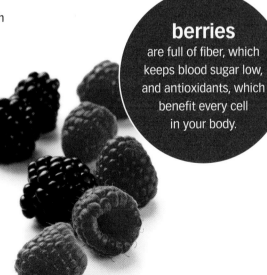

berries are full of fiber, which keeps blood sugar low, and antioxidants, which benefit every cell in your body.

bran

GL *LOW*

When you eat grains—and of course, they should be a regular part of your diet—you can't do better than bran. In fact, a bowl of bran cereal has just one-third the GL of a bowl of cornflakes. (Check out "How Cereals Rate" at right.) That means your blood sugar will go up only a third as much, so it doesn't have far to fall. (Remember, it's those precipitous drops that cause trouble and make you hungry again.)

There's really no better way to get one of the three daily servings of whole grains we recommend than starting your day with bran cereal. Top it with berries, and you've really hit your Magic eating stride.

Think of bran as the heavy "overcoat" worn by kernels of whole grain oats, wheat, or rice. It contains the highest concentration of fiber of any part of the grain (12 grams per 1/2 cup for wheat and rice bran; 7 grams per 1/2 cup for oat bran). As you know, fiber helps you feel fuller on fewer calories, smoothing the way for weight loss.

Bran also helps tame those wild blood sugar surges after meals. When researchers gave obese children either a sugar solution or a sugar solution plus 15 grams (about 4 tablespoons) of wheat bran, the kids' blood sugar levels were much lower when they ate the bran. If you add bran to your diet regularly, you could really lower your blood sugar over the long term—by as much as 22 percent. At least that's the drop experienced by people in a study who ate rice bran for two months as part of a heart-healthy diet.

Oat bran is high in soluble fiber, which gives it extra power over blood sugar. Adding oat bran to the mix— meaning pancake, muffin, or cookie mix—can significantly change the food's effect on your blood sugar. Researchers found that for each gram of beta-glucan, the type of soluble fiber found in oat bran, added to snack bars, the Glycemic Index of the bar

dropped by 4 points. A lower GI translates into a lower GL—which means a milder blood sugar response after you gobble down the goody. It takes only 1/3 cup of oat bran to provide 1.5 grams of beta-glucan.

As you can tell, we're big on bran!

Health Bonus

Oat bran can bring down high cholesterol and reduce the risk of heart disease, and it has an FDA-approved health claim to prove it. In one study, men who consumed the most wheat bran (about 9 grams per day) were 30 percent less likely to develop heart disease than those who consumed the least (not quite 2 grams per day).

Rice bran can also lower cholesterol, and early research in animals suggests it may help tame high blood pressure as well. The natural oils in rice bran may be the Magic ingredient. Rice bran is also gluten-free, a real plus for people who have a sensitivity to gluten.

Wheat bran may help reduce the risk of colon and breast cancer. And of course, bran helps keep you regular.

Cooks Tips

Because bran contains oils that can become rancid, be sure to store it in the refrigerator or freezer once it's been opened. Many bran cereals, on the other hand, contain preservatives that will keep them fresh for several months in the pantry.

---

don't fall for it

Bran muffins may appear to be health food, but they're usually anything but. Most store-bought muffins are loaded with sugar, fat, and calories. Make your own for a much healthier treat (see the Apple-Bran Muffins recipe on page 197).

This much bran cereal should fill you up.
Use less if you sprinkle it over yogurt.

HOW cereals RATE

Some cereals are "fast acting" and send blood sugar on a rollercoaster ride, while others are digested slowly—more at the speed of an old-fashioned merry-go-round. Bran is among the slowest-acting cereals of all.

Cereal	Serving (equal to 30 g)	Glycemic Load
Quaker Oat Bran	1/16 cup	3
Kellogg's Bran Buds	1/3 cup	7
Kellogg's All-Bran	1/2 cup	9
Kellogg's Raisin Bran	1 cup	12
Kellogg's Bran Flakes	1 cup	13
Kellogg's Special K	1 cup	14
General Mills Cheerios	1 cup	15
Nabisco Cream of Wheat	1 cup	17
Kellogg's Corn Flakes	1 cup	24
Kellogg's Crispix	1 cup	22
Kellogg's Rice Krispies	3/4 cup	22
Nabisco Instant Cream of Wheat	1 cup	22

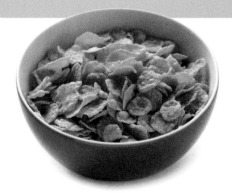

Menu Magic

❂ Make meat loaf more Magic by using oat bran or another bran as a binder in place of bread. It will help blunt the effect of the mashed potatoes you eat with it by lowering your blood sugar response to the entire meal.

❂ Sprinkle bran flakes on casseroles.

❂ Use bran in muffin recipes in place of half the flour for muffins that are high in fiber and loaded with nutrients. If you don't have bran flour on hand, try using bran cereal. Some brands have muffin recipes right on the box. Add fruit and nuts for truly Magic muffins.

❂ Start your day with plain bran cereal, hot or cold (look for Quaker and other brands). It's one of the lowest-GL cereals you can choose.

❂ Make pancakes or waffles with rice flour and rice bran or try adding different types of bran and experimenting with the taste and texture. Top with fresh blueberries to squeeze in a serving of fruit.

Smart Substitution

Instead of Cream of Wheat: Have a bowl of cooked bran cereal topped with dried cranberries or fresh strawberries.

RELATED recipes

Apple-Bran Muffins *197*
Fudge Brownies *280*

broccoli

GL
VERY LOW

Because it's big on volume and small on calories, broccoli is a great way to bulk up carb dishes (think pasta, casseroles, and baked potatoes) to lower their GL.

Not only does broccoli have very little impact on your blood sugar, it's one of the best food sources of chromium, a mineral required for insulin to function normally (remember, insulin helps the body use up blood sugar so there's less in the bloodstream). One cup of broccoli provides almost half of your daily chromium requirement. Fiber, at a hearty 4 grams per stalk, is also part of broccoli's "benefits package."

Broccoli also packs a wallop of vitamin C. One cup contains more than 100 percent of the RDA for this vitamin. If you're fighting diabetes—or even if you already have it—that's important. According to a British population study, people with the highest blood levels of vitamin C were less likely to have elevated levels of glycated hemoglobin, a long-term indicator of high blood sugar. The researchers concluded, "Dietary measures to increase plasma vitamin C may be an important public health strategy for reducing the prevalence of diabetes." Even if vitamin C can't protect you from diabetes (the jury is still out), it and other antioxidants can certainly lower your risk of diabetes-related complications such as eye and nerve damage.

Health Bonus

Broccoli is known for its cancer-fighting compounds. Numerous studies over the past 20 years have found that people who eat plenty of broccoli have a significantly lower risk of several cancers, including breast, colon, cervical, lung, prostate, and bladder cancer. Broccoli's also a good source of calcium, which may help lower high blood pressure, common in people with diabetes.

Cooks Tips

Don't overcook broccoli; it will turn pale and mushy and lose some of its nutrients.

PERFECT portions: 1/2 cup

The GL of broccoli is based on a 1/2-cup serving, but feel free to eat as much as you want.

Menu Magic

- For creamy soup without the cream, puree cooked broccoli, cauliflower, and onion with salt and white pepper. Add low-fat milk for a creamier texture.

- Add chopped broccoli florets to omelets, vegetable lasagna, and pizza.

- For a super-low-GL meal, make a beef and broccoli stir-fry and serve over a modest portion of brown rice.

- Whip up a broccoli salad to tote on your next picnic. Mix broccoli florets, sliced carrots, sliced green olives, diced pimientos, and chopped walnuts and marinate in Italian dressing.

- Top steamed broccoli with a spoonful of low-fat sour cream and some slivered almonds for a healthy side dish.

- Dip raw broccoli in light ranch or Italian dressing as a snack or an addition to lunch.

RELATED recipes

Broccoli and Cheese Omelet *194*
Broccoli with Lemon Vinaigrette *272*
Orange Beef Stir-Fry with Broccoli and Red Pepper *226*
Whole Wheat Pizza with Broccoli and Olives *259*

Hate Broccoli? Blame It on Your Genes

Does the taste of broccoli on your tongue make you recoil in disgust? You may be able to blame your genes. Researchers have discovered a gene that makes some people hypersensitive to the bitter-tasting compounds in broccoli, Brussels sprouts, and cabbage.

brown rice

Brown rice doesn't have the wonderfully low GL of some other grains, like barley or oats. Nevertheless, it's a far better choice for your blood sugar than most white rice. So, if rice is on the menu, better make it brown.

As a nutrient-packed, fiber-rich whole grain, brown rice has many of the good qualities you expect in a Magic food. Not only does it boast six times the fiber of white rice, it's packed with vitamins, minerals, and natural plant compounds made by nature to protect

PERFECT portions: 1/2 cup

Stick with one serving, or 1/2 cup, per meal, since rice is, after all, a high-carb food.

your health. And, as a whole grain, brown rice is part of the formula for lowering your risk of diabetes and heart disease. Remember, we want you to aim to eat three servings a day of whole grains, which protect against metabolic syndrome, diabetes, heart disease, stroke, and cancer. A serving of brown rice is 1/2 cup.

(continued)

RICE glossary

Who knew rice could be so complicated? Here's a rundown of rice terms to help get you through the rice maze.

Brown rice: Still has the bran and the germ of the whole rice kernel, so it contains all the nutrition of a whole grain. Has a longer cooking time and a higher fiber content. Has a nutty flavor and a hearty texture.

Converted rice: The rice is steamed before it's husked, allowing the individual grains to absorb more nutrients. Takes about the same amount of time to cook as white rice, but less time than brown rice.

Wild rice: Not a rice at all, but the seeds of a marsh grass. It's high in protein and fiber and several B vitamins. Has a pungent, earthy flavor.

Basmati rice: A long-grain, aromatic white rice grown in the Himalayas. It cooks up dry and fluffy. You can get brown or white basmati rice. The GL of brown basmati is lower, closer to that of brown rice.

Long-grain white rice: The most common rice used in cooking. The nutritious bran and germ have been processed out, taking fiber and natural

plant compounds with them. As with most refined products, some nutrients, such as iron, thiamin, niacin, and folate have been added back. Has a bland flavor.

Long-grain quick-cooking rice: The rice is completely cooked and dehydrated, so cooking time is short, usually 10 to 15 minutes. Comes as white or brown rice.

Sticky rice: Also called glutinous rice, though it doesn't contain gluten, this is a short-grain, white, refined rice that sticks together. Though it's sometimes called "sweet rice," it has a bland flavor like most white rice.

Arborio rice: A plump, refined, short-grain white rice that absorbs water without developing a mushy texture. Used in risotto and noted more for its ability to absorb flavors.

Jasmine rice: A long-grain white rice that has a subtle flower-like aroma.

brown rice continued

Regular brown rice takes about 35 minutes to cook. When time is of the essence, don't opt for instant rice, white or brown, which has been partially cooked and dehydrated and has a high GL. You'd do better to opt for converted white rice, which has a GL similar to that of brown rice and many of the nutrients, too. While brown rice should always be your number one rice choice (more nutrients and fiber), converted white rice is the next best thing.

All rice starts off as brown rice. Only when it's been refined and the bran and germ have been removed is white rice born. Different types of rice vary in their GL depending on the type of starch they naturally contain (see Rice Rankings). Three rices to avoid: jasmine, Arborio (the kind used in risotto), and "sticky rice."

Health Bonus

Brown rice offers more than just fiber. It's rich in the bone-building mineral magnesium, the immune-boosting antioxidant selenium, and manganese, a mineral important for keeping up the body's natural defenses.

Cooks Tips

Because brown rice contains some fat naturally found in the whole grain, it won't stay fresh as long as white rice. You can store uncooked brown rice in the cupboard for up to 6 months. Put it in the refrigerator to make it last longer.

Menu Magic

✪ Substitute brown rice for white rice in casseroles, stir-fries, and side dishes to lower the GL of a meal while adding a chewy texture and nutty flavor.

RELATED recipes
Brown Rice Pilaf with Flaxseeds, Lime and Cilantro *265*
Brown Rice Pilaf with Toasted Flaxseeds *265*

rice RANKINGS

There's much more to rice than just white or brown. And different varieties vary as much in their effect on your blood sugar as they do in flavor. Take a look.

Rice	Glycemic Load per 2/3 cup (150 g)
Medium	
Converted white rice	16
Brown rice	18
Wild rice	18
Cajun style rice mix	19
Long and wild rice blend	20
Mexican style rice mix	22
High	
Basmati rice	23
Long grain white rice	23
Long grain quick cooking	27
Very High	
Sticky rice (used in sushi rolls)	31
Arborio risotto rice	36
Jasmine rice	46

brussels sprouts

GL *VERY LOW*

Like most vegetables, these mini-cabbages have a very low GL, which means they're kind to your blood sugar. But Brussels sprouts also have something special: soluble fiber (2 grams in 1/2 cup). This stuff forms a gel in your stomach that acts as a barrier between food and the enzymes that break it down, making your meal "slow acting" instead of "fast acting" when it comes to digestion. And that goes for everything in the meal—even the roll. Remember, where blood sugar is concerned, a slow rise is better.

One study found that women who ate cruciferous vegetables, including Brussels sprouts, most often reduced their risk of developing diabetes by two-thirds compared to those who ate cruciferous veggies least often. So get your fill!

Another surprising bonus: Almost one-third of the calories in Brussels sprouts come from protein, meaning that even though they seem substantial, these veggies are blessedly low in carbs.

If you have diabetes or any other risk factor for heart disease, take note: Brussels sprouts are a top source of vitamin C (50 milligrams per 1/2 cup), a must-have nutrient for keeping arteries healthy and fending off complications of diabetes. A large European study found that adults with the highest blood levels of vitamin C had only half the risk of dying from cardiovascular disease compared to those with the lowest levels.

Health Bonus

Like their cousins cabbage and broccoli, Brussels sprouts are powerful anticancer foods. They're also rich in lutein and zeaxanthin, members of the carotenoid family that are celebrated for their ability to keep your eyesight sharp as you age. And sprouts are an underappreciated source of bone-building vitamin K, with six times the recommended daily amount.

PERFECT portions: 1/2 cup

A serving is 1/2 cup, but there's no reason not to eat more.

Cooks Tips

Like cabbage, Brussels sprouts can really stink up your kitchen. Cooking time equals odor intensity, so keep it short (steaming is a good option). Store leftovers in a well-sealed container, or else you'll smell the consequences when you open the fridge.

Menu Magic

Brussels sprouts are one of those all-or-nothing foods; either you love 'em or you hate 'em. But before you decide once and for all, give these Brussels sprout dishes a try.

- Steam sprouts, then sauté them in olive oil along with any or all of the following: crushed mustard seed, cumin, fennel seed, cayenne pepper, finely chopped ginger, fresh lime juice, and salt. Top with slivered almonds.

- Get two Magic foods in one dish by combining baby carrots and halved Brussels sprouts. Sauté them in olive oil (a third Magic food), then add chicken broth and simmer. Add some lemon juice (another!) and dill just before they're done.

- Pair the strong taste of Brussels sprouts or other cruciferous vegetables with a sweet-tasting side dish such as applesauce or sweet potatoes.

- To make Brussels sprouts even more blood sugar-friendly, add vinegar. Marinate cooked sprouts overnight in vinegar (try tarragon vinegar), crushed garlic, minced onion, salt, and a bit of honey.

RELATED recipe

Sautéed Brussels Sprouts with Red Pepper and Caraway Seeds *273*

bulgur

GL MEDIUM

If you're following the Seven Secrets of Magic Eating, you're trying to get three servings of whole grains a day. For chewy texture and a slightly nutty taste, try bulgur as a deliciously filling side dish or hot cereal. It can even be used to make stuffing. Best of all, it cooks quickly.

Bulgur ranks right up there with whole wheat bread, wheatberries, and bran—all Magic foods, and all forms of the same nutritious wheat grain. That's right, bulgur isn't an individual type of grain. It's wheat grain that's been partially cooked by boiling or steaming, then dried and cracked.

Eating more whole grains has been shown to cut diabetes risk by 35 percent in men and women and reduce heart disease risk by 25 percent in women and 18 percent in men. Just six weeks on a whole grain diet can markedly improve insulin sensitivity, according to one study.

Health Bonus

As with all whole grain foods, eating more translates into lower risk not only of diabetes and heart disease but also of certain cancers. In a Swedish study of more than 61,000 women, researchers found that those who ate at least 4 1/2 servings of whole grains a day had a 23 percent lower risk of developing colon cancer compared to women who ate fewer than 1 1/2 servings a day. The lignans in bulgur may also help protect against breast cancer.

Cooks Tips

You'll find bulgur in different textures. Coarse bulgur is used for pilaf and rice dishes, medium is used as breakfast cereal, and fine is used for tabbouleh (a Middle Eastern salad made with bulgur, chopped parsley, cucumbers, tomatoes, olive oil, and lemon juice). The finer the grain, the quicker bulgur cooks up.

PERFECT portions: 1/2 cup

A typical serving size is 1/2 cup, but you can have as much as 3/4 cup of cooked bulgur and the GL will still be in the medium range.

Menu Magic

- Try bulgur pilaf as a side dish. There are a million different recipes, some including dried fruit and some with vegetables and/or herbs. Grab a good cookbook and take your pick. You can also enjoy bulgur in cold salads.

- Throw together some tabbouleh as an excellent, portable summertime lunch salad or side dish. Toss in chopped vegetables from your garden, such as tomatoes and cucumbers, and add some goat or feta cheese or chicken for extra protein.

- Cook up hot bulgur cereal in salted water as you would oatmeal. Top with fresh fruit or with chopped walnuts, dried cranberries, cinnamon, and a drizzle of honey. Some manufacturers make bulgur cereals with extra ingredients, such as soy, which adds extra protein.

- Stuff zucchini with bulgur and extra-lean ground beef or pork.

Smart Substitutions

Instead of rice: Use cooked bulgur in stir-fries.

Instead of Cream of Wheat: Have bulgur as your hot cereal in the morning (Cream of Wheat has a relatively high GL).

RELATED recipe

Bulgur with Ginger and Orange *264*

cabbage

GL VERY LOW

For centuries, Russian peasants sustained themselves on this leafy veggie. But even if your fridge is full of other foods, you should still consider eating cabbage. It's very low in calories (just 16 calories per 1/2 cup cooked) and high in fiber. Together, these two attributes spell weight loss, which should benefit your blood sugar. Add to that the fact that cabbage is way low on the GL scale, and you've got a Magic winner. And eating cabbage doesn't mean spooning up pale stew; if you prepare it right, cabbage can be a culinary delight.

This veggie doesn't just help you lose weight. Cabbage (especially the red variety) is also a surprisingly excellent source of vitamin C, which some experts believe may reduce the risk of developing diabetes. Red cabbage offers another bonus: It's rich in natural pigments called anthocyanins, which new research suggests may help boost insulin production and lower blood sugar levels.

Finally, cabbage is often prepared with vinegar, which can help lower the GL of your whole meal.

Health Bonus

Cabbage contains sulphoraphane, which has potent anticancer properties. One study of women found that those who ate the most cabbage and its cruciferous cousins, like broccoli and Brussels sprouts, had a 45 percent lower breast cancer risk than women who ate the least.

Cabbage may also help guard against lung cancer. Fermented cabbage, a.k.a. sauerkraut, may have even higher levels of anticancer compounds, a result of the fermentation process. Just beware of sauerkraut's high sodium content; rinse it before heating.

Cooks Tips

Overcook cabbage, and you'll regret it when the smell lingers. Overcooking also destroys cabbage's stores of vitamin C, which can't stand the heat. Steam cabbage until limp, stir-fry it quickly, or chop it raw for salads

PERFECT portions: 1/2 cup

A serving is 1/2 cup of cooked cabbage (1 cup raw), but consider the sky the limit.

and slaws. Older cabbage or cabbage that's been in the fridge for a while may have a stronger smell. To minimize the odor, cook the cabbage quickly in an uncovered pan with as little water as possible. Try adding a tablespoon of vinegar to the cooking water to further cut the odor.

Menu Magic

- Enjoy cabbage in coleslaw.
- Add sliced or chopped cabbage to soups and stews.
- Place sautéed cabbage underneath a small serving of steak to add gourmet appeal.
- Braise red cabbage with chopped apples, walnuts, and red wine.
- Sauté cabbage and onions to serve as a side dish.
- Use shredded cabbage in place of lettuce on sandwiches and burgers.
- Combine cooked shredded cabbage with low-fat sour cream and caraway seed, then heat and serve as a side dish.
- Wrap thick fish fillets in cabbage leaves and steam over seasoned broth.

RELATED recipes

Asian Noodle Hot Pot *225*
No-Mayonnaise Creamy Coleslaw *216*
Pork Chop and Cabbage Skillet Dinner *232*

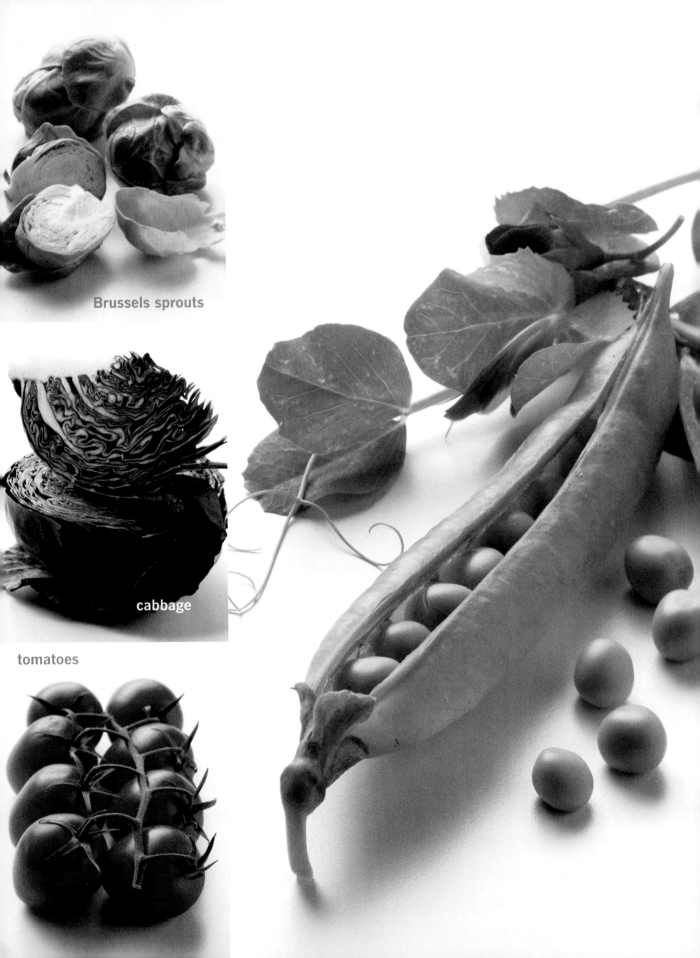

Brussels sprouts

cabbage

tomatoes

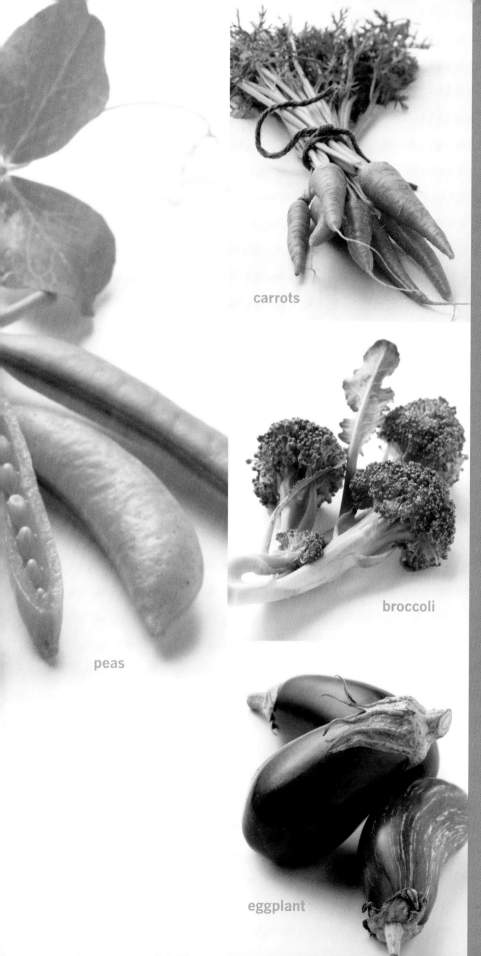

carrots

With low or very low glycemic loads, vegetables are one food group that won't play havoc with your blood sugar—and will help you fight diabetes and weight gain. We've chosen these veggies as Magic foods because of their impressive nutritional profile, and in the case of eggplant, the ability to stand in for meat.

❖ broccoli

❖ Brussels sprouts

❖ cabbage

❖ carrots

❖ cauliflower

❖ eggplant

❖ onion

❖ peas

❖ spinach

❖ tomato

broccoli

peas

magic
vegetables

eggplant

carrots

GL *VERY LOW*

Carrots perfectly illustrate the difference between the glycemic index (GI) and the glycemic load (GL). When the GI first made waves among health enthusiasts, carrots got a bad rap for raising blood sugar. That's because the type of sugar they contain is transformed into blood sugar very rapidly—almost as fast as table sugar. But since the amount of sugar is low, carrots are still on the menu.

Thank goodness they are, because they're one of the richest sources of beta-carotene, which is linked to a lower risk of diabetes. One study found that people with the highest blood levels of beta-carotene had 32 percent lower insulin levels (suggesting better blood sugar control) than those with the lowest beta-carotene levels. Like most vegetables, carrots are also a good source of beneficial fiber.

Health Bonus

Carrots won't help you throw away your reading glasses, but they will help protect against two sight-robbing conditions, macular degeneration and cataracts. They're also rich in soluble fiber, which helps lower cholesterol. One study found that volunteers who ate about a cup of carrots a day had an average 11 percent reduction in their cholesterol after three weeks.

Cooks Tips

Cut off the green carrot tops before storing, or they'll pull moisture from the carrots and make them wither.

don't fall for it

"Raw foods" proponents would have you believe that all foods are most healthful in their uncooked state. Not true. In the case of carrots, you get different benefits depending on whether they're raw or cooked. During cooking, the carrot's cell walls break down, releasing the beta-carotene inside. Raw carrots, on the other hand, contain more vitamin C.

PERFECT portions: 1/2 cup

A serving is 1/2 cup of cooked carrots or 1 cup raw. The GL of cooked is slightly higher.

Menu Magic

- Add grated carrots to sandwiches. For a decidedly different sandwich spread, mix finely grated carrots with low-fat whipped cream cheese and add chopped green olives and grated onions.

- Munch on baby carrots and hummus as a snack or with lunch.

- Mix up spicy carrot soup by pureeing cooked carrots and adding them to sautéed onions and garlic along with vegetable broth and either soy milk or fat-free yogurt. Include chopped celery, salt, white pepper, and curry powder if you like.

- For a salad with Middle Eastern flair, combine cooked sliced carrots, olive oil, chopped parsley, minced garlic, fresh lemon juice, and salt. The lemon juice reduces the GL of the dish even more.

- Cook baby carrots with rosemary and thyme, olive oil, chopped onions, and black pepper. Squeeze the juice of orange wedges over the top.

RELATED recipes

Asian Noodle Hot Pot *225*
Barley Salad with Snow Peas and Lemon Dressing *211*
Bean and Barley Soup *222*
Beef and Veggie Meat Loaf *230*
Chicken Pot Pie with a Whole Grain Biscuit Crust *236*
Garden Pasta Salad *217*
Hearty Split Pea Soup with Rye Croutons *223*
Moroccan Spiced Carrots *274*
No-Mayonnaise Creamy Coleslaw *216*
Pork Chop and Cabbage Skillet Dinner *232*
Slow-Cooker Beef and Vegetable Stew *228*
Spring Vegetable Stir-Fry with Tofu *260*
Tuna and Carrot Sandwich on Rye *222*
Whole Wheat Noodles with Peanut Sauce and Chicken *214*

cauliflower

GL VERY LOW

Not many vegetables are as filling and low in calories as cauliflower. While it's an acquired taste for some, cauliflower is perfect for your Magic diet if you like it, most obviously because it has so few calories, so much fiber, and so little carbohydrate. But we also like it because, when cooked the right way, it can substitute for mashed potatoes! It even stands in for rice.

Cauliflower's loaded with vitamin C—1 cup raw supplies 75 percent of what you need for the day. That makes it an ideal food for helping protect cells against damage from high blood sugar.

One caveat: If cauliflower is drowned in fatty cheese sauce, it's no longer a Magic food.

Health Bonus

Cauliflower, like its cousins broccoli, cabbage, and Brussels sprouts, is rich in anticancer compounds. A review of 80 studies found that people who ate the largest amounts of these foods had the lowest risk of all types of cancer, particularly lung, stomach, colon, and rectal cancers. In a test-tube study, juice extracted from cauliflower blocked growth of breast cancer cells.

Cooks Tips

Cook cauliflower in an uncovered pan to avoid trapping its strong odor. Add a couple of tablespoons of lemon juice to preserve its color. Overcooking not only intensifies the aroma, it also destroys much of the vitamin C.

If you're not a fan of cauliflower, try broccoflower, a milder hybrid of broccoli and cauliflower.

Menu Magic

- Instead of mashed potatoes, try this tasty cauliflower puree. Boil a head of cauliflower cut into florets, one diced peeled potato, and six peeled garlic cloves until tender. Drain and puree (in batches) in a food processor and thin with enough warm milk to make it velvety. Drizzle olive oil on top and season with salt and pepper.

PERFECT portions: 1/2 cup

A serving of cauliflower, 1/2 cup cooked, provides a slim 17 calories and 2.5 grams of fiber. Not a bad deal at all.

- Serve cauliflower raw or lightly steamed with seasoned yogurt dip.

- Combine cauliflower with broccoli in quiches, omelets, and casseroles.

- Toss florets with olive oil and garlic and roast in the oven.

- Bake a whole head of cauliflower to serve with dinner. Place a trimmed and rinsed head in a steamer, cover, and cook until firm but tender. Place in a baking dish and coat with a mixture of whole wheat bread crumbs, olive oil, garlic powder, salt, dried oregano, and minced garlic. Sprinkle a bit of Parmesan cheese on top and bake for 10 to 15 minutes at 350°F (176°C).

- Stir-fry cauliflower and broccoli florets with water chestnuts and season with a dash of soy sauce and sesame oil.

- Make a cauliflower salad by combining florets with tarragon vinegar, Dijon mustard, salt, white pepper, and olive oil. Cover and marinate overnight.

Smart Substitution

Instead of rice: Shred cauliflower in a food processor until the texture is similar to rice. Lightly steam it and use in recipes that call for cooked rice.

RELATED recipes

Cauliflower and Spinach Casserole *270*
Spiced Cauliflower with Peas *272*

cheese

GL
VERY LOW

With virtually zero carbs and loads of protein, cheese is a "better blood sugar" food for sure, because it won't budge the blood sugar needle even a bit, and it will make you feel plenty full. Cheese is also an excellent source of calcium, and studies show that getting plenty of calcium from food may help prevent insulin resistance, a harbinger of diabetes. According to a recent study, women who get plenty of calcium from dairy products also have a significantly lower risk of developing metabolic syndrome, which is linked to both diabetes and heart disease.

That doesn't mean you can load up on all the mac 'n' cheese you want, though. It's packed not only with calories but also with cheese's big "design flaw"— saturated fat, the kind that clogs arteries and reduces your body's sensitivity to insulin. That's why it pays to choose, whenever possible, lower-fat cheeses, such as low-fat cottage cheese, low-fat string cheese, part-skim mozzarella, skim ricotta, farmer cheese, and soft goat cheese. Otherwise, the drawbacks of cheese could easily outweigh its benefits. Soft cheeses have less fat per ounce (30 g) than hard cheeses (usually about 6 or 7 grams instead of 8 or 9).

When you do use a hard cheese like cheddar, you'll want to eat less of it and/or choose a low-fat version (see "The Art of Using Low-Fat Cheese" on the opposite page). You probably won't want to snack on low-fat cheddar, though, so give another cheese a try for nibbling. We suggest goat cheese sprinkled with herbs and drizzled with lemon juice. The acidic juice offers an added benefit, since the acid has the power to lower blood sugar. Another way to cut cheese calories is to choose a strong-flavored type like Parmesan, Romano, feta, or Muenster because a little goes a long way, and you can use less.

Cheese wouldn't be so bad if we didn't tend to use so much of it, as in lasagna or pizza that's downright gooey with the stuff—but that's easy to remedy! When making lasagna, you can use the usual amount of ricotta (part skim) and Parmesan but only half the mozzarella (part skim). Add a little extra spaghetti

CHEDDAR & BETTER cheese

Cheese 1 oz (30 g) except where noted	Calories	Fat (g)	Calcium (mg)
Blue	100	8	175
Brie	95	8	52
Camembert	85	7	110
Cheddar	114	10	205
Cottage cheese, 1% (1 cup)	164	3	138
Feta	74	6	140
Goat, soft	76	6	40
Gruyére	117	9	287
Limburger	93	8	141
Muenster	105	9	204
Mozzarella, part skim	72	5	183
Neufchâtel	74	7	22
Parmesan, grated	129	9	390
Romano	110	8	302
Swiss	107	8	273

sauce to keep the lasagna moist. For pizza, you can ask for half the cheese at any pizzeria.

Health Bonus

If you think milk is good for you, consider this: It takes about 10 pounds (4.5 kg) of milk to create a single pound (450 g) of cheese, making it a concentrated source of all the good stuff in milk, including phosphorus, zinc, vitamin A, riboflavin, vitamin B$_{12}$, and calcium. Probably because of their calcium content, low-fat dairy foods can also help bring down high blood pressure. (If you're a cottage cheese fan, though, note that it's one type of cheese that's *not* high in calcium.)

Cheese can even help prevent cavities, especially if you eat it after meals or as a between-meal snack.

Cooks Tips

To make cheese last longer in the fridge, wrap it tightly in plastic wrap or aluminum foil to prevent it from drying out and change the wrapping each time you use the cheese to keep mold from taking hold.

Menu Magic

- ☺ Serve cheese and fruit as an appetizer or a snack or even dessert. Mix and match flavors and textures. Try cheddar with sliced apples, Brie with pears, shaved Parmesan with Asian pears, or cottage cheese with peaches.

- ☺ Pack string cheese in your briefcase or purse for a low-fat, high-protein hunger tamer.

- ☺ Add feta or goat cheese to omelets.

- ☺ Create a salad with shredded Swiss, diced seedless grapes, chopped pecans, and chopped fresh basil. Serve with whole wheat crackers.

- ☺ Make an easy toaster-oven pizza by topping a whole wheat pita with tomato sauce, part-skim mozzarella, and a vegetable of your choice and cooking until the cheese melts.

PERFECT portions: 1 ounce (30 g)

A serving of cheese is a scant 1 ounce (30 g). For hard cheese, that's about the size of two board-game die. Cheese calorie counts range from a low of about 72 per serving for part-skim mozzarella to a high of about 130 per serving for Parmesan.

RELATED recipes

All-New Chicken Cordon Bleu *235*

Cauliflower and Spinach Casserole *270*

Cherry Tomatoes Filled with Pesto Cream Cheese *200*

Chocolate-Raspberry Cheesecake *284*

Greek Lentil Salad *217*

Greek Pasta and Beef Casserole *230*

Lemony Blueberry Cheesecake Bars *279*

Macaroni and Cheese with Spinach *255*

Mediterranean Salad with Edamame *215*

Mushroom and Herb Pizza *258*

Penne with Asparagus, Ricotta and Lemon *252*

Penne with Tomato and Eggplant Sauce *256*

Quick Spinach and Sausage Lasagna *253*

Shrimp and Orzo Casserole *251*

Spinach and Goat Cheese Omelet *194*

Zucchini-Basil Frittata *193*

The Art of Using Low-Fat Cheese

At their worst, low-fat cheeses taste pretty much like cardboard. But used smartly, they're perfectly good stand-ins for their full-fat brethren.

- ☺ Fat-free cheeses are best used as is (uncooked) for sandwiches and salads. They can be difficult to shred, so consider buying them shredded.

- ☺ Don't melt low-fat cheeses under the broiler or in a toaster oven. They tend to toughen and get rubbery under direct heat. They do work, however, in casseroles and heated sandwiches and burgers.

- ☺ To melt low-fat cheeses for sauces, use low heat and stir slowly in one direction. Cook for about 25 percent longer than you would to melt full-fat cheese.

cherries

GL VERY LOW

Remember secret number 3 of Magic eating, Eat More Fruits and Vegetables? These foods from the produce aisle are full of disease-fighting plant compounds, and they barely budge your blood sugar thanks to their very low GL. Cherries may be an especially good choice. Besides plenty of sugar-lowering soluble fiber, they contain red pigments that may increase your body's insulin output, which ultimately lowers your blood sugar. And they're low in calories to boot.

When you get a snack attack, reach for a handful of cherries instead of higher-GL foods like crackers or pretzels. At dessert time, pile them on a half portion of ice cream, and your bowl will look just as full but with far fewer calories.

Sorry, though, maraschino cherries don't cut it. These so-called cherries have been bleached, processed, and injected with sugar and red dye, taking all the magic out of a once-healthy food. Also skip cherry juice, which is usually sweetened and lacks the fiber of whole cherries.

Health Bonus

Cherries pack a real antioxidant punch, rivaling even oranges. Their stash of vitamin C and other antioxidants helps fend off heart disease, cancer, and many complications of diabetes. One study found that the antioxidant compounds in cherries help protect brain cells, while other plant compounds can put a dent in your cholesterol.

The type of soluble fiber cherries contain, called pectin, is also great at lowering cholesterol.

Cooks Tips

If chewing around the cherry pit and spitting it out is a little too messy for your taste, check into buying a cherry pitter. Some can pit olives as well. Instead of serve and spit, you'll pit and serve!

PERFECT portions: 1/2 cup

The GL of cherries is based on 1/2 cup's worth, but since the GL and the calorie count are so very low, feel free to eat more.

Caution: One bad cherry in a bag can truly spoil the whole bunch. Sort your cherries and pick out the bad ones before putting them in the fridge.

Menu Magic

- Add finely chopped cherries to ground meat; you'll cut the fat, boost the nutrition, and add unexpected zip to meat loaf and burgers.
- Add frozen tart cherries to your next smoothie.
- Add chopped fresh cherries to low-fat yogurt for a fantastic midday snack.

Smart Substitution

Instead of hot fudge with ice cream: Add cherries to your frozen treat.

RELATED recipes
Cherry-Almond Gratin *288*
Cherry Clafouti *283*

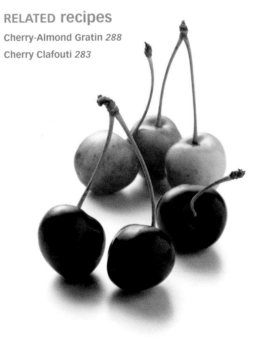

chicken AND TURKEY

GL
VERY LOW

"A chicken in every pot" was a great political slogan back in the days of the Depression. It's also a good approach to Magic eating. Because chicken is full of all-important protein, low in fat, incredibly versatile, and cooks up fast, we consider it the ultimate convenience food.

Remember, protein foods don't raise blood sugar a bit. And chicken has a leg up (pun intended) on beef in the fat and calorie departments. A 3-ounce (85-g) serving of skinless chicken breast has 95 percent less saturated fat—the stuff that hampers insulin sensitivity—than an equal serving of beef tenderloin. It also has 40 percent fewer calories. (As you know, a wide waistline contributes to insulin resistance, which makes blood sugar control difficult.)

Because protein foods like chicken take a while to digest, they slow the digestion of the whole meal, including the carbs it contains (like the mashed potatoes on the plate with your roasted chicken breast and the bread holding your turkey sandwich fillings), making for a slower rise in blood sugar. Getting enough protein also helps keep you full longer, which in turn helps with weight loss. The plan: Serve up chicken as a main dish as often as you like, but also use it to add protein to salads and pasta.

Enjoy your chicken grilled, baked, sautéed, or broiled, but skip the fried chicken, or you'll be eating more fat than chicken. One extra-crispy fast-food chicken breast, for example, can contain close to half of a day's total recommended fat intake (28 grams), including 8 grams of saturated fat and 4.5 grams of trans fat—a virtual heart attack in a bucket. If you want the taste of fried chicken, try our Oven-Fried Chicken recipe on page 238.

What about turkey? If you serve it only at Thanksgiving, it's time to invite the big bird in more

PERFECT portions: 3 ounces (85 g)

A serving of chicken is 3 ounces (85 g) if you eat it twice a day or 6 ounces (170 g) if you eat it once a day. For easy portion control, try chicken breast tenders, small strips of skinless chicken breast perfect for stir-frying. Typically, two or three tenders equal about a 3-ounce (85-g) serving. Bulk up your stir-fry with plenty of vegetables—and serve it over brown rice, of course.

often. Turkey breast is actually lower in fat and cholesterol and higher in protein than chicken breast. Adding ground turkey is a great way to use less ground beef when making meat loaf, meatballs, and chili and thus lower the fat. Be sure to look for ground turkey *breast,* though; regular ground turkey is much higher in fat.

Health Bonus

Chicken is a good source of the antioxidant mineral selenium. Low levels of selenium in the blood have been linked with poor blood sugar control and complications in people with diabetes, and selenium may offer some protection against the cell damage caused when blood sugar is out of control.

Chicken is also a good source of B vitamins, which play a role in preventing and treating many diseases, including asthma and nerve damage. They also support the immune system.

Got a cold? Homemade chicken soup really can help. Researchers have discovered that it can boost levels of immune cells that lessen inflammation, possibly cutting short a cold.

Cooks Tips

To keep chicken moist, cook it with the skin on, then remove it before serving.

(continued)

Menu Magic

A boneless chicken breast is like a blank canvas. Get as creative as you like! The possibilities are endless, but here are a few easy suggestions.

- Marinate your chicken in three other Magic foods—olive oil, lemon or lime juice, and minced garlic—to make it tasty and tender. Add chopped green chiles to take it up a notch. Marinate for at least 2 hours, then grill or sauté.

- Sauté sliced chicken tenders in olive oil and garlic and add to pizza.

- Keep grilled chicken breast or turkey slices from the deli in the fridge so you can throw them over salad greens for an easy, high-protein lunch.

- Stir-fry or sauté your chicken and add any of these other Magic foods: curry powder (its Magic ingredient is turmeric); broccoli; peaches; apples; almonds, peanuts, or cashews; sesame seeds; spinach; tomatoes; onions; and garlic.

Lean protein foods like **chicken** are at the crux of Magic eating, because they balance out the carbs in a meal and also make weight loss easier.

- Whip up a tasty bowl of chicken fried rice with cooked brown rice, chicken breast strips, egg, sliced scallions, chopped red bell pepper, soy sauce, ground ginger, and crushed garlic. Quickly stir-fry in canola oil.

- Make a light version of chicken salad by using half low-fat mayo and half fat-free yogurt. Add scallions, dill, mustard, and lemon juice for extra flavor. Serve over fresh crunchy lettuce.

Smart Substitutions

Instead of beef meatballs: Make yours turkey meatballs, and you'll get great taste with fewer calories and less saturated fat.

Instead of beef chili: Try turkey chili.

RELATED recipes

All-New Chicken Cordon Bleu *235*

Chicken Breasts with Peaches and Ginger *234*

Chicken Pot Pie with a Whole Grain Biscuit Crust *236*

Chicken Sauté with Apple *235*

Grilled Chicken Salad with Oranges *210*

Honey-Mustard Turkey Burgers *240*

Oven-Fried Chicken *238*

Peanut Chicken Soup *224*

Roasted Moroccan Chicken Thighs with Squash and Pearl Onions *238*

Turkey and Bean Chili with Avocado Salsa *243*

Turkey Meatballs *242*

Turkey Shepherd's Pie with Sweet Potato Topping *241*

Turkey-Noodle Casserole with Spinach *239*

Whole Wheat Noodles with Peanut Sauce and Chicken *214*

Whole Wheat Pasta with Sausage, Beans and Greens *254*

cinnamon

GL
VERY LOW

When you think of cinnamon, you might conjure up images of hot apple pie or warm-from-the-oven oatmeal cookies. And of course, there wouldn't be cinnamon toast without it. You'd probably never imagine, though, that cinnamon has health benefits. In fact, researchers recently discovered that this warming spice can actually help lower your blood sugar. Some of the natural compounds in cinnamon have the ability to mimic insulin, helping glucose get into cells, where it can be used for energy, and significantly lowering blood sugar in the process.

One study involving 60 men and women found that taking as little as 1/4 to 1/2 teaspoon of cinnamon a day lowered blood sugar by 18 to 29 percent. It also reduced bad LDL cholesterol by 7 to 27 percent in people with diabetes.

You probably also wouldn't guess that cinnamon is a good source of fiber (although actually, it's not so surprising when you consider that it comes from the bark of the cinnamon tree). Two teaspoons provides 2.5 grams of fiber—more than 1/2 cup of raw cabbage or bell peppers or two dried apricot halves.

Cinnamon also contains the mineral manganese, which may help improve the way your body uses blood sugar. Just 2 teaspoons can set you up with more than one-third of the manganese you need for the day.

Health Bonus

The natural chemicals in cinnamon can help prevent blood platelets from clumping together and forming dangerous clots that can trigger a heart attack. And studies show that a mere whiff of cinnamon can boost brain activity and improve concentration.

Menu Magic

There are more ways than you can imagine to sprinkle cinnamon into your diet.

- Add cinnamon to applesauce as the apples are cooking or use it to spice up baked apples.

PERFECT portions: 1/2 teaspoon

Just 1/2 teaspoon a day can benefit your health. If you like cinnamon, go ahead and eat a couple of teaspoons a day, but don't go overboard. Cinnamon contains natural compounds that can be toxic in high doses.

- Shake it on whole grain toast or whole grain English muffins.

- Add a half teaspoon or so of cinnamon to ground coffee before starting the pot. You can also add it to tea or drink chai, which contains cinnamon and other spices.

- Mix it into hot cereals, especially oatmeal.

- Sprinkle a little cinnamon on top of ice cream or frozen yogurt or add it to plain yogurt along with a little honey.

- Mix some with low-fat cream cheese for a tasty bread spread.

- Flavor winter squash or sweet potatoes with cinnamon.

RELATED recipes

citrus fruits

GL VERY LOW

Orange you in the mood for a sweet snack? (Sorry, we couldn't resist.) Whether you grab an orange, a tangerine, or half a grapefruit, citrus fruits have an amazing ability to help steady your blood sugar.

First, they're packed with pectin, a type of soluble fiber that helps keep blood sugar—and cholesterol—low. Pectin, like most types of fiber, also leaves you feeling full longer, taming the temptation to overeat at your next meal. How high in soluble fiber are these fruits? Out of the 20 most-eaten fruits and vegetables, oranges and grapefruit come out on top.

Citrus fruits are naturally low in calories (80 for an orange, 41 for half a grapefruit, and 45 for a tangerine). And speaking of calories, it seems we may have mis-judged the much-maligned Grapefruit Diet. Apparently, grapefruit really can help you lose weight. A study at the Scripps Clinic in San Diego looked at 100 obese people and found that those who ate half a grapefruit or drank grapefruit juice before each meal lost an average of 3.3 to 3.6 pounds (1.5 to 1.6 kg) over 12 weeks compared to a loss of only 0.5 pound (225 g) by the people who didn't have the fruit. Grapefruit probably works by reducing insulin spikes after meals. (The smaller the spike in insulin, the better your body is able to process sugar.) Obviously,

eating grapefruit before a meal also dampens your appetite so you eat less of the higher-calorie main dish.

Citrus fruits are most renowned for their vitamin C, an antioxidant that can help fight heart disease and complications of diabetes, such as nerve damage and damage to the retina of the eye. You'll get more than a whole day's vitamin C requirement in a single orange; half a grapefruit will give you 78 percent.

Now, a few words about fruit juice. First, while it's a whole lot more nutritious than soda, you'll need to pour yourself a small glass. Four to 6 ounces (125 to 180 ml) is appropriate—that's why they make juice glasses. Without the fiber found in the whole fruit, fruit juice packs a lot more calories, and it has a greater effect on your blood sugar. The GL of a whole orange, for example, is very low at 5. The GL of 4 ounces (125 ml) of O.J., however, is a much higher 12—and most of us drink more than that.

Don't think that orange juice with pulp contains more fiber; it doesn't. Fresh-squeezed juice, however,

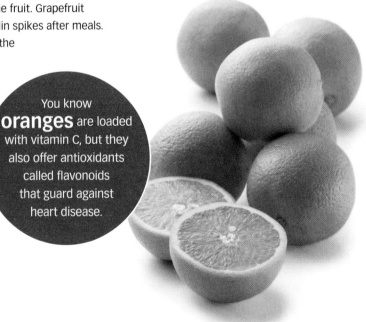

You know **oranges** are loaded with vitamin C, but they also offer antioxidants called flavonoids that guard against heart disease.

may be higher in fiber than high-pulp O.J., since the fruit's membranes go into the juice.

If you choose grapefruit juice, check the label to be sure you're buying an unsweetened brand. Sound too bitter? Stick with red or pink grapefruit juice for a naturally sweeter taste.

Health Bonus

Because citrus fruits can help lower your cholesterol, they deserve a starring role in your diet. You'll get some cancer protection, too, for your effort. Research shows that compounds in citrus fruits can help prevent cancerous changes from occurring in colon cells, and pink and red grapefruits contain lycopene, which studies show may help reduce the risk of developing breast and prostate cancer.

Cooks Tips

Do you shun grapefruit because it's a pain to eat? Make it easy on yourself and buy a grapefruit knife or a special tool for citrus sectioning. This gizmo looks like a cross between salad scissors and a pizza cutter and lets you remove sections or leave them in place (it works for oranges, too.) A good old grapefruit spoon, the kind with serrated edges, is handy to have, too.

At the store, don't judge an orange by its color. That bright hue that looks so appealing may be due to dye rather than ripeness. Instead, look for fruit that's firm and heavy for its size.

Menu Magic

- ❂ Start breakfast with half a grapefruit.
- ❂ Add grapefruit or orange sections to green salads.
- ❂ Garnish your dinner plate with orange sections—and eat them.

PERFECT portions: 1 medium orange

If you're eating a grapefruit, a serving is half of one fruit.

Grapefruit and Meds May Not Mix

If you take prescription medication, watch your grapefruit intake or discuss it with your doctor. Researchers have found that the natural compounds in grapefruit can interfere with the action of some prescription drugs, making them either stronger or weaker than they're supposed to be. A case in point: Grapefruit and grapefruit juice can increase the action of statins, cholesterol-lowering drugs commonly prescribed for people with diabetes. The result? An increased risk of developing toxic side effects from the medication.

- ❂ Whip up an orange smoothie with peeled, seeded oranges; low-fat plain yogurt; frozen strawberries; and vanilla. Blend and pour.

RELATED recipes

Grilled Chicken Salad with Oranges *210*

Orange and Pomegranate Compote *278*

Pink Grapefruit Brulée *277*

Spinach, Grapefruit and Avocado Salad with Poppy Seed Dressing *216*

coffee

GL *VERY LOW*

Health experts have gone 'round and 'round on the coffee issue—is it bad for you or good for you? Our answer: In moderation, coffee, especially decaf, may have beneficial effects on your blood sugar. A study from Finland, which boasts the highest coffee consumption in the world, found that the risk of developing type 2 diabetes went down as coffee consumption went up; the biggest benefits were to people who drank a whopping six cups a day (although we don't recommend that you follow suit). And a recent study from the Harvard School of Public Health found that among more than 88,000 women, drinking just one cup of coffee a day (caffeinated or decaffeinated) was associated with a 13 percent lower risk of developing type 2 diabetes compared with non–coffee drinkers; drinking two to three cups a day was associated with a 32 percent lower risk.

Coffee contains a long list of natural plant compounds, including polyphenol antioxidants called chlorogenic acids, that may contribute to its beneficial effect on blood sugar.

That said, *caffeine* does tend to cause blood sugar to spike, not to mention giving you the jitters. One clinical study found that among nine people who drank a single large cup of caffeinated coffee after an overnight fast, blood sugar was significantly higher for half an hour afterward than it was after drinking a sugar solution; not so after drinking decaffeinated coffee. The answer: Switch to decaf.

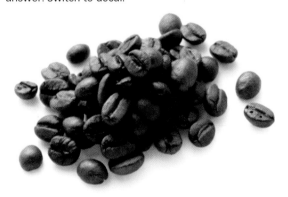

PERFECT portions: 1 to 2 cups

Choose decaf for better blood sugar.

Coffee's not only our morning wakeup call, it's also the number one source of antioxidants in our diets, outpacing even cranberries and red grapes, according to a recent study. Mind you, cranberries, grapes, and other fruits and vegetables are much higher in antioxidants than coffee is, but we don't consume them the way we do coffee too bad for us.

Health Bonus

Several studies show that the antioxidants in coffee offer protection against disease of the liver and colon and Parkinson's disease. And a recent Canadian study found that as coffee drinking increased, the risk of developing Alzheimer's disease decreased.

Menu Magic

A cup of coffee with your breakfast or after dinner, especially if it's decaf, is a good alternative to soda and may even reduce your craving for a sugary doughnut or dessert if you add a little flavor twist. Here are but a few.

- Make your own version of Irish coffee by adding a tablespoon each of orange juice and lemon juice. (Remember, lemon juice, which is acidic, lowers the effect of a food or drink on your blood sugar.) Top with a spoonful of whipped cream.

- Create a delicious grog by adding cloves, nutmeg, cinnamon, grated lemon, and orange peel to coffee. Stir in fat-free half-and-half and lightly sweeten.

- Make Mexican mocha with coffee, chocolate syrup, cinnamon, and nutmeg.

- Mix strong coffee and sugar-free hot chocolate. Add a dash of cinnamon and grated orange peel.

RELATED recipe
Iced Coffee Frappé *209*

eggplant

GL
VERY LOW

Aside from eggplant Parmesan, which contains more fat than two large servings of fast-food French fries, eggplant dishes aren't exactly regulars on most of our tables, but they should be. Voluminous and almost meaty in texture, eggplant is a great addition to pasta because it lets you use less pasta, lowering the GL of the meal, and still fill your plate. It's also a fabulous filling for lasagna in place of meat, reducing calories and saturated fat.

When it's not deep fried (eggplant acts like a sponge, soaking up four times as much fat as French fried potatoes), it's low in calories (it's almost 95 percent water) and carbs. Because its spongy flesh is also a good source of soluble fiber, eggplant makes the list of foods that can help lower both your blood sugar and your cholesterol.

Health Bonus

While it's not a powerhouse of vitamins and minerals, eggplant is one of the richest plant sources of antioxidants you can find in the supermarket, ranking right up there with spinach and sweet potatoes.

Cooks Tips

Eggplants come in an unexpected variety of sizes, shapes, and colors. Look for a type called Black Magic; it has nearly three times the antioxidants found in other eggplants.

don't fall for it

Eggplants are members of the nightshade family, rumored to aggravate arthritis symptoms. But according to the Arthritis Foundation, there is no evidence that any member of the nightshade family has any effect on arthritis.

PERFECT portions: 1/2 cup

Since eggplant has very few calories and a very low GL, feel free to eat more than this, especially if you don't add a lot of oil.

To limit the amount of oil eggplant soaks up, salt eggplant slices and lay them out on a cooling or cookie rack over the sink for at least 15 minutes. Turn the slices, salt the other side, and leave for at least 15 minutes more. Rinse off the excess salt, pat the slices dry, and you're ready to go.

Menu Magic

- As an appetizer, whip up blood sugar–friendly baba ghanoush, a Middle Eastern dish made with pureed roasted eggplant, minced garlic, tahini (sesame paste), lemon juice, and olive oil. Serve it with a whole wheat pita or whole wheat crackers. It's also good as a sandwich spread.

- For dinner, make ratatouille, a hearty vegetable dish featuring eggplant and many other Magic foods, including onions, garlic, tomatoes, and olive oil.

- Sauté eggplant with onion and garlic and use it to replace some of the ground beef in beef dishes to cut fat and calories and add an antioxidant boost.

- Substitute eggplant and mushrooms for ground beef the next time you make lasagna.

- For a quick, easy side dish, grill small Japanese eggplants brushed with olive oil, minced garlic, and salt and pepper. There's nothing quite as good as grilled eggplant.

RELATED recipes

Caponata *202*

Grilled Eggplant Sandwiches with
Red Pepper-Walnut Sauce *220*

Penne with Tomato and Eggplant Sauce *256*

eggs

GL
VERY LOW

If there's one food that's developed an undeserved reputation over the years for being bad for your health, it's eggs. Let's reveal the realities.

Eggs are an excellent, inexpensive source of high-quality protein—so high, in fact, that egg protein is the gold standard nutritionists use to rank all other proteins. What makes the protein in eggs so superior? It contains all of the essential amino acids (the ones your body can't make on its own) in just the right proportions.

Because they're all protein and fat, eggs have no impact on your blood sugar, making them a much better breakfast choice than, say, a stack of white-flour pancakes. And like all protein foods, they may help control your appetite by keeping you full longer. One study found that women who ate two eggs with toast at breakfast felt less hungry before lunch and ate significantly fewer calories during the rest of the day than those who ate a bagel and cream cheese that provided the same number of calories.

Now, about eggs and cholesterol. Yes, it's true, eggs have a lot of it—about 213 milligrams—all in the yolk. It's also true that if you have diabetes, your heart health should be a top priority. But dozens of studies have found

Scrambled, poached, or hard boiled, **eggs** keep your blood sugar steady and provide many of the vitamins and minerals you need.

PERFECT portions: 1 to 2 eggs

A large egg serves up about 75 calories and 5 grams of fat, less than 2 grams of it saturated. The fat and cholesterol are all in the yolk. You can enjoy a two-egg omelet with a piece of whole grain toast, and your breakfast will still be reasonably low in calories as long as you don't load it up with butter and cheese. Studies find that even two eggs a day have no effect on cholesterol in most people. Replace one of the eggs with two egg whites if you like.

that it's saturated fat, not cholesterol, that has the greatest effect on blood cholesterol, so eating eggs in moderation is just fine. For people with elevated cholesterol or those who are especially sensitive to the cholesterol in foods (for some people, cholesterol levels do rise after eating a cholesterol-rich meal), experts recommend eating no more than three or four egg yolks a week. Egg whites, which contain no cholesterol, don't count.

Health Bonus

Egg yolks are one of the few foods naturally rich in vitamin D, a much-needed vitamin that few of us get enough of. Vitamin D helps the body absorb calcium and has recently been linked with lower risks of various cancers to boot. Eggs are also a surprisingly good source of bone-building vitamin K. Plus, they're loaded with lutein (the chickens get it from their feed), which helps protect against macular degeneration, a leading cause of blindness in older folks.

Eggs also contain choline, a compound that animal studies suggest could help improve your memory as you age. Some studies found that giving extra choline to

(continued on page 108)

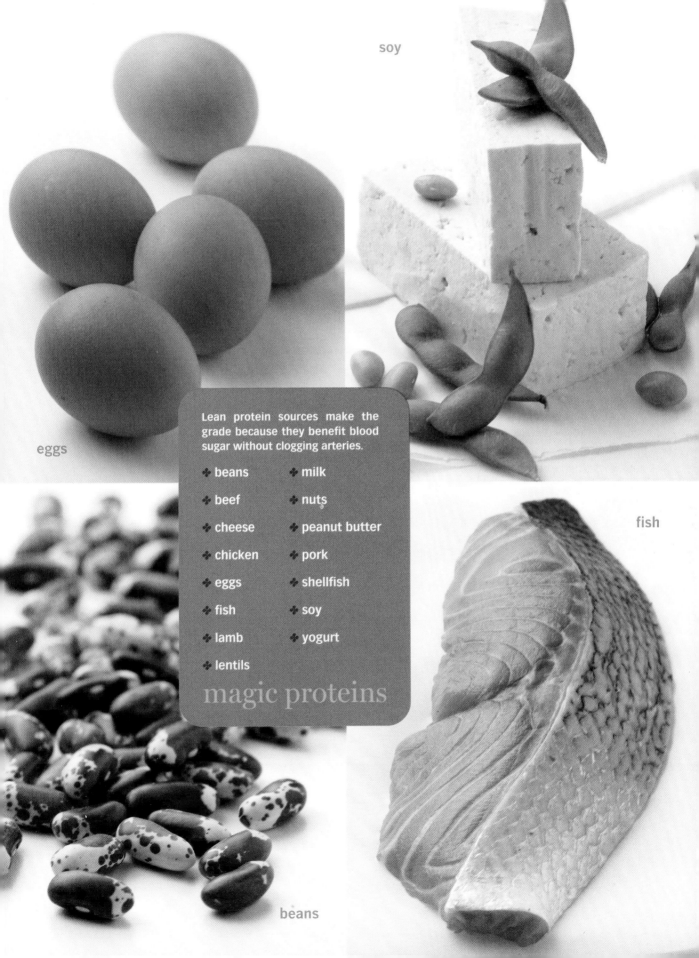

soy

eggs

Lean protein sources make the grade because they benefit blood sugar without clogging arteries.

- ❖ beans
- ❖ beef
- ❖ cheese
- ❖ chicken
- ❖ eggs
- ❖ fish
- ❖ lamb
- ❖ lentils
- ❖ milk
- ❖ nuts
- ❖ peanut butter
- ❖ pork
- ❖ shellfish
- ❖ soy
- ❖ yogurt

magic proteins

fish

beans

pregnant rats created better-functioning brain cells in their babies.

Cooks Tips

If you have an egg tray in your refrigerator door, ignore it. Eggs stay fresh best if you keep them in their original container, pointed ends down. Don't buy eggs sold at room temperature at the store. Eggs age more in a single day at room temperature than they do in a week when stored in the fridge.

You know that eating raw or undercooked eggs carries a risk of salmonella poisoning. The risk is lower than you might think (about 1 in 20,000 eggs carries the gut-wrenching bacteria), but it's not worth taking a chance. You have two options: Eat only thoroughly cooked eggs (that means no eggs "over easy" and no Caesar salad made with raw eggs) or buy pasteurized eggs, which have been warmed enough to kill any salmonella bacteria but not enough to cook the egg.

Menu Magic

Like the chickens they come from, eggs are one of nature's most versatile foods. And they're not just for breakfast.

- ✪ Keep hard-boiled eggs in the fridge for a perfect protein-rich snack.

- ✪ For lunch, have an egg salad sandwich (made with low-fat mayonnaise) on whole wheat bread. Add chopped pickles to lower the glycemic effect of the bread. Or sprinkle on some turmeric, another Magic food (also good on scrambled eggs).

- ✪ Serve a frittata for dinner (think of it as Italian egg pie). We provide one recipe on page 193, but you can add almost anything to your frittata, such as lean ham, diced tomato, spinach, and goat cheese. Use 1 to 2 cups of filling for every four or five eggs.

- ✪ Prepare deviled eggs with low-fat mayonnaise, chopped pickles, chili powder or paprika, and mustard powder.

- ✪ Grill some French toast for breakfast. Dip whole wheat bread in a mixture of egg, cinnamon (another Magic food), vanilla, and milk, then spray the skillet with oil, add the bread, and cook. The protein and fat in the egg will help blunt the blood sugar impact of the bread.

- ✪ Pickle some eggs in vinegar, another Magic food. You get the benefit of high protein plus the blood sugar–lowering power of vinegar.

RELATED recipes

Lemony Blueberry Cheesecake Bars *279*
Pumpkin Custards *278*
Spinach and Goat Cheese Omelet *194*
Zucchini-Basil Frittata *193*

Designer Eggs: Worth the Price?

Environmental and ethical issues of chicken housing and feeding aside, eggs vary little in nutrition from one brand to the next, with two exceptions. One is eggs fortified with heart-smart omega-3 fatty acids. Usually, this is accomplished by adding flaxseed to the chickens' feed. Each egg typically provides 150 to 200 milligrams of omega-3s—a small fraction of the amount you'd get from eating a piece of fish, but some is better than none. The other exception is reduced-cholesterol eggs, which contain 25 percent less cholesterol than regular eggs. These eggs are usually produced by feeding the chickens a vegetarian diet high in canola oil.

fenugreek

GL VERY LOW

This penetrating, pungent spice is not only a standout ingredient in strong, flavorful dishes like Indian curries, it's also proven to help tame blood sugar. In fact, fenugreek supplements are sold for that reason. Here's why fenugreek works: New research suggests it has an uncanny knack for mimicking insulin, which brings down blood sugar.

The yellowish brown seeds, which smell like celery but taste more bitter, also pack a soluble-fiber punch, and you know by now that this type of fiber helps lower blood sugar. One study in animals even suggested that fenugreek could help prevent weight gain, in part by preventing the absorption of fat calories— a definite plus for lowering your diabetes risk. All that makes fenugreek seeds a sweet deal.

Fenugreek leaves are often used in traditional Indian dishes. While they're packed with healthy plant compounds, they haven't been studied as much as the seeds for their ability to lower blood sugar.

Health Bonus

With 1 gram of fiber in only 1/2 teaspoon, fenugreek seeds are a fabulous source of cholesterol-lowering soluble fiber. Plus, the natural antioxidant compounds they contain may help counteract some of the damaging effects of diabetes.

Cooks Tips

For milder flavor, roast fenugreek seeds before grinding them (a coffee bean or spice grinder works well) for recipes. Don't overcook them, or they'll turn bitter.

PERFECT portions: 1/2 teaspoon

It takes only about 1/2 teaspoon of fenugreek seeds a day to make a big difference in blood sugar. In one study, people with diabetes were even able to cut back on their blood sugar–lowering medications by consuming this amount.

Menu Magic

Because of fenugreek's strong, some might say peculiar, flavor, the spice won't work with all your favorite recipes. But there are some dishes in which its flavor is a natural.

- Add ground seed to bread dough to make a spicy loaf.

- Sprinkle ground seed into eggs along with coriander, garlic, cardamom, and cumin for a taste of India in your omelet.

- Stir seeds into lentil dishes. Dahl is an Indian lentil or split-pea dish that wouldn't be complete without fenugreek among the ingredients.

- Find a favorite curry recipe; fenugreek is a common ingredient, either in the curry or in Indian spice mixes.

- Use a combination of fenugreek, cinnamon, ginger, and cumin as a spice rub for chicken. You could also add turmeric, another Magic food, or celery seeds. Store the mixture in a tightly closed container in a dark, cool place.

- Make an after-dinner tisane (a tea that requires straining) using 1/2 teaspoon fenugreek seeds. Steep for 5 to 10 minutes in freshly boiled water, then strain and drink.

RELATED recipes

Curried Butternut Squash Puree *269*
Dahl with Spinach *261*

fish

GL
VERY LOW

The Greenland Inuit eat an incredibly high-fat diet with few vegetables, yet their rate of heart disease is stunningly low. Chalk it up to all the fatty fish they eat: The staple food in their diet is fish rich in omega-3 fatty acids. You've probably heard by now that omega-3s fend off heart disease—something that could be right around the corner if your blood sugar is stuck in overdrive. It's no wonder fish makes our list of Magic foods.

A study at the Harvard School of Public Health found that women with diabetes who ate fish just once a week had a 40 percent lower risk of dying from heart disease than did women with diabetes who ate fish less than once a month.

FISHING FOR
Omega-3s

Some fish are richer in heart-healthy omega-3 fatty acids than others. See for yourself.

Fish	Omega-3s g per 3 oz (85-g) serving
Herring	1.71-1.81
Salmon, Atlantic farmed	1.09-1.83
Sardines	0.98-1.70
Mackerel	0.34-1.57
Salmon, Chinook	1.48
Salmon, Pacific farmed	1.04-1.43
Trout, rainbow, farmed	0.98
Trout, rainbow, wild	0.84
Tuna, white, canned in water	0.73
Salmon, chum or sockeye	0.68
Flounder/sole	0.42
Tuna, light, canned in water	0.26

Source: Circulation, November 19, 2002.

But omega-3s do more than protect your heart. They also quell inflammation in the body, a major contributor to numerous chronic diseases of aging, including insulin resistance and diabetes. It may even play a role in brain diseases such as Alzheimer's as well as certain cancers.

Of course, fish is also a protein food, and protein foods have virtually no impact on blood sugar. We suggest that you aim to eat fish for dinner once or twice a week when you might otherwise have chicken or beef. Make it baked, broiled, pan-fried, stewed, or grilled. Just don't make it fast food or deep fried, like fish and chips or a fish sandwich. Loaded with bad-for-you fats, this fare just isn't the same kettle of fish. One study found eating fried fish and fish sandwiches offered no heart benefits at all.

All fish contain some omega-3s, but fatty types such as albacore tuna, salmon, mackerel, lake trout, herring, and sardines are richest in them (see "Fishing for Omega-3s" at left).

Health Bonus

While the strongest proof of the health benefits of fish points to the heart, there's also plenty of research showing that food with fins can cut the risk of prostate cancer and help maintain brain power as you age. There's also evidence that fatty fish may help defend against depression.

Cooks Tips

One of the keys to successful fish dishes is buying the freshest fish possible. Here's what to look for.

For whole fish

- Shop at a busy fish counter. Lots of customers mean lots of turnover and fresher fish.

- The fish's eyes should be clear, not cloudy.

- The inside of the gills should be bright red, not grayish or even pink.

- It shouldn't smell bad. Fish should have a moist, almost musky smell like a cucumber or melon's.

Safer Salmon

Salmon and other fatty fish, such as tuna and swordfish, have a tendency to store environmental pollutants like mercury by absorbing them into their fat tissue. Experts have debated whether the benefits of eating these fish outweigh the risks and whether wild or farmed fish is the best way to go.

A recent analysis involving a handful of researchers from different institutions came to this bottom line: Whenever you can, choose wild Pacific salmon instead of farmed salmon, which is typically higher in several chemical contaminants. If you really prefer farmed salmon, which has higher levels of omega-3s and is usually cheaper, opt for farmed salmon from Chile. It's the healthiest and safest by far. Canned salmon happens to come from wild varieties, making it a safe choice.

For fish fillets

- They should be moist and firm.
- If there are gaps or separations in the flesh, it's not fresh.
- They shouldn't smell fishy.

Fresh fish will keep in the fridge for a day or two, but cook it as soon as possible or freeze it for up to six months.

Don't bypass frozen fillets. Vacuum-packed sole, cod, or salmon fillets are the next best thing to fresh.

Menu Magic

Fish makes a perfect weeknight meal because it's done before you know it.

- Fire up the grill; almost any type of fish tastes fabulous grilled, especially salmon. Brush it with a little olive oil to keep it from sticking. Throw some zucchini strips on the grill, too, and you have a blood

PERFECT portions: 3 ounces (85 g)

If you are having fish as your main meal of the day, a serving of up to 6 ounces (170 g) is acceptable.

sugar–friendly meal. (Add a side of whole grains such as a bulgur dish.)

- Wrap trout in foil with lemon slices, dill, thyme, salt, and pepper and bake. Serve over quinoa.
- Squeeze fresh lemon juice over fish seasoned with rosemary and sautéed on the stove. Serve with brown rice pilaf.
- Stuff a tomato with tuna salad made with low-fat mayonnaise or plain yogurt, hard-boiled eggs, chopped apples, celery, and onion. Serve with whole wheat crackers.
- If you're a fan of sardines, try this: Sauté some onion and garlic in olive oil, then add sardines canned in tomato sauce. When thoroughly heated, pour the mixture over whole wheat pasta and toss. Top with lemon juice and grated Parmesan.
- Pickled herring is another acquired taste, but it may be worth acquiring—check out its extraordinarily high omega-3 content in the chart on the facing page. As an appetizer, try pickled herring on small squares of whole grain rye toast, sprinkled with chopped parsley and hot paprika.

RELATED recipes

flaxseed

GL
VERY LOW

Teeny-tiny, shiny brown flaxseeds are a godsend to your blood sugar as well as your heart, so if you haven't tried them yet, it's time for a trip to the store. Buy ground flaxseed or grind it yourself in a food processor or coffee grinder. If you don't see it in your supermarket, look in a natural foods store. Using flaxseed may be a mystery to you now, but it's simple once you know how. It has a pleasant, nutty flavor.

Flaxseed is rich in both protein and fiber (more than 2 grams per tablespoon of ground seeds). It's also a good source of magnesium, a mineral that's key to good blood sugar control, because it helps cells use insulin. Several large studies have found that the risk of developing type 2 diabetes skyrockets when magnesium intake is low, so get your fill. Even if you already have diabetes, getting plenty of magnesium can help.

Don't eat enough fish? Load up on flaxseed. It's rich in alpha linolenic acid (ALA), which the body uses to make the same type of omega-3 fatty acids you get from fish. Like fish, flaxseed keeps your heart healthy by lowering cholesterol, keeping your heart pumping normally,

and preventing dangerous blood clots from forming. Also like fish, it guards against inflammation in the body, which is linked to many age-related disorders, including insulin resistance and diabetes.

Health Bonus

Because flaxseed protects against inflammation, it also helps guard against inflammatory conditions such as rheumatoid arthritis, asthma, Crohn's disease, eczema, and psoriasis.

The omega-3 fats in flaxseed help prevent and even help treat breast cancer, thanks to hormone-like plant compounds called lignans. In the body, these convert to compounds that are similar to the body's own estrogen but have much weaker activity. By occupying estrogen receptors on cells, they block the effects of natural estrogen and thus may provide protection against hormone-fueled cancers such as breast cancer. Flaxseed has several hundred times more lignans than any other plant food.

Like fish, flaxseed may also offer protection from Alzheimer's and depression.

Constipated? Flaxseed should do the trick. (Eat too much, and you'll quickly discover the laxative effects.)

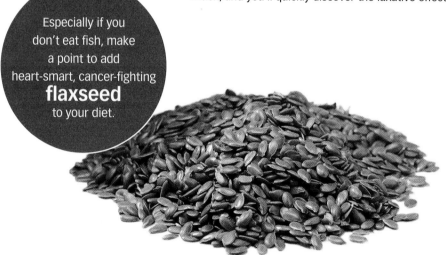

Especially if you don't eat fish, make a point to add heart-smart, cancer-fighting **flaxseed** to your diet.

Cooks Tips

The lignans in flaxseed are much better absorbed by the body if the seeds are eaten ground or crushed. (Whole seeds, on the other hand, tend to pass right through your body undigested.) But because of its high fat content, flaxseed will spoil if you grind it but don't use it right away. The solution: Buy whole seeds in bulk and grind them only as you need them. Whole seeds will last up to a year stored at room temperature. If you buy ground flaxseed, keep it in the fridge.

Menu Magic

You can easily make ground flaxseed part of almost any meal.

- Sprinkle on hot or cold cereal.
- Add to meat loaf, meatballs, burgers, and casseroles.
- Stir into yogurt or add to granola or trail mix.

What about Flaxseed Oil?

Flaxseed oil provides the omega-3 fatty acids that flaxseed does, but not the fiber or lignans. If heart health is your main concern, you may want to consider taking either flaxseed oil or fish oil daily to get more "good fats" into your diet. Because flax thins the blood, talk to your doctor before taking it if you're on aspirin therapy or taking blood-thinning medication. Dosages range from 1 teaspoon to 1 tablespoon once or twice a day.

The oil goes rancid easily, so keep it refrigerated. You can use it in salad dressings, add it to steamed vegetables after cooking, or sprinkle it over grain dishes, but don't cook with it, since heat destroys its nutrients.

PERFECT portions: 1 to 2 tablespoons

A tablespoon or two a day, ground and blended into other foods, could do wonders for your blood sugar control and overall good health. You can also mix 1 or 2 tablespoons of ground flaxseed into a glass of water and drink it.

- Add a tablespoon or two to doughs and batters for pancakes, waffles, muffins, and breads. Just keep an eye on baked goods in the oven; the flaxseed could make them brown quicker than usual.
- Use as a topping for ice cream or frozen yogurt.
- Add to smoothies.
- Use to replace one-fourth of the flour in muffin or pancake batter.
- Add to cooked fruit desserts like baked apples or blueberry compote.
- Sprinkle in your favorite sandwich filling, such as tuna or chicken salad.
- Add to cream cheese or sprinkle on a soft cheese and enjoy with some whole grain crackers for a blood sugar–friendly snack.

RELATED recipes

Berry-Flaxseed Smoothie *208*
Brown Rice Pilaf with Flaxseeds, Lime and Cilantro *265*
Brown Rice Pilaf with Toasted Flaxseed *265*
Oatmeal with Apple and Flaxseeds *193*
Whole Wheat Flaxseed Bread *196*

garlic

GL *VERY LOW*

You probably know garlic is good for your cholesterol. And if you like garlic, you wouldn't even think of making your favorite recipes without it—which is a good thing because this pungent herb may also be good for your blood sugar.

According to early research with animals, garlic may increase insulin secretion, which would lower blood sugar, and improve insulin sensitivity, in effect helping to reverse diabetes. Since supplements show no blood sugar benefits, enjoy garlic the old-fashioned, tasty way. A recent animal study found that high doses of raw garlic significantly reduced blood sugar levels.

"The stinking rose" offers other health benefits as well. Study after study shows it can help keep cholesterol under control by lowering "bad" cholesterol (LDL) and pumping up "good" (HDL). In an analysis of five trials in which participants received either garlic supplements or placebos, the authors concluded that you could lower your total cholesterol by about 9 percent with the equivalent of 1 1/2 to 3 cloves of garlic daily for two to six months. Garlic also thins the blood, making it less likely to form artery-clogging clots.

Health Bonus

A diet rich in garlic could mean a lower risk of several types of cancer, including cancer of the stomach and colon. Garlic also has the ability to bring down high blood pressure.

Cooks Tips

Unless you enjoy chopping, buy a garlic press. Keep your garlic in a cool, dark place, either in a plain old cup in your cabinet or in a fancier garlic keeper—the kind made of terra cotta or pottery with a lid to keep light out and holes in the sides to let air in. Don't keep it in the fridge, or it will sprout quickly.

To peel garlic with minimal hassle, bang the side of the clove with the side of a large knife. The peel will practically slip off at that point.

PERFECT portions: all you can eat

The more, the better.

Menu Magic

- Add sautéed garlic to just about any chicken, fish, beef, or tofu dish.

- Use roasted garlic as a spread for bread instead of butter or add it to mashed potatoes or pasta. To roast, break the heads into cloves but don't peel them. Spread them on a baking sheet, drizzle with a bit of olive oil, sprinkle with salt, and bake at 375°F (190°C), shaking the pan occasionally, until tender, about 30 minutes. Then simply squeeze the cloves out of their skins.

- Add minced garlic to rice or other grain dishes before cooking.

- Add minced garlic to vinaigrette dressing.

- Sauté vegetables such as spinach or mushrooms in olive oil and garlic.

- Make a garlic/mustard marinade for beef by mixing spicy mustard, olive oil, balsamic vinegar, black pepper, and chopped garlic (lots of it). Add the beef to the marinade and refrigerate for at least 2 hours.

- If you're grilling, feel free to add the whole garlic bulb to the grill. Turn it so all sides are exposed to the heat. It's ready to eat when the skin is dark brown and peels easily.

RELATED recipes

jerusalem artichokes

GL *VERY LOW*

This Magic food, also known as the sunchoke, is unusual in more ways than one. Not only does it have no connection with Jerusalem or artichokes (it's actually related to the sunflower), it looks more like a small gnarly potato than an artichoke, and it grows underground. But the similarity with potatoes ends there. Decidedly unlike potatoes, Jerusalem artichokes (which are crunchy and slightly sweet) have an amazingly beneficial effect on your blood sugar. That's because the starches they contain, called fructans (specifically types of fructans called inulin and oligofructose), aren't readily digested the way typical carbs are. In fact, they're barely digested at all.

Because these starches can't be broken down by enzymes in the small intestine, they travel to the large intestine (colon), where they are digested by intestinal bacteria and eventually excreted. In the end, they supply less than 40 percent as many calories as regular carbohydrates.

Along with being a low-GL food, Jerusalem artichokes may have another advantage. Foods that contain inulin, as 'chokes do, may help smooth out blood sugar and insulin levels after a meal. Preliminary studies are investigating whether higher doses of inulin may also increase fullness and help cut calorie intake.

Health Bonus

Jerusalem artichokes may help improve the health of your colon. The fructans they contain act as prebiotics, meaning that they provide fodder for beneficial bacteria in the intestinal tract. Fructans also help increase the amount of water and bacteria in the stool, helping to relieve constipation.

Looking to boost your heart health? Jerusalem artichokes can help there, too. The same indigestible carbs that help smooth out blood sugar and relieve constipation may signal the liver to produce fewer triglycerides and fatty acids that can clog your arteries.

PERFECT portions: 1/2 cup

A half cup contains only 57 calories and few blood sugar–raising carbs.

Cooks Tips

Jerusalem artichokes are in season between about October and April, although some stores carry them year-round. Look for firm 'chokes with a smooth, unblemished surface, and avoid those that feel soft, look dried out, or have sprouts. Scrub them well with a vegetable brush to get rid of grit and dirt (remember, they grow underground). Peeling is optional. You can drizzle on a little lemon juice or vinegar to help retain their white color.

A note of caution: Start with small servings; inulin can cause flatulence.

Menu Magic

- Boil and mash a Jerusalem artichoke just like a potato, or if you prefer, add to regular mashed potatoes to decrease the GL.

- Toss thin raw slices into salads.

- Slice a 'choke and use in place of water chestnuts in stir-fries.

- Steam cubes or slices on the stove or in the microwave, then drizzle with olive oil and lemon juice.

- Grate into a vegetable slaw.

- Slice and serve a sunchoke with dip, along with other crudités.

Smart Substitutions

Instead of grated potatoes: Use grated in potato pancake recipes.

Instead of pureed potatoes: Use as a thickener in soups.

RELATED recipe

Jerusalem Artichoke Pancakes *268*

lamb

GL
VERY LOW

Lamb may very well have been the first meat eaten by humans. Today, in some parts of the world, people eat lamb as we eat beef—as a staple food. If you choose the right cuts, lamb is a Magic source of protein, just as beef is.

The leg—the classic spring roast—is the leanest of all, especially if you buy the shank as opposed to the butt, a.k.a. sirloin. (Actually, the foreshank is even slightly leaner but must be tenderized, usually by cooking in liquid for hours.) Loin chops are a bit fattier, and the shoulder is a bit fattier still. The ribs (rack of lamb) are the fattiest, along with ground lamb. If you want lean ground lamb, you'll have to ask the butcher to grind it for you from one of the leaner cuts.

Fortunately, lamb isn't marbled the way beef is; most of the fat is on the outside and is easily trimmed.

Health Bonus

Like beef, lamb is rich in B vitamins, iron, and zinc. Zinc is essential for a healthy immune system. A shortfall of iron can sap anyone's energy and concentration. As for the B vitamins, they help improve cholesterol ratios and lower levels of homocysteine, an amino acid linked with increased risk of heart attack, stroke, and Alzheimer's disease.

Cooks Tips

Lamb is meat from sheep less than a year old, so it's generally moist and tender. Get the most for your money by purchasing fine-textured, pink meat with a minimum of firm white fat. Always trim visible fat from fresh lamb and remove any pieces of fell, a papery membrane that covers surface fat. Meat from sheep more than a year old is called mutton and has a stronger taste. It tends to be leaner, though less tender, than lamb. To keep it tender, allow enough time to cook it slowly over medium heat.

PERFECT portions: 3 ounces (85 g)

If this is your main meat for the day, a serving of up to 6 ounces (170 g) is appropriate.

Menu Magic

Lamb stew, lamb chops, lamb curry, leg of lamb… there are so many different, delicious ways to enjoy this Magic food.

- Make a big pot of lamb stew on the weekend and freeze the leftovers or enjoy them during the week. Include plenty of vegetables, such as carrots, squash, onions, peas, and sweet potatoes.

- Make some lamb kebabs by alternating chunks of uncooked lamb and vegetables such as zucchini, tomatoes, and onions on skewers. Grill and serve over whole wheat couscous.

- Braise lamb shanks slowly (2 to 3 hours) in a combination of red wine, minced garlic, and rosemary for a tender entrée. You'll want to brown the shanks before braising.

- Serve roasted or grilled lamb with a dollop of mint yogurt sauce made with low-fat plain yogurt, chopped mint leaves, minced garlic, and a dash of cayenne pepper.

- Use chopped leftover lamb to add protein to tabbouleh, or add it to bulgur cooked in chicken broth, sautéed celery and onions, and slivered almonds. Season with cinnamon, another Magic food.

RELATED recipes
Lamb Stew with Spring Vegetables 229
Mustard-Crusted Lamb Chops 232

lemons

GL
VERY LOW

When life hands you lemons, eat 'em! That's right, get ready to pucker up, because lemon juice helps lower blood sugar, thanks to its incredible acidity (just thinking about lemons starts your salivary glands gushing). Because of that acidity (see Chapter 2 in Part 1 to brush up on the acid effect), even a little lemon juice can lower the GL of any meal. Lime juice should have a similar effect.

Health Bonus

Four tablespoons of lemon juice will give you almost half the vitamin C you need for the day. Remember, antioxidants like vitamin C make cholesterol less likely to stick to your artery walls. Lemons are also packed with a natural disease-preventing compound called limonene that may help lower cholesterol and is even being studied for its potentially potent anti-cancer powers.

The citric acid in lemon juice also helps stave off kidney stones by reducing the excretion of calcium in the urine. Lemon rind is rich in a compound called rutin, which strengthens the walls of veins and capillaries, potentially reducing the pain and severity of varicose veins.

Cooks Tips

Looking for a juicy lemon? Give it a squeeze. The softer the lemon, the thinner the skin and the juicier the fruit is. To maximize juice output, bring lemons to room temperature and roll them firmly back and forth on the counter a few times with the palm of your hand before cutting.

Menu Magic

- Use lemon juice in salad dressings.
- Serve plenty of lemon slices alongside fish, which wouldn't be the same without them.

PERFECT portions: 1 to 2 tablespoons

If the effects of lemon juice are anything like those of vinegar—and we think they are—1 to 2 tablespoons should be enough to lower the blood sugar impact of a meal by as much as 30 percent.

- Add it to tuna the next time you make yourself a tuna sandwich.
- Spritz your water or seltzer with lemon juice to add flavor (possibly encouraging you to drink more water) and lessen the blood sugar impact of whatever you're eating.
- Think lemon chicken!
- Use lemon juice in marinades for meat or poultry. Combine lemon juice, balsamic vinegar, olive oil, fresh rosemary, and minced garlic, then add the meat and refrigerate overnight, if possible.
- Squeeze fresh lemon juice on vegetables, pasta, soups, rice, and stews. It will add so much flavor, you'll be able to cut back on salt.

RELATED recipes

lentils

GL
VERY LOW

Lentils are the perfect slow-acting food, with an ideal mix of slow-digesting protein and complex carbohydrates. And since they cook quickly—no presoaking required—there's little excuse not to use them in soups, salads, and main dishes even on weeknights. If you add them to rice dishes, you'll be able to use less rice and significantly lower the GL of the dish.

Their secret weapon against blood sugar spikes is soluble fiber, and plenty of it. A cup of cooked lentils carries a whopping 16 grams of fiber, most of it the soluble type. Of course, soluble fiber is also the stuff that lowers cholesterol. It's little wonder that lentils are a staple in the Mediterranean diet, famous for protecting the heart.

Lentils are also a good source of protein (18 grams per cup, cooked), which makes them wonderfully filling and weight-loss friendly.

Health Bonus

One recent study found that women who included lentils or beans in their diets at least twice a week had a 25 percent lower risk of breast cancer compared to women who ate them less than once a month. Lentils are also unusually rich in folacin, a B vitamin proven to lower blood levels of homocysteine, an amino acid linked with an increased risk of heart disease and dementia. The fiber in lentils also helps keep you regular.

Cooks Tips

Stored in a cool, dry, dark place, lentils will keep for up to six months. Hang on to them any longer, and they'll dry out. Don't mix new lentils with older ones, since the older ones will take longer to cook.

PERFECT portions: 1/2 cup

Since the GL is very low, and lentils are among the most nutritious plant foods around, you can enjoy a bit more.

Menu Magic

- Add cooked lentils to green salads or pasta dishes.

- Mash cooked lentils and blend with fresh salsa or with garlic, yogurt, and lemon juice for an easy and terrifically healthy dip or spread.

- Cook a pot—or open a can—of lentil soup. Interesting options include red lentil and tomato soup, lentil-barley soup, lentil and Swiss chard soup with lemon (chock full of Magic foods!), and chicken and lentil stew.

- Make lentils a main dish by cooking them with smoked turkey sausage, onion, tomatoes, and herbs.

- Reinvent rice by adding lentils. Cook and season a variety of colored lentils and serve over brown or converted rice.

RELATED recipes

Curried Red Lentil Soup *224*
Dahl with Spinach *261*
Greek Lentil Salad *217*
Lentil and Bean Chili *262*
Mustard-Glazed Salmon with Lentils *247*

melons

GL
VERY LOW

Despite their mouthwatering sweetness, melons are surprisingly blood sugar friendly, making them perfect with breakfast, as snacks, or in fruit salads and even salsas. Yes, the sugar they contain is quickly converted to glucose, or blood sugar, but melons are mostly water (as much as 90 percent), so they don't have as much sugar as you'd think. Because of their water content, melons are also remarkably low in calories.

Watermelon perfectly illustrates the difference between the glycemic index (GI) and the glycemic load (GL). Because the sugar it contains is fast acting, it has a sky-high GI—but since you get very little sugar when you eat a serving of watermelon, its GL is low.

The vitamin C in melons (cantaloupes are the real C standouts) makes them top-notch for preventing some of the damage high blood sugar can cause to cells as well as to arteries and blood vessels. And melons' potassium helps guard against high blood pressure, a real risk of diabetes. As one of the richest sources of lycopene (a natural compound that's close kin to beta-carotene), it may also help keep heart disease at bay, which is important since heart disease risk runs high for people with diabetes.

Health Bonus

Lycopene-rich foods such as watermelon may offer protection against certain kinds of cancer, including prostate, breast, endometrial, lung, and colon cancers. The strongest evidence has been regarding prostate cancer. One study of 47,000 men found that those who ate two to four servings of tomatoes (another lycopene-rich food) a week had a 26 percent reduced risk of prostate cancer compared to those who ate none.

PERFECT portions: 1 cup cubed

Since melons are mostly water, feel free to have a bit more.

Remember Mom's admonition to eat your carrots for good eyesight? It's the beta-carotene in carrots that makes them good for your eyes, and cantaloupe is rich in this nutrient, too.

Cooks Tips

If only melons came with tags indicating how ripe they were, you'd never pick a bad one again. They don't, but you can use these clues.

Watermelon: Thump it to see if it's ripe. If it sounds a bit hollow, it should be ready. You can also shake it to see if the seeds are loose, an indication of ripeness.

Cantaloupe: If it smells too sweet and musky, it's past its prime. Unlike watermelon, cantaloupe will continue to ripen at room temperature, so if you buy one that's not quite ripe, keep it on the counter until it's ready.

Honeydew: Look for a smooth outer peel and softness at the stem end of the melon (press it with your thumb).

Be sure to rinse melons well before you cut them. Since melons are grown on vines that lie on the ground, they come in contact with all kinds of bacteria

(continued)

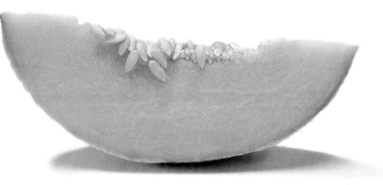

melons continued

from dirt, water, and animals. When you slice through the peel, you could move that bacteria from the outside to the inside on the knife.

For convenience, consider buying a melon baller. These come in various sizes and make it easy to serve melon as an appetizing snack or dessert. They're also good for coring pears and apples.

Bitter Melon—More Like Medicine

Bitter melon, also part of the melon clan, is anything but sweet. As its name implies, this light green vegetable (yes, all melons are vegetables), which looks more like a cucumber with warts than a melon, has a very bitter taste due to a high concentration of quinine. Animal research shows that the natural compounds in bitter melon can lower blood sugar levels as much as some prescription drugs, possibly by boosting insulin secretion, improving the ability of cells to absorb glucose, blocking the absorption of sugar in the intestine, and hindering the release of glucose from the liver.

One of the largest studies of bitter melon in people with type 2 diabetes lasted only two days, but it showed significant drops in blood sugar for 100 participants within hours after they drank a liquid containing suspended pulp from the melon. A number of smaller but longer trials have had similar results.

Most people who try bitter melon use supplements, but if you want to eat the melon itself (it's very much an acquired taste), cut the white fibrous seed core in half and remove the seeds. Don't eat them! The red seed covering can be toxic. Blanching the melon before cooking will help reduce the bitter flavor. It can then be used in soups or stir-fries.

Menu Magic

- Make melons part of any fruit salad. Use a scooped-out watermelon shell to serve the salad at a picnic.

- Try a salad with watermelon chunks and feta cheese, topped with fresh mint leaves and, if you like, some toasted pumpkin seeds or toasted pine nuts.

- Make a refreshing watermelon slush by mixing cubed watermelon and ice in the blender. Add a bit of honey at the end.

- Garnish plates with a slice of watermelon—and eat it!

- Serve honeydew with vanilla ice cream.

- Mix small melon cubes with chicken or seafood salad.

- Make watermelon salsa by blending watermelon, sweet onions, black beans, jalapeños, chopped cilantro, minced garlic, and salt.

- Keep melon cubes or balls in the fridge for handy, refreshing snacks.

- Blend cantaloupe, orange juice, lime juice, and cinnamon for a cold soup appetizer.

- Make a melon smoothie with cantaloupe, honeydew, lime juice, and a little honey.

- Place chunks or balls of several different types of melon on skewers for a fun, colorful appetizer. Add grapes between the melon pieces if you like.

- Eat thinly sliced cantaloupe or honeydew on top of Swiss cheese for a colorful snack.

RELATED recipe

Cantaloupe and Blueberry Compote with Green Tea and Lime *276*

milk

VERY LOW

There's something rather mysterious about milk in relation to blood sugar. It moves the needle only a smidge, which isn't surprising since it's fairly low in carbohydrates and rich in protein (a perfect combination for steadying blood sugar). But researchers think there's some natural component in milk that may help directly protect against insulin resistance, a forerunner of type 2 diabetes.

Two Harvard studies found that people who made dairy foods part of their daily diets were 21 percent less likely to develop insulin resistance and 9 percent less likely to develop type 2 diabetes for each daily serving of dairy they had. Pretty impressive! (Apparently not everyone has gotten the word, though: Some Web sites actually tell you that milk *causes* diabetes.)

Choose fat-free milk over whole or even 2 percent, which still has a fair amount of saturated fat, the kind that increases insulin resistance and clogs arteries.

Health Bonus

Milk is, of course, rich in calcium and vitamin D, both important for shoring up bone. Fat-free milk actually has more calcium than whole, and it's also virtually the only good source of vitamin D you're likely to find in your kitchen. D is a "don't miss" vitamin: Experts are realizing not only that our needs for it are higher than previously thought—and our blood levels woefully

don't fall for it

Almost everyone has seen the commercials advertising dairy foods as an aid in losing weight. The trouble is, the results of studies on dairy and weight loss have been inconsistent, with the latest showing that people who eat a lot of calcium-rich dairy foods don't in fact have an easier time losing weight. There's no harm in getting more fat-free milk into your diet; just don't bank on dairy foods to solve your poundage problems.

PERFECT portions: 1 cup

Three 8-ounce (250-milliliter) servings a day of low-fat milk or other dairy products, such as yogurt, may help tame insulin resistance and also provide much of the calcium you need.

low—but also that it may play a key role in preventing certain cancers if we get enough.

Low-fat dairy foods such as fat-free milk are also a cornerstone of the doctor-recommended DASH diet proven to help control high blood pressure.

Cooks Tips

If you're not a fan of fat-free milk because it's too thin, try ultra-pasteurized fat-free milk, also called UHT (ultra-high temperature). Brands include Parmalat. It tends to have a creamier texture than regular fat-free milk but no more fat or calories.

Menu Magic

- Pretend you're a kid again and drink a cold glass of fat-free milk with lunch or dinner.

- Make yourself a banana-strawberry smoothie with frozen strawberries, a frozen banana, fat-free milk, and a dash of vanilla extract.

- Create "cream" of carrot or tomato soup using fat-free milk. Thicken it with a small amount of flour.

- Enjoy a soothing cup of chai once in a while instead of coffee.

RELATED recipes

Cauliflower and Spinach Casserole *270*
Chai *208*
Cherry Clafouti *283*
Greek Pasta and Beef Casserole *230*
Macaroni and Cheese with Spinach *255*
Oatmeal with Apples and Flaxseeds *193*
Sole Florentine *247*

nuts

GL VERY LOW

There's a good reason that people put nuts in trail mix to take with them when they're hiking. Nuts provide sustained energy because, thanks to their mix of fat and protein, they're a "slow-burning" food. For the same reason, they're friendly to your blood sugar. In fact, Harvard researchers discovered that women who regularly ate nuts (about a handful five times a week) were 20 percent less likely to develop type 2 diabetes than those who didn't eat them as often.

Yes, nuts are high in fat—but it's mostly "good" fat. Remember secret number 5 of Magic eating, Favor Good Fats? Good fat may reduce insulin resistance, and in the case of most nuts, 85 percent of their fat is this kind.

Good fats, of course, also improve heart health, even boosting levels of "good" HDL cholesterol. In studies, people who ate as few as 5 ounces (150 g) of nuts a week as part of an overall heart-healthy diet lowered their risk of developing heart disease by 35 percent compared to those who ate nuts less than once a month. (This doesn't apply to macadamia nuts, though, because of their high saturated fat content.) In fact, one study found that a diet that includes unsaturated fats from almonds and walnuts may have 10 percent more cholesterol-lowering power than a traditional cholesterol-lowering diet.

If you eat nuts frequently, you may also be damping down chronic inflammation in your body, which can help reduce your risk of both diabetes and heart disease. And the protein in most nuts is unusually rich in the amino acid arginine, which may help relax blood vessels, making a heart attack less likely.

Some nuts, including peanuts, walnuts, and almonds, also contain plant sterols, which have been shown to lower cholesterol, and a natural compound called resveratrol, the same one found in red wine and shown to lower heart disease risk. Like fish, walnuts are a good source of omega-3 fats, another shot in the arm against heart disease.

Peanuts aren't technically nuts at all, but legumes. Unlike nuts that grow on trees, they grow underground, but for health, they rank right up there with all the aboveground nuts (also see the peanut butter entry on page 136).

HOW MANY nuts IN A SERVING?

Nut	Serving Size 1 oz (30 g)
Almonds	20-24
Brazil nuts	9 or 10
Cashews	16-18
Hazelnuts	18-20
Peanuts	40
Pine nuts	150-157
Pistachios	45-47
Walnuts	8-11 halves

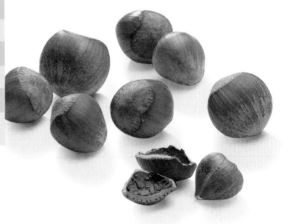

Health Bonus

Nuts provide a hard-to-find nutrient—vitamin E, an important antioxidant that may help fight prostate and lung cancers. Brazil nuts are selenium superstars, providing a whopping 200 times more of the mineral than any other nut. Selenium has been linked to prevention of both cancer and heart disease. Almonds provide bone-building calcium. Hazelnuts and cashews boast the most copper, a much-needed nutrient for people with diabetes.

Cooks Tips

To squirrel away nuts, store them in an airtight container in the fridge for up to six months; in the freezer, they'll last for up to a year.

Roasting nuts brings out their flavor. Preheat the oven to 300°F (150°C). Place 1/2 cup of shelled nuts on a baking sheet in a single layer and roast for 7 to 10 minutes. Check near the end of the roasting time to make sure they don't burn.

Menu Magic

Pick a dish, almost any dish—adding nuts can make it a real standout in terms of both taste and nutrition. Here are but a few simple suggestions to take your recipes to the next level.

- Stir chopped walnuts or pecans into rice dishes.
- Add pistachios to chicken salad.
- Mix pine nuts or chopped walnuts into pasta dishes along with olive oil, basil, and sun-dried tomatoes.
- Create your own trail mix for snacking with dried fruit, high-fiber cereal, and your favorite nuts.
- Top off pumpkin, squash, or tomato soup with chopped roasted nuts.
- Sprinkle your favorite chopped nuts and some dried cranberries on green salads.
- For better-tasting waffles, pancakes, and muffins, add chopped nuts to the batter.

PERFECT portions: 1 ounce (30 g)

Nuts are high in calories, so a serving is small. Because nuts come in all shapes and sizes, the number that equals a serving varies quite a bit (see "How Many Nuts in a Serving?" on opposite page). Macadamia nuts contain a whopping 1,000 calories per cup, so indulge sparingly.

- For a single-serving, low-GL snack in place of chips or crackers, place 1 ounce (30 g) of nuts in a self-sealing bag to carry with you.
- Sprinkle pecans into unsweetened applesauce.
- Stir nuts into stir-fry dishes.

Smart Substitution

Instead of white flour: Use ground nuts to replace some of the white stuff called for in a crust or cake batter.

RELATED recipes

Apple-Bran Muffin *197*
Asian Peanut Dip *204*
Bulgur with Ginger and Orange *264*
Caponata *202*
Cherry-Almond Gratin *288*
Cherry Tomatoes Filled with Pesto Cream Cheese *200*
Chocolate-Raspberry Cheesecake *284*
Fudge Brownies *280*
Grilled Chicken Salad with Oranges *210*
Maple-Walnut Roasted Apples *282*
Oatmeal-Peanut Butter Trail Bars *207*
Quinoa with Chiles and Cilantro *266*
Spiced Almonds *203*
Spinach with Pine Nuts and Currants *274*
Upside-Down Nectarine Muffins *199*
Wheatberry Salad with Dried Apricots and Mint *266*
Whole Wheat Noodles with Peanut Sauce and Chicken *214*

oats

GL MEDIUM

A steaming bowl of oatmeal—sprinkled with Magic cinnamon, of course—is more than comfort food. Studies show that oats can reduce postmeal blood sugar and insulin levels in people with and without diabetes.

Soluble fiber is the reason oatmeal is top-notch for steady blood sugar. This type of fiber turns into a gel in your stomach, slowing the digestive process and blunting the rise in blood sugar that normally goes with it. Oats are also an excellent source of the mineral manganese, which plays a role in blood sugar metabolism.

Dozens of studies have concluded that eating oatmeal five or six times a week can reduce your risk of developing type 2 diabetes by as much as 39 percent. And, since oatmeal's a whole grain, starting your day with a bowl will take you one step closer to living the second secret of Magic eating, Make Three of Your Carb Servings Whole Grains.

Oats also fight heart disease, as it says right on the oatmeal box. This has been proven beyond a shadow of a doubt in more than 40 studies over 30 years of research. It's largely because of the special type of soluble fiber, called beta-glucan, in oatmeal.

One more benefit of this flaky food: It fills you up and keeps you full. In one study, people who ate oatmeal for breakfast consumed one-third fewer calories at lunch than those who ate a sugared flaked cereal. (The bran of the oat is just as good for your blood sugar as flakes, so be sure to read the bran entry on page 84.)

Health Bonus

The soluble fiber called beta-glucan not only helps tame blood sugar and cholesterol, it may also help boost your immune system's ability to fight off infection, as well as reduce high blood pressure. Oats are also a good source of natural plant compounds that may help reduce the risk of breast cancer by mimicking estrogen and preventing the natural hormone from triggering the growth of cancer cells. And they're packed with powerful disease-fighting antioxidants called polyphenols and saponins.

OATS glossary

While all oats have the power to tame your blood sugar, there are differences in taste and texture among types.

Oat groats: Oats that have been cleaned, toasted, hulled, and cleaned again. These are the most minimally processed of all the oat varieties and must be soaked and cooked for a long time.

Steel-cut oats: Whole grain groats that have been cut into two or three pieces using steel disks. These take 30 to 45 minutes to cook and have a hearty oat flavor and a chewier texture than rolled oats.

Rolled (old-fashioned) oats: Oats that have been steamed, rolled, resteamed, and toasted. They take about 15 minutes to cook.

Instant oats: These are prepared the same way as rolled oats but cut into smaller pieces so they cook faster. No actual cooking is required; just pour boiling water over them and stir.

Oat flour: Flour made by grinding groats and separating out the bran. It is gluten free.

Oat bran: This is made by grinding oat groats and separating the bran from the flour. It's higher in insoluble fiber than whole oats and can be prepared as a hot cereal like oatmeal.

Are Some Oats Better than Others?

Some oats have been processed more or less than others. On the "less" end of the scale are steel-cut oats (see "Oats Glossary" on the facing page). The GL of less processed oats is about 20 percent lower than that of more processed forms, but even instant oats are a good source of fiber and have a moderate GL. Shop carefully for instant oatmeal, though; most brands have added sugar—as much as 4 teaspoons per packet. Generally, only "regular" (unflavored) instant oatmeal is sugar free.

Cooks Tips

Don't substitute instant oats in a recipe that calls for quick-cooking or old-fashioned oats. The texture is different, and instant oats usually have other flavors added.

Menu Magic

- ✪ Grind oats in the blender and use them to coat fish and chicken.

- ✪ Make a batch of oat bran muffins and keep them on hand for tasty breakfast treats.

- ✪ Next time you make pancakes or waffles, replace up to one-third of the flour in the batter with oatmeal ground to a fine powder in the blender.

- ✪ Bake up a tray of oatmeal cookies (using whole wheat flour in place of one-third of the white flour) and include Magic cinnamon, of course!

- ✪ Make fresh oat biscuits.

- ✪ Use oat flour as a thickener for stews and soups.

PERFECT **portions:** 1/2 cup, cooked

Oats are slow-acting carbs that are good for your blood sugar—if you keep the portion size reasonable. Eat more than a cup, and the GL moves into the high range. Fill up the rest of your bowl with fresh fruit and a sprinkling of nuts.

- ✪ For dessert, serve oat-rich fruit crisps and cobblers. Just watch the butter content. It's better to use a good-for-you brand of margarine such as Smart Balance instead.

Smart Substitutions

Instead of sugary cereal: Have steel-cut or old-fashioned oatmeal with raisins and walnuts for a hearty and filling breakfast.

Instead of bread crumbs: Use oats in meat loaf and meatballs.

Instead of wheat flour: Substitute oat flour for a third of the wheat flour in baked goods.

olive oil

GL
VERY LOW

It's a wonder olive oil isn't more expensive, because in the world of Magic eating, it's liquid gold.

Remember secret number 5 of Magic eating, Favor Good Fats? Well, olive oil is the flagship of the good-fats fleet. In fact, we recommend using olive or canola oil (when you need a neutral-tasting oil) most of the time instead of other oils.

Good fats like those in olive oil work miracles for your blood sugar—and your health in general. Unlike butter, these unsaturated fats don't increase insulin resistance and may even help *reverse* it, helping your body steady its blood sugar.

Olive oil also "spikeproofs" your meals by slowing digestion so carbs take longer to break down into blood sugar. Simply tossing your salad with olive oil and vinegar will help blunt the blood sugar impact of whatever else you're eating (see page 159 to find out why the vinegar's also important).

One recent Australian study found that when six men were given either olive oil, water, or a mixture of water and oil before a high-carb meal, it took almost three times as long for their stomachs to begin emptying—significantly delaying the subsequent rise in blood sugar—when they had the olive oil. You may also remember from the first chapter that meals that raise blood sugar quickly result in feeling hungrier before the next meal. Slower rises in blood sugar equal feeling full longer, which in turn equals weight loss!

As for heart health, eating generous amounts of olive oil is one of the main reasons that people who follow the Mediterranean diet have less heart disease and far fewer heart attacks. One study found that when 28 men and women added 2 tablespoons of extra-virgin olive oil a day to their usual diets for six weeks, they experienced a 12 percent drop in total cholesterol and a 16 percent drop in LDL ("bad") cholesterol. Numerous studies over the years have shown that olive oil not only lowers LDL but also raises HDL, the good kind. The oil is also rich in antioxidants called phenols, which help protect artery walls from cholesterol buildup.

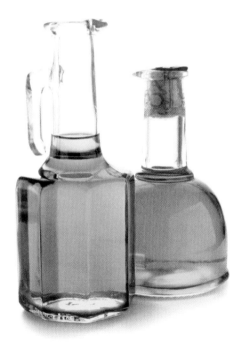

Olives: Magic Fruits

Olive oil, of course, comes from olives, the mother lode of good-for-you fats. So consider olives a Magic food, too. For true olive taste, buy fresh ones from the deli section, not canned. (Once you get used to them, you'll never go back to canned.) If you use quality, flavorful olives, a little will go a long way.

Like olive oil, olives pack a lot of calories (about 6 per medium black olive), so try to use them in place of other fats in your diet, not in addition to them.

Health Bonus

Olive oil contains an anti-inflammatory component so strong that researchers liken it to aspirin. This may be another reason that people who follow the Mediterranean diet have such low rates of heart disease, which is linked to inflammation. So, by the way, is type 2 diabetes, not to mention other chronic diseases like Alzheimer's.

In contrast, a diet heavy in corn, safflower, and sunflower oils can actually promote inflammation in the body, which can damage arteries and lead to heart disease and other health problems. We recommend against using any of these types as your main cooking oil.

Olive oil also contains natural compounds called lignans, which may reduce the risk of cancers of the colon, breast, prostate, pancreas, and endometrium.

Cooks Tips

Olive oil isn't like wine; it doesn't improve with age. In fact, it can become rancid. Store it in a tightly sealed dark container in a cool place. If your oil turns cloudy, it's time to throw it away and buy a new bottle.

Menu Magic

Great cooks use olive oil in just about everything. Use it whenever you can in place of other vegetable oils, margarine, or butter. Here are a few suggestions.

- Serve a dish of good olive oil with cracked black pepper for dipping fresh bread (whole grain, of course!).

- Instead of using butter on bread or mashed potatoes, try olive oil mixed with roasted garlic (see the garlic entry for tips on roasting).

- Use it as a base for marinades for beef, chicken, fish, or pork.

- Add it to pasta, chopped tomatoes, crumbled feta cheese, chopped fresh basil, and capers for a fast and oh-so-simple supper.

PERFECT portions: 1 tablespoon

Use olive oil whenever you can in place of other oils, but pour lightly. At 120 per tablespoon, those healthy calories could easily turn into unhealthy pounds.

- Use it to replace the smoked meats and sausage typically used to flavor bean and pea soups.

- In recipes that call for butter or margarine, use 3/4 teaspoon olive oil in place of 1 teaspoon butter or margarine.

- Dice olives into sauces, especially tomato-based types.

- Top your pizza with olives along with other vegetables of your choice.

- Add olives to green salads, pasta salads, and tuna sandwiches.

RELATED recipes

Barley Salad with Snow Peas and Lemon Dressing *211*
Black Bean and Barley Salad *213*
Caponata *202*
Garden Pasta Salad *215*
Greek Lentil Salad *217*
Grilled Chicken Salad with Oranges *210*
Marinated Olives *202*
Mediterranean Salad with Edamame *215*
Mediterranean Split Pea Spread *205*
Seared Fish Steaks with Tomato-Olive Sauce *246*
Spinach, Grapefruit and Avocado Salad with Poppy Seed Dressing *216*
Tuna and Cannellini Salad with Lemon *213*
Warm Salmon Salad with Olive Toasts *249*
Wheatberry Salad with Dried Apricots and Mint *266*
Whole Wheat Pizza with Broccoli and Olives *259*

onions

GL VERY LOW

Don't cry for onions—embrace them! They may be synonymous with tears and onion breath, but they're essential to cooks everywhere for their unique flavor. They're also good for you. It's true that these underground globes don't offer a whole lot of nutrients, but what they have in bulk are powerful sulfur-containing compounds, which are responsible for their pungent odor—and many of their health benefits.

According to several studies, onions may help bring down high blood sugar in diabetic animals. In one Egyptian study of diabetic rats, onion juice reduced blood sugar levels by an amazing 70 percent. One of few published studies in humans, from India, dates back some 30 years, but it found that people with diabetes who ate 2 ounces (60 g) of onions a day experienced a significant drop in blood sugar levels.

Researchers credit these effects to the sulfur compounds in onions as well as their flavonoids. These powerful antioxidant compounds also help fight some of the side effects of high blood sugar, not to mention heart disease.

Onions even seem to boost HDL, the "good" cholesterol. One study found that people who ate the most onions, along with other foods rich in flavonoids, had a 20 percent lower risk of heart disease. Thanks to their sulfur compounds, onions, like aspirin, also help prevent dangerous blood clots. And they're known to help lower high blood pressure.

Finally, onions are one of the richest food sources of chromium, a trace mineral that improves the body's ability to respond to insulin.

Health Bonus

Onions' sulfur compounds and flavonoids may help fend off several forms of cancer. One Chinese study found that men who ate at least 1 tablespoon of chopped onions and other related vegetables (garlic, scallions, chives, and leeks) a day had about half the risk of developing prostate cancer compared to men who ate less than 1/4 tablespoon of these veggies daily. There's also a link between a high intake of flavonoids and reduced risk of lung cancer.

Evidence suggests that onions may help preserve bone and prevent osteoporosis. And because the sulfur compounds are strongly anti-inflammatory, onions may also help relieve the pain and swelling of arthritis.

The green tops of scallions, or spring onions, are rich in vitamin C and beta-carotene.

Cooks Tips

The more tears they cause, the more health benefits onions have. To stem the flood while you're chopping, try chilling onions for about a half hour before cutting, and slice them from the top, leaving the root end intact; it has the strongest concentration of eye-burning compounds.

Be sure to wash onions well before chopping, especially if you're going to eat them raw. Onions grow underground and can harbor nasty bacteria. Store onions in a cool, dry place, not in the fridge, and not near potatoes. Potatoes give off moisture and a gas that causes onions to spoil faster.

Antioxidant-Rich Onions

To reap the most benefit from onions, choose varieties with the most antioxidants. Here they're ranked from highest to lowest (we've included shallots, which are related to onions). If you don't recognize some of the names, don't worry. Just know that sweeter or milder-tasting onions have fewer antioxidants than their more pungent counterparts.

❶ Shallots
❷ Western yellow
❸ Northern red
❹ Empire sweet
❺ Western white
❻ Imperial Valley sweet
❼ Vidalia

Menu Magic

Like garlic, onions can be added to just about anything. Here are just a few suggestions.

☺ Add onions to almost any stew or stir-fry.

☺ To get a bit of raw onion into your diet, combine chopped onions, tomatoes, avocado, and jalapeño peppers for a blood sugar–friendly chip dip. Finish with a splash of lime juice.

☺ Sauté chopped onions in olive oil and add to corn, potatoes, or peas.

☺ Add chopped scallions to rice dishes.

☺ Add sliced onions to green salads.

☺ Use chopped onions to add crunch to any sandwich salad, such as chicken, tuna, or egg salad.

☺ Make fruit chutney with peaches, mangos, pears, apples, or apricots and plenty of chopped onion. Serve with meals as a condiment that won't upset your blood sugar balance.

☺ Roast some onions to serve as a savory side dish. Cut the root and top from a large onion. Place root side down on a foil-covered baking sheet and bake for about an hour at 400°F (200°C). When it's done, remove it from the oven and make a deep criss-cross cut in the top. Season with flavored vinegar, herbs, sea salt, coarse-ground pepper, and olive oil.

☺ Enjoy French onion soup, but go easy on the bread and cheese topping. Try adding a few whole grain croutons instead.

☺ Use caramelized onions to add wonderful flavor to any vegetable and pasta dish. To caramelize an onion, thinly slice onion, then heat 1 tablespoon olive oil in a heavy skillet over medium heat. Add onion and cook, covered, 10 minutes, stirring often. Remove cover and cook for 10 more minutes, stirring occasionally.

PERFECT portions: 1/4 cup

Onions have very few calories, so add them cooked or raw to as many dishes as you can think of. Minced raw onions offer the greatest health benefits.

RELATED recipes

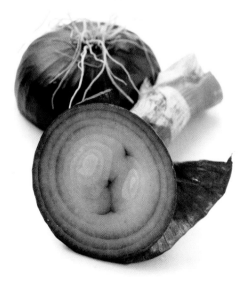

pasta

GL MEDIUM

You might think there's nothing worse for your blood sugar than a bowl of pasta. Surprisingly, you'd be wrong. As it turns out, pasta has only a moderate effect on blood sugar levels. (The Italian bread you may eat with your pasta, however, is a different story.)

Yes, pasta is high in carbs. But the type of wheat it's made from (durum wheat) appears to be digested more slowly than similar white flours used to make bread. You can also thank the special protein structure of the dough for pasta's moderate GL. It's a protein "latticework" that traps the starch molecules so it takes more time for your stomach's digestive enzymes to get to them and turn them into blood sugar. (Want to know more? You'll need a degree in food chemistry.) The more thoroughly you cook pasta, though, the easier it is for your body to break it down, so if you like your pasta al dente, or slightly firm the way Europeans eat it, all the better.

Choose whole wheat pasta instead of regular old white pasta, and you'll have a serving or two of whole grain—and about three times as much fiber per serving. Remember, you're aiming to make three of your daily carbohydrate servings whole grains, which will lower your risk of diabetes.

Pasta is pretty much as good—or as bad—for you as what you eat with it. Pile on vegetables like tomatoes and spinach or steamed broccoli, add a little olive oil and garlic, and you've got a terrific low-GL meal. Drown your pasta in cream sauce, and you might as well eat cheesecake.

If you're watching your cholesterol, you might go a little easy with egg noodles. It's no secret that they're made with eggs, and since eggs contain cholesterol, so do the noodles. (As we pointed out in the egg entry on page 106, though, dietary cholesterol isn't the main contributor to high cholesterol levels.) Another option? Eggless "egg" noodles.

Health Bonus

All white pasta is enriched with iron and B vitamins (pasta that's 100 percent whole grain is not). Pasta also contains some protein, although it's not a "complete" protein source, meaning that it's missing some of the amino acids that make up a complete protein. You can easily remedy this by sprinkling a little grated cheese on your pasta.

pasta is actually smart for your blood sugar if you choose the whole grain kind and keep your portions moderate.

Cooks Tips

Yes, pasta *can* last longer than some marriages, up to three years. Store it in a closed pasta canister so you can easily toss it into boiling water on short notice.

After you've cooked your pasta (taste it; it should be firm when you bite it), drain it immediately or it will keep cooking.

Menu Magic

Pasta has to be one of the most versatile foods ever invented. All you need to do is pick your pasta; for toppings, the sky's the limit. Think herbs, sautéed vegetables, beans, chicken, perhaps a bit of olive oil, and a sprinkling of Parmesan cheese. If you include garlic and onions, you could get as many as six Magic foods on one plate!

- Grab a bag of frozen vegetables, cook them, and toss them with hot pasta, some olive oil, sautéed garlic, and a bit of cheese for a healthy dinner in no time flat.

- Cook any vegetable you like and puree it in the blender. Serve on hot pasta and top with herbs and spices of your choice.

- Top pasta with meatballs made with ground turkey breast or extra-lean ground beef and some no-sugar-added tomato sauce. Serve with a nice big green salad.

- Add pine nuts or chopped walnuts to your pasta dish. Remember, nuts and seeds are Magic, too.

- Add beans, chickpeas, or lentils to a modest portion of pasta to fill up your plate and lower the GL of the meal. You'll also get more protein.

Smart Substitution

Instead of mashed potatoes: Make pasta with olive oil and zucchini as a side dish with dinner.

PERFECT portions: 1/2 to 1 cup

Serve 1 cup of pasta as a main dish or 1/2 cup as a side dish to keep the GL within the medium range.

RELATED recipes

Asian Noodle Hot Pot *225*

Garden Pasta Salad *215*

Greek Pasta and Beef Casserole *230*

Macaroni and Cheese with Spinach *255*

Penne with Asparagus, Ricotta and Lemon *252*

Penne with Tomato and Eggplant Sauce *256*

Quick Spinach and Sausage Lasagna *253*

Shrimp and Orzo Casserole *251*

Turkey-Noodle Casserole with Spinach *239*

Whole Wheat Noodles with Peanut Sauce and Chicken *214*

Whole Wheat Pasta with Sausage, Beans and Greens *254*

Powered-Up Pasta

For pasta that's even friendlier to your blood sugar, go with one of the many new high-fiber, high-protein options that have popped up on supermarket shelves. Some are multigrain pastas, made from grains such as oats, spelt, and barley in addition to durum wheat. Since these are higher in soluble fiber, they have less impact on your blood sugar than regular or even whole wheat pasta. Some contain flaxseed as a source of heart-healthy omega-3 fatty acids. Some have added protein—40 or 50 percent more than regular pasta—from sources like soy flour, milk solids, or egg whites. This also makes them more blood sugar friendly. One brand with many of these bells and whistles is Barilla Plus.

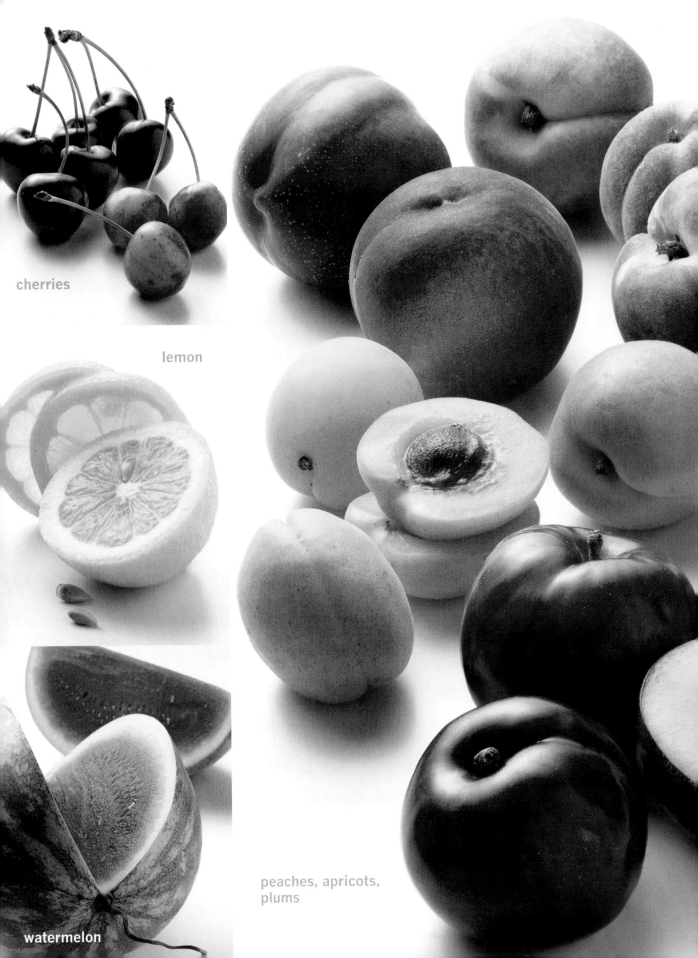

cherries

lemon

watermelon

peaches, apricots,
plums

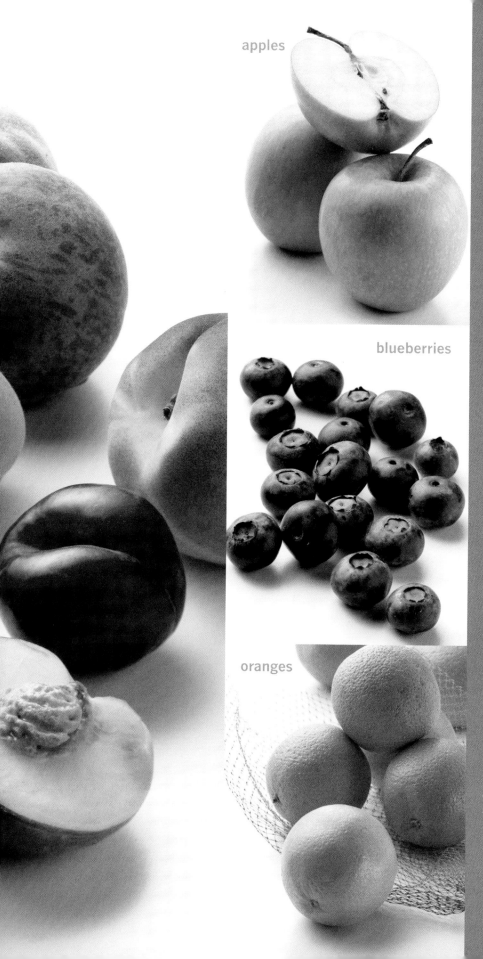

apples

blueberries

oranges

Despite their sweetness, most fruits have a low glycemic load and fit in perfectly with a Magic diet. Lemons even directly lower blood sugar.

* apples

* berries

* cherries

* citrus fruits

* lemons

* melons

* peaches, apricots, plums

magic fruits

peaches, apricots, plums

GL
VERY LOW

Apricots, peaches, and plums … oh my! Like apples, citrus fruits, and berries, these stone fruits (so named because of the stone-like seed inside) make perfect low-calorie snacks or sweet additions to entrées and desserts. Chalk up their low GLs to their high water content and their stash of blood sugar–taming, cholesterol-busting soluble fiber.

Peaches boast the most fiber of the three. Apricots, which are close cousins to peaches, are richest in beta-carotene, linked with protection from heart disease and cancer. Plums are chock-full of several disease-fighting antioxidants, and dried plums outrank more than 20 other popular fruits and vegetables in antioxidant power, which is important for staving off heart disease and preventing damage caused by high blood sugar.

Fruit you bite into wins hands-down over fruit you spoon from a can. A peach contains only 35 calories, whereas a cup of peaches canned in heavy syrup has 190. If you buy canned, go for peaches packed in their own juice (110 calories per cup).

You may as well cross peach and apricot nectars or fruit juice blends off your grocery list. They usually contain a lot of added sugar or high-fructose corn syrup and little or no fiber—a devastating combo

stone fruits make delectable snacks that just happen to benefit your blood sugar thanks to their stash of soluble fiber.

What's in a Name?

You may have seen fruits called pluots in the store. What the heck are they? A pluot looks much like a plum, but it's a cross between a plum and a plumcot. And what's a *plumcot*? A cross between an apricot and a plum. What about the plum sauce in some Chinese foods? It's not really made from plums at all. It's made from Umeboshi plums—a type of Japanese apricot!

Finally, you may have noticed that you don't see or hear the word *prune* as much these days. That's because of a major multimillion-dollar marketing effort to rename prunes *dried plums* in an effort to boost sales.

that could send your blood sugar through the roof. If you like nectars, dilute them with an equal amount of seltzer for a fizzy and still-sweet beverage. (Our Peachy Iced Tea on page 209 calls for 2 cups of peach nectar but serves eight people and has only 52 calories per cup. It's our way of weaning you off sugary fruit drinks.)

Health Bonus

Stone fruits contain compounds that may help keep those baby blues (or browns or greens) crystal clear and free of cataracts. And study after study has pronounced that people who eat more fruits and vegetables are healthier all around, with less diabetes, heart disease, cancer, and obesity. Stone fruits also offer potassium, a mineral that helps defend against high blood pressure and stroke. And we would be remiss not to mention the unique intestinal benefits of dried plums (or prune juice)—consume them, and you will go, end of story.

Cooks Tips

Apricots are delicious raw, but when they're cooked, their beta-carotene and soluble fiber are made more available to the body. For a savory accompaniment to grilled meat or poultry, pit and quarter fresh apricots and gently sauté them in olive oil with a touch of minced garlic.

Menu Magic

- Top off whole grain pancakes and waffles with peach slices.

- Give chicken dishes or stews a taste of the Middle East by adding diced dried apricots or plums.

- Poach plums in red wine and sprinkle with grated lemon zest for a healthy dessert.

- Sprinkle cinnamon and nutmeg on sliced peaches and use them to top low-fat ice cream or yogurt.

- Sauté sliced, peeled peaches in a small amount of good-for-you margarine like Smart Balance (and some ginger, if you like) and serve alone or as a dessert topper.

- Blend up a peach smoothie with low-fat vanilla yogurt, diced peaches, frozen strawberries, and vanilla.

PERFECT portions: 1 peach or plum

Because apricots are smaller, consider two of them a serving.

- Add diced peaches to chicken salad for a sweet twist.

- Add chopped dried plums to poultry stuffing.

- Top off oatmeal with sliced peaches, dried plums, or diced apricots.

- Add chopped dried apricots to cold cereal.

- Dip dried apricots in dark chocolate for a decadent but still relatively healthy treat (but remember to keep portions small!).

- Add chopped apricots to wild rice before cooking.

- Create your own trail mix with nuts, pieces of bran cereal, and chopped dried apricots.

- Make plum sauce by blending juice-packed plums with cinnamon and spices. Pour over grilled chicken breast or pork tenderloin.

Smart Substitution

Instead of cream cheese and jelly: Spread bread with Neufchâtel (reduced-fat cream cheese) and top with thin slices of ripe plums.

RELATED recipes

Chicken Breasts with Peaches and Ginger *234*
Mixed Berry and Stone Fruit Soup *276*
Orange-Glazed Roasted Plums *282*
Peachy Iced Tea *209*
Plum-Walnut Crumble *287*
Spice-Crusted Pork Tenderloin with Peach Salsa *233*
Upside-Down Nectarine Muffins *199*

peanut butter

GL VERY LOW

Think peanut butter is just for kids? Well, perhaps the classic PB&J (peanut butter and jelly on sticky white bread that melts in your mouth) is best left as part of childhood, but don't throw out the baby with the bathwater. Peanut butter is actually a smart addition to a Magic diet, and it makes perfect sense since peanuts are a Magic food, too.

Peanut butter packs a one-two punch against blood sugar spikes: protein and "good" (unsaturated) fat. In fact, the famed Nurses' Health Study found that women who ate peanut butter at least five times a week were as much as 30 percent less likely to develop diabetes.

On a related note, you may have heard of the peanut butter diet. Crazy? Maybe not. It seems that peanut butter sticks to your ribs as well as the roof of your mouth, thanks to its winning combo of good fat, protein, and fiber. A study at Purdue University found that eating it can dampen appetite for up to 2 hours longer than a low-fiber, high-carb snack. (Try our Oatmeal–Peanut Butter Trail Bars as the perfect between-meal stomach satisfier.)

The Good News Spreads

Peanut butter doesn't stand alone when it comes to health benefits. Other nut butters, such as almond, walnut, and pistachio butters, are healthy choices, too. (Cashew and macadamia nut butters are higher in saturated fat.) Seed butters, including sunflower seed and pumpkin seed butter, fit the better-blood-sugar bill as well. Check out health food supermarkets and online stores for some of the more unusual varieties.

Like nuts, peanut butter is also a potent protector of the heart. Its good fat helps to tame high cholesterol—after all, it's the same type of fat found in olive oil. One study found that diets that got most of their monounsaturated fat from peanut butter provided almost the same reduction in heart disease risk as diets that got most of their monounsaturated fats from olive oil.

Like the peanuts it comes from, peanut butter is rich in plant compounds called sterols, one of the top proven cholesterol busters. (In fact, sterols are added to some cholesterol-lowering margarines.) Plus, it has a gram of fiber per tablespoon. You really couldn't pack many more benefits into something you can spoon out of a jar.

Watch what brand you buy, though. Many are sweetened with corn syrup or sugar—1/2 teaspoon per 2 tablespoons of peanut butter. We don't quite understand why, since ground peanuts taste great on their own. Natural and organic brands generally have no added sugar and less sodium than regular brands.

Health Bonus

The stash of sterols in peanut butter not only helps control cholesterol, it may also help fend off colon, prostate, and breast cancers. Peanut butter is also a rich source of the heart-healthy antioxidant compound resveratrol, the one for which red wine is most famous. Natural brands of the spread contain even more resveratrol than other types of peanut butter.

Eating peanut butter (or nuts) several times a week is a proven way to keep high blood pressure under control. And peanut butter ranks right up there with most nuts for its stash of vitamin E, important for a healthy immune system.

Peanut butter as a bone builder? Yep. It's one of the top sources of the bone-building mineral boron. Finally, eat peanut butter and/or nuts at least five times a week, and you could lower your risk of developing gallstones, according to one study.

Cooks Tips

Some natural peanut butters need to be refrigerated after you open them (check the label). If the oil separates, let the jar come to room temperature, then stir it up. Most national brands, however, can be sealed tightly and stored in the pantry.

Menu Magic

- ☼ Spread peanut butter on whole grain waffles or pancakes for breakfast.

- ☼ Make a peanut butter and banana sandwich on whole grain bread for a pack-and-go lunch. Or smear half a banana with some peanut butter as a snack.

- ☼ For a nibble that won't make your blood sugar go haywire, spread peanut butter on whole grain crackers or triangles of toasted whole wheat pita bread.

- ☼ For an even lower-GL snack that will stave off hunger longer, spread peanut butter on apple slices, celery sticks, or carrots.

- ☼ Be adventurous and try different types of nut butters with different types of fruit and vegetables. Almond butter on sliced pears (Anjou, Bartlett, or Asian) is a delicious combination.

PERFECT portions: 1 tablespoon

Peanut butter won't raise your blood sugar, but it does contain almost 100 calories per tablespoon. When you're spreading bread, a cracker, or a bagel, be sure you practice portion control and stick with that amount.

Smart Substitution

Instead of jam: Spread peanut butter on your whole grain toast or bagel. You'll get more calories but also more hunger-satisfying protein and less sugar.

RELATED recipes

Asian Peanut Dip *204*

Oatmeal–Peanut Butter Trail Bars *207*

Peanut Chicken Soup *224*

Whole Wheat Noodles with Peanut Sauce and Chicken *214*

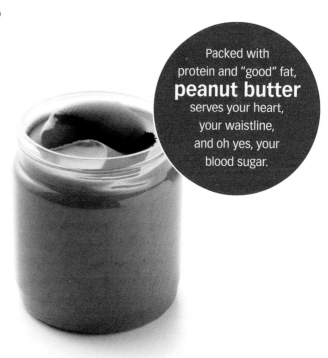

Packed with protein and "good" fat, **peanut butter** serves your heart, your waistline, and oh yes, your blood sugar.

peas

GL VERY LOW

Want a high-protein food that's low in calories? Eat peas! That's right, peas.

Since they're on the starchy side as far as vegetables go, peas seem like a bad idea for blood sugar. But if you passed up peas, it would be a mistake.

You may not realize it, but peas are a super source of protein, one reason they leave blood sugar unscathed. A half cup contains an impressive 4 grams of protein and only 60 calories. Peas also have a low GL thanks in part to their stash of soluble fiber, the kind that lowers blood sugar. At almost 4.5 grams of total fiber per 1/2 cup (about a third of which is soluble), a small side of peas will help get you to the recommended 25 grams of fiber per day.

For heart protection, you can't beat these green legumes. The type of soluble fiber they contain, pectin, is top-notch for lowering cholesterol. Peas also pack potassium, which helps lower high blood pressure, and they fork over quite a bit of the B vitamin folate, which experts think may play a role in keeping arteries clear—extra-important for people with diabetes.

Health Bonus

Green peas are an outstanding source of lutein and zeaxanthin; they contain even more than some supplements. These members of the carotene family lower the risk of cataracts and macular degeneration, the leading cause of blindness in older adults.

Cooks Tips

Frozen peas are handy, but avoid canned peas, which usually contain added sodium and have much less flavor. Steer clear of frozen peas swimming in cheese or cream sauce. They'll overload you with calories before you can say, "Pass the peas, please."

Cook peas in as little water as possible, just until tender, to retain their nutrients. Use a steamer for the best results.

PERFECT portions: 1/2 cup

Peas are firmly in the very low GL category, so don't be too concerned about eating a little more than half a cup.

Menu Magic

- Serve up a classic peas-and-carrots side dish.

- Add peas to any soup with noodles or other grain products in it. Peas are a complete protein when combined with grains.

- Top off salads with peas.

- Make peas part of just about any stew or casserole.

- Mix up a cold green pea salad for your next picnic. Recipes abound. One version uses frozen early peas, chopped pimientos, chopped scallions, a small amount of low-fat sour cream, chopped apple, lemon juice, salt, and pepper. Another combines peas with toasted almonds, scallions, feta cheese, low-fat mayonnaise, and balsamic vinegar.

- Toss peas in with pasta or noodles.

- Snack on snow peas or sugar snaps. The pods give you even more fiber, although the peas contain less protein than more mature, out-of-the-pod types.

RELATED recipes

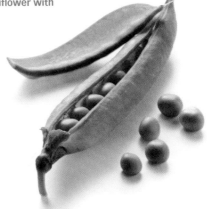

pork

GL VERY LOW

You can't eat like a pig and stay healthy, but you can *eat pig,* a.k.a. pork. Like other protein foods, pork won't bump up your blood sugar a bit. And the leanest cuts, such as tenderloin, are almost as low in fat as chicken! That's why advertisers dubbed pork "the other white meat," even though it is in fact red meat.

Over the past 20 years, changes in feeding and breeding practices have produced much leaner cuts of pork, making them appropriate in a Magic diet. Less fat means fewer calories, which means less excess weight and better blood sugar control.

Health Bonus

Like all other animal foods, including beef and eggs, pork is a good source of vitamins B_6 and B_{12}, which help keep homocysteine in check. High levels of this amino acid raise the risk of heart disease and dementia. Pork is also a standout for riboflavin (vitamin B_2), important for metabolizing carbohydrates and for producing red blood cells.

Cooks Tips

To keep pork as lean as possible, trim off any excess fat before you cook. One of the biggest mistakes made with pork is overcooking it. That's a recipe for a tough, dried-out dish. To keep lean cuts moist during roasting and to bring the GL of the meal even lower, try using a marinade that contains vinegar, wine, or citrus juice. The acid from the marinade will soften the meat, making it juicier and tastier.

Years ago, people worried about getting trichinosis, caused by intestinal parasites, from pork. Today, because of changes in the way animals are fed and raised, it's much less of a concern. And as was the case all along, cooking pork properly—to an internal temperature of 160°F (71°C)—will kill any trichina parasites that may be present.

PERFECT portions: 3 ounces (85 g)

If this is your only meat of the day, up to 6 ounces (170 g) is appropriate. Be sure to choose a lean cut.

Menu Magic

Think of using pork just as you would beef or chicken, and the possibilities are endless.

☺ Use pork strips or cubes in stir-fries along with plenty of vegetables (try a frozen stir-fry mix).

☺ Try pork tenderloin on the grill.

☺ Create hearty pork and wild rice soup with cubed pork loin, white beans, chickpeas, cooked wild rice, chopped onion, chicken broth, olive oil, cumin, chopped parsley, and coriander.

☺ Make pork and black bean chili with cubed pork, black beans, chopped red bell peppers, diced tomatoes, chunky salsa, minced garlic, chopped onion, and chili powder. Cook in a slow cooker for 7 hours.

☺ Throw a lean pork chop on the grill along with sliced summer squash and halved tomatoes.

☺ Use extra-lean ground pork, labeled 97% lean, in place of regular or even extra-lean ground beef for meat loaf, meatballs, or burgers. You may have to go to a health food supermarket to get such lean pork, or order it online, but it's worth the effort since it's significantly lower in fat than pork labeled "lean" (and often lower than ground pork whose label says "extra lean" but doesn't include a number).

☺ Use pork in kebabs, along with cherry tomatoes and pieces of onion and yellow bell pepper.

RELATED recipes

Pork Chop and Cabbage Skillet Dinner *232*
Spice-Crusted Pork Tenderloin with Peach Salsa *233*

pumpernickel bread

GL
LOW

Pumpernickel bread combines the benefits of two other Magic foods: rye bread and sourdough bread. That's because traditional pumpernickel is made with coarsely ground rye flour (and perhaps some wheat flour) and is fermented with sourdough starter. The acetic acid from the starter (see the sourdough entry on page 147) and the soluble fiber in rye (see the rye entry on page 141) keep the GL of the bread low—much lower than that of white or even whole wheat bread.

One Canadian study found that pumpernickel bread had four to eight times as much resistant starch as breads made with wheat or barley. Resistant starch benefits blood sugar because it doesn't digest easily. Like dietary fiber, it travels right past the stomach and small intestine and settles in the colon, where it's broken down by bacteria and eventually expelled.

Not all store-bought pumpernickels have the same benefits as traditional German pumpernickel, though. Many get their dark color from molasses, not from whole rye kernels and a special baking process that takes many hours. These types usually contain more wheat flour than rye, and some are made using yeast instead of sourdough starter. Your best bet is to shop at a place that sells "artisan" breads. Such bakeries tend to use more traditional pumpernickel recipes. If the bread feels heavy for its size, it's probably the real thing. Commercial brands, if you can find them, include Mestemacher (imported from Germany) and Rubschlager, which makes cocktail rye breads.

Health Bonus

As with rye bread, pumpernickel loads you up with lignans, the naturally occurring plant compounds that may help reduce the risk of breast and prostate cancers.

Cooks Tips

If you buy traditional pumpernickel bread from the bakery or make it yourself, it's preservative free, so

PERFECT portions: 1 ounce (30 g)

A serving is about the size of a small slice. Obviously, you'll need two servings to make a sandwich.

you'll need to store it in a plastic bag and use it within a few days.

Menu Magic

- For appetizers, top small squares of pumpernickel bread with cream cheese, sliced onion, and tomato.

- Serve strong-flavored sandwich fillings, such as aged cheese, on pumpernickel.

- Mustard goes well with pumpernickel, so spread this Magic food (actually, the vinegar in mustard is the Magic ingredient) on your next ham and Swiss sandwich on pumpernickel.

- Serve a slice of pumpernickel as a hearty, satisfying accompaniment to soup or chili instead of crackers.

RELATED recipes

Salmon Sandwiches with Wasabi Mayonnaise *220*
Smoked Salmon Canapés *203*

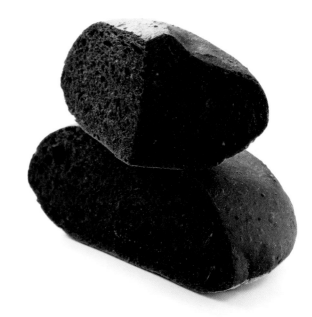

rye bread

GL
LOW

Why rye? Because research shows that unlike white bread, which is one of the worst foods for your blood sugar, whole grain rye bread (or whole grain rye crackers or cereal) can help smooth out blood sugar swings and actually reduce the risk of developing type 2 diabetes. Rye bread is even superior to whole wheat bread when it comes to blood sugar control.

In one study, on days when women ate whole-rye bread, their blood sugar levels were 10 percent lower than on days when they didn't eat it. Another study found that eating rye bread reduced the release of insulin compared to eating refined wheat bread, meaning that less insulin was needed to keep blood sugar in check. That's a good thing, because when the body regularly churns out a lot of insulin, the risk of insulin resistance goes up (and so does the risk of diabetes).

A third study found that men who ate whole grain rye bread, crackers, and cereal (they got 18 grams of fiber a day from rye) for four weeks saw a drop in blood sugar of up to 19 percent compared to their levels at the start of the study.

What's so special about rye? The structure and size of the starch particles in the bread certainly play a role. Another explanation: Rye contains about three times as much soluble fiber as wheat—also a plus for lowering high cholesterol.

There's one major caveat. By "rye" bread, we mean bread made from whole rye flour. Most of the rye breads you find in stores is made with a combination of refined rye and wheat flour, so they don't have the same fiber content or health benefits. Get out the magnifying glass if you have to and look for "whole grain rye flour" at the top of the ingredients list. Real rye bread is heavy and dense and bears little resemblance to white sandwich bread.

PERFECT portions: 1 ounce (30 g)

A serving is one slice. Obviously, you'll need two servings to make a sandwich.

Health Bonus

Rye is loaded with lignans, plant compounds that may help reduce the risk of breast and prostate cancers. And researchers have found that some of the unique plant compounds in whole grain rye are helpful for intestinal health. One study from Finland (the Finns love their rye) found that people who ate 4 1/2 slices of whole grain rye bread a day had 26 percent lower levels of compounds linked to colon cancer.

Cooks Tips

If you feel a baking spree coming on, and you want to make your own whole grain rye bread, check out your local health food store or shop online for mail-order whole grain rye flour.

Menu Magic

- Serve your favorite sandwich fixins' on whole grain rye bread.

- When you reach for cheese and crackers, make the crackers whole grain rye. Classic brands are Ryvita and Wasa.

- Try whole grain rye rolls at dinner instead of white rolls, if you can find (or make) them.

- For something different at breakfast, try a multi-whole grain hot cereal that contains rye. Look in a natural foods store for the widest selection.

RELATED recipes

Hearty Split Pea Soup with Rye Croutons *223*
Smoked Salmon Canapés *203*
Tuna and Carrot Sandwich on Rye *222*

seeds

GL VERY LOW

Send in the seeds! Like nuts, they are emerging as nutritional superstars. Packed with protein, "good" fat, and fiber, they're just what the doctor ordered for steadying your blood sugar, whether you add them to dishes or eat them as snacks.

Although seeds are indeed high in fat—about 12 to 14 grams per ounce (30 g)—almost all of that fat is the heart-healthy monounsaturated and polyunsaturated kinds. Another plus? Seeds also pack plenty of protein, to the tune of 4 to 9 grams per ounce (30 g). For that same ounce you'll also get 2 to 10 grams of fiber (pumpkin seeds have the most).

Break open that package of pumpkin or sunflower seeds, and sprinkle on those sesame seeds. When you do, you may also lower your cholesterol. Seeds are rich in the natural plant compounds called sterols, which are proven cholesterol busters. (Sterols derived from other sources are even added to some cholesterol-lowering margarines.)

One recent study found that when people with high levels of "bad" LDL cholesterol ate about 1.5 ounces (40 g) of sesame seeds a day for four weeks as part of an already heart-healthy diet, their LDL levels dropped by almost 10 percent more than when they followed the same diet without sesame seeds. Not surprisingly, their LDL levels went back up after they stopped eating the sesame seeds.

Researchers in another study tested 27 varieties of nuts and seeds and found that sesame seeds had the highest sterol content. Sunflower seeds also ranked high in sterols.

Health Bonus

By weight, both pumpkin and sesame seeds have more iron than liver does! And a single ounce of sesame seeds has almost as much calcium as a glass of milk. Sunflower seeds serve up selenium, a mineral that's been linked to a lower risk of both heart disease and cancer. Most seeds are also real vitamin E finds. Sunflower seeds, for example, provide most of the

---

PERFECT portions: 1 to 2 tablespoons

Seeds are high in calories, so don't go overboard. A 1/4-cup serving of sunflower seeds, for example, contains 210 calories. For snacks, stick with a handful of pumpkin seeds or a palmful of sunflower seeds. A tablespoonful will do if you're topping off a salad or sprinkling seeds on veggies.

---

day's needs for E, a nutrient that helps protect against everything from cataracts to cancer. Seeds are also good sources of immune-boosting zinc.

Pumpkin seeds are a traditional kitchen-cabinet treatment for prostate enlargement, and research suggests there may be good reason. Their zinc, vitamin E, selenium, and sterol content probably all help toward this end. The nutrients in seeds may even protect against prostate cancers.

Smart Substitution

Instead of chips: When you crave a crunchy, salty snack, reach for a handful of seeds (or nuts). Your blood sugar and your arteries will thank you.

(continued on page 144)

How to Perfectly Roast Seeds

You can make your own roasted seeds once you've eaten your fill of squash, pumpkin, or watermelon. Here's how.

Separate the seeds from the flesh and strings, wash them well, and let them dry. Then mix them in a bowl with a small amount of vegetable oil and salt. Spread them in a single layer on an ungreased baking sheet and sprinkle on some seasonings (take your pick of cumin, celery salt, cinnamon, paprika, or chili powder). Place the baking sheet in an oven preheated to 300°F (150°C) for about 45 minutes, shaking and stirring the seeds occasionally to prevent burning.

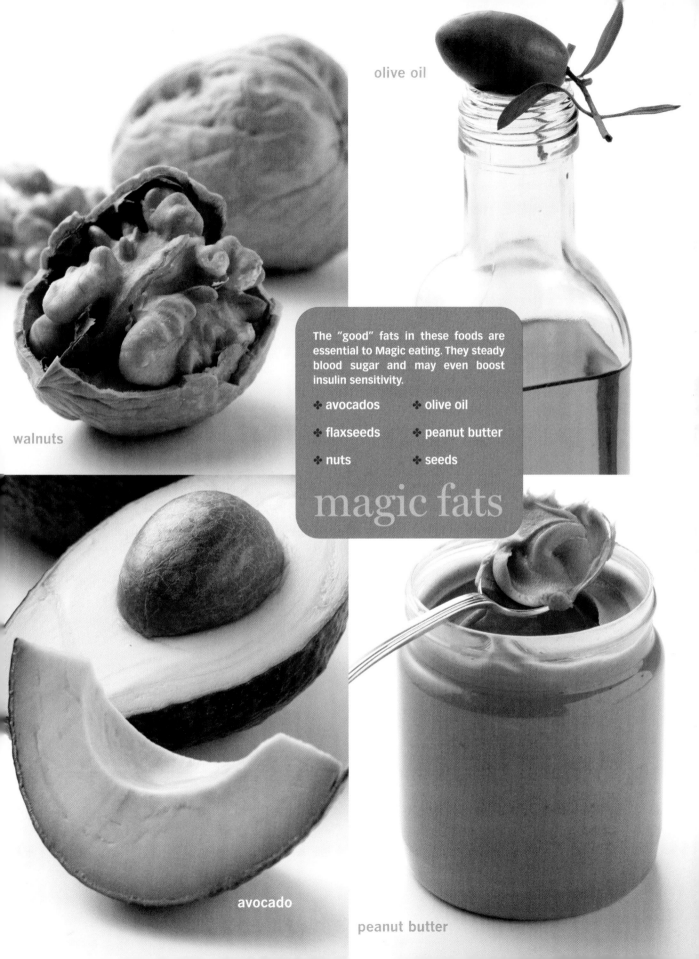

olive oil

walnuts

The "good" fats in these foods are essential to Magic eating. They steady blood sugar and may even boost insulin sensitivity.

✤ avocados ✤ olive oil

✤ flaxseeds ✤ peanut butter

✤ nuts ✤ seeds

magic fats

avocado

peanut butter

seeds continued

Cooks Tips

Seeds can go rancid if you store them too long. To keep them fresh for several months, store them in an airtight container away from heat.

A note of caution: Although peanut allergies are better known, reactions to sesame seeds are among the fastest-growing allergies. They are still relatively rare, but if you notice a rash, swelling, or trouble breathing after eating the seeds, you may be allergic.

Menu Magic

- Add seeds to steamed or sautéed vegetables.
- Sprinkle sesame seeds over brown rice.
- Coat thin fish fillets or chicken cutlets with a mixture of crushed sunflower and pumpkin seeds, then pan fry.
- Chop pumpkin or sunflower seeds and add to hot or cold cereal.
- Add toasted sesame seeds to ground meat for meatballs. They add crunch as well as boosting the nutrition quota of your meal.
- Toss some sesame seeds into bread dough or muffin or pancake batter. You can also add them to piecrusts.
- Spread tahini (ground sesame paste) on toasted whole grain bread.
- Top off your favorite salad greens with pumpkin seeds.
- Add sunflower seed kernels to tuna salad.
- Blend sunflower seeds into scrambled eggs or a vegetable omelet.
- Sprinkle your favorite seeds on top of tomato, carrot, or squash soup.
- Add sesame seeds to fruit salad for crunch.

RELATED recipes

No-Mayonnaise Creamy Coleslaw *216*

Oven-Fried Chicken *238*

Quinoa with Chiles and Cilantro *266*

Salmon Sandwiches with Wasabi Mayonnaise *220*

Sautéed Brussels Sprouts with Red Pepper and Caraway Seeds *273*

Sautéed Spinach with Ginger and Soy Sauce *275*

Spinach, Grapefruit and Avocado Salad with Poppy Seed Dressing *216*

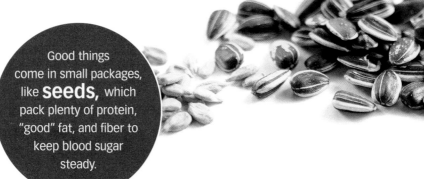

Good things come in small packages, like **seeds,** which pack plenty of protein, "good" fat, and fiber to keep blood sugar steady.

shellfish

GL
VERY LOW

When it comes to Magic eating, the underwater world is your oyster. It's not just food with fins that benefit your blood sugar; shrimp, lobster, and their crabby and clammy cohorts all count, too. They're rich in protein and low in calories, making them Magic foods indeed.

Shrimp and lobster are almost completely devoid of saturated fat, and they're good sources of omega-3 fatty acids. These are the same heart-smart fats found in fatty fish and renowned for their ability to reduce the risk of heart disease, a goal that's at the top of the list for anyone with diabetes. It's true these crustaceans are relatively high in cholesterol, but as we explained in the eggs entry (page 106), it's saturated fat, more than dietary cholesterol, that raises levels of cholesterol in the body. An average serving of shellfish has about one-third the cholesterol found in one egg, so moderate consumption generally isn't a problem. In fact, shellfish helps protect against heart disease.

Lobster, the upper crust of the crustacean world, happens to be a particularly rich source of a little-known mineral called vanadium, which some studies suggest may enhance insulin's effect in the body, helping to keep an anchor on blood sugar. (In human studies at Harvard's Joslin Diabetes Center, vanadium improved insulin sensitivity and lowered cholesterol, too. In another study, at Temple University in Philadelphia, vanadium supplements were shown to lower blood sugar.)

Despite how rich it tastes, lobster is one of the lowest-fat shellfish as long as you don't plunge it into a pool of melted butter. It's lower in fat than beef, pork, and even chicken.

Health Bonus

Most shellfish are rich in copper and zinc, both important for your immune system to function at its peak. They also pack an astounding amount of vitamin B_{12}, which may help ward off depression, heart disease, and even Alzheimer's. And they're super sources of selenium, an anti-cancer mineral.

Clams are stuffed (pun intended) with sterols, the cholesterol-lowering compounds we've mentioned elsewhere.

Cooks Tips

Clams, oysters, mussels, and scallops should be alive when you buy them. That means the shells will be tightly closed or should close when you tap them. You can store them in the fridge in a container covered loosely with a damp cloth, but don't store them in water. The shells will open during cooking (discard any that don't). Steam for 4 to 9 minutes or boil for 3 to 5 minutes after the shells open.

Eating shellfish raw (think oysters on the half shell) or less than well done is risky business. They may harbor bacteria, viruses, and parasites, all of which are killed by cooking.

Many large supermarkets now carry large bags of frozen shrimp, so stock your freezer. Thaw them according to package directions, and you have the makings of a fast, high-protein meal. Think shrimp stir-fry.

Menu Magic

Keep it simple. Too often, shellfish are topped off with butter or creamy sauce or dipped in bread crumbs and fried. A generous squeeze of lemon juice (another Magic food) will usually suffice, especially if you don't overcook the shellfish; overcooking makes them dry.

- Serve boiled shrimp with cocktail sauce as a health-smart party appetizer.

- Use shrimp in stir-fries instead of chicken or beef. Add them in the last 5 minutes to avoid overcooking.

- Add cooked shrimp, clams, or mussels to your favorite pasta sauce.

(continued)

shellfish continued

- Chop some cooked shrimp and sprinkle over a green salad to add low-fat protein. Use a lemony dressing.

- Make crab salad by mixing lump crabmeat (canned is fine) with vinaigrette dressing. Serve over greens.

- Top pizza with minced cooked clams.

- Toss some shrimp, scallops if you have them, and even fish chunks with olive oil and lemon juice, skewer them, pop them on the grill, and you're ready to eat in 5 minutes.

- Place a cooked medium shrimp, some small chunks of avocado and tomato, and a bit of salsa onto a lettuce leaf. Roll it up and eat!

- Put together shrimp tacos by combining shrimp, lettuce, tomato, a bit of shredded cheese, and green salsa in a corn taco shell.

- Order steamed clams as an appetizer.

- Instead of creamy, high-fat clam sauce like you'd get at a restaurant, make linguini with clams using canned clams (minced), garlic, olive oil, chopped hot peppers, and chopped tomatoes.

RELATED recipes
Shrimp and Orzo Casserole *251*
Shrimp and Scallop Stew *250*

Shellfish BY THE NUMBERS

Because shellfish are virtually devoid of carbohydrates, their GL is virtually zero. All shellfish are low in saturated fat, but different types offer slightly different nutritional advantages, as you'll see below.

Shellfish 3 1/2 oz (100 g)	Calories (g)	Protein (g)	Total Fat (mg)	Cholesterol	Vitamins and Minerals
Clams	74	12.77	0.97	34	Excellent source of iron and potassium.
Crab, Alaska King	84	18.29	.60	42	Good source of zinc.
Crab, Blue	87	18.06	1.08	78	Good source of zinc and calcium.
Crab, Dungeness	86	17.41	.97	59	Good source of zinc and potassium.
Lobster	112	20.6	1.51	70	Excellent source of vitamin B_{12} Good source of zinc.
Mussels (steamed)	86	11.9	2.24	28	Good source of iron.
Oysters Pacific Eastern farmed Eastern wild	81 59 68	9.45 5.22 7.05	2.30 1.55 2.46	50 25 53	Excellent source of zinc. Good source of iron and selenium.
Scallops	88	16.79	.76	33	Good source of vitamin B_{12}.
Shrimp	106	20.31	1.73	152	Fair source of various vitamins and minerals and omega-3 fatty acids.

sourdough bread

GL
LOW

This is one bread that won't hit a sour note when it comes to your blood sugar. Even though it's made from white flour (typically a no-no for Magic eating), sourdough bread has a relatively mild effect on blood sugar compared to other white breads.

Sourdough is an ancient bread with thousands of years of bread-making history behind it. It has a distinctive taste, the result of lactic acid produced by bacteria used to ferment the dough. A sourdough "starter" is made from a combination of yeast and bacteria growing in a paste of flour and water. Some is used for making a loaf, and the rest is saved to grow and use for future baking.

It's the acid produced by the bacterial culture that makes a poor blood sugar choice into a better one. One small Swedish study involving 12 healthy people found that when the volunteers ate a breakfast that included bread with added lactic acid in an amount found in sourdough bread, the rise in their blood sugar was 27 percent less after 1 1/2 hours than it was when they ate the same breakfast but with a bread made with a combination of whole grain flour and processed white flour.

Health Bonus

One study using sourdough bread made with specific strains of bacteria found that it could reduce gluten intolerance in people sensitive to wheat gluten. While that doesn't mean that people diagnosed with gluten intolerance can eat sourdough bread with impunity, it does suggest that the bread is more easily digested than other breads made with wheat flour.

PERFECT portions: 1 ounce (30 g)

A serving is about the size of one small slice, depending on the brand. Eat two slices, as you would in a sandwich, and the bread becomes a medium-GL food—still reasonable.

Cooks Tips

You can either make your own sourdough bread using a sourdough starter or buy a loaf at the local bakery. Note that all rye breads made with whole grain rye are by nature sourdough. (For bread to rise, yeast reacts with the gluten in the wheat. Rye doesn't contain enough gluten to rise with yeast, so sourdough starter is used to get the same effect.)

Some breads are called sour breads because they have sour flavoring agents added. While it's possible they could have a beneficial effect on blood sugar (say, if the souring agent is vinegar), they haven't been studied as sourdough bread has.

Menu Magic

Sourdough bread has a distinctive tart taste, but you can use it whenever you might use regular bread. Try it for sandwiches and hamburgers, as a crunchy accompaniment to al dente spaghetti and sauce, or to go with soup.

RELATED recipe

Grilled Eggplant Sandwiches
   with Red Pepper–Walnut Sauce 220

soy foods

GL *VERY LOW*

Congratulations! If you've turned to this entry, it probably means you've already discovered soy foods and want to know more about their health benefits, or you have an open mind and are willing to try them. That's good for you—because so is soy.

For starters, soy has more protein, by volume, than beef and almost none of the saturated fat. Right off the bat, this earns it a secure spot on the list of Magic foods. Soybeans have an extraordinarily low GL of 1, which makes foods made from them, such as tofu, tempeh, miso, edamame, and roasted soy nuts (see "Soy Glossary" below) excellent additions to your Magic diet.

Studies suggest that soy may have special power to help lower blood sugar, beyond its low glycemic load. In a recent study on meal-replacement drinks that involved overweight people, those using soy-based drinks lost slightly more weight than those using milk-based drinks, and they also saw their blood sugar levels drop (the milk group didn't).

This result may be thanks to the type of protein in soy. When Swedish researchers fed study subjects meals containing protein from fish (cod), milk (cottage cheese), and soy, they discovered that the soy-protein meal was the friendliest to blood sugar.

Like many other foods, soybeans are best enjoyed in their most unadulterated forms. Products like soy protein bars and flavored soy milk often contain way too much added sugar or fat to be worth eating. Some flavored soy milks, for instance, are sweetened with as much as 6 teaspoons of sugar per 8 ounces (250 ml).

Health Bonus

Soy is smart for your heart. It seems its cholesterol-lowering powers aren't quite as strong as we once thought, but soy is still good for overall heart health thanks to its "good" fats, its fiber, and its cholesterol-lowering plant sterols.

Eating soy can also help reduce the risk of a serious diabetes complication: kidney disease. In a small study of people with type 2 diabetes and kidney disease, those who were given about one-third of their protein intake as soy protein saw their urinary albumin excretion (UAE) drop by 9.5 percent, a sure sign that their kidneys were functioning better. In another study, the participants' kidneys were better able to filter blood when they followed a soy-based diet for eight weeks.

SOY glossary Soy is a bean, but out of that bean comes many different products.

Edamame: Fresh green soybeans, available shelled or in the pod. You can eat them raw, but most people prefer them steamed with a bit of salt. You don't eat the pods.

Mature soybeans: You can buy these canned. Just rinse them before adding to casseroles, soups, or chili.

Soy nuts: Roasted mature soybeans, usually eaten as a snack.

Tofu: As one manufacturer put it, tofu is to the soybean as cheese is to milk. Cheese is made when milk separates into curds and whey.

Soybeans produce soy milk, which can also be separated into curds and whey; tofu is the bean curd. It comes in different textures, with silken tofu being the very softest and extra-firm the firmest.

Tempeh: Made from fermented soybeans and formed into a chewy cake, tempeh is used as a meat substitute in recipes.

Miso: Fermented soybean paste, used as a seasoning or soup base.

Soy milk: The creamy liquid that's pressed out of soaked, cooked soybeans.

Population studies suggest soy can lower the risk of several kinds of cancer, including prostate, breast, and endometrial cancers, and ease menopausal discomforts, all likely due to soy's estrogen-like compounds, called isoflavones. More research is needed before any specific recommendations on soy intake can be made.

Cooks Tips

Keep tofu and tempeh refrigerated and use them within two or three days of opening them. Opened tofu should be stored in water that is changed daily. Miso will last in the refrigerator for several months. Fresh edamame should be eaten within a day or two. Roasted soy nuts can be kept in a cool, dry place for up to six months.

Menu Magic

Soy products are a mystery to many people, but once you get to know them, you'll find they're easy to use and quite handy.

Edamame

- Steam edamame in their pods, then shell them. Add the beans to grain or vegetable salads.

- Keep a bag of frozen edamame in the freezer and steam some for a high-protein Magic snack.

Soy nuts

- Snack on these out of hand or sprinkle them into stir-fries. They have less fat and more fiber than true nuts (but they're still high in calories, so watch portion sizes).

Soy burgers

- Crumble and add to pasta sauces in place of meat.

Silken tofu

- Stir into low-fat sour cream for vegetable dip.

- Replace all or some of the cream in cream soups with silken tofu.

- Blend silken tofu with banana and peaches and a touch of honey to make a protein-rich smoothie.

PERFECT portions: 1/2 cup tofu

If you're eating fresh soybeans, a serving is 1/2 cup shelled. For dry-roasted soybeans, which are higher in calories, a serving is 1/4 cup.

Tofu

- Use diced tofu to replace some of the cheese in lasagna or macaroni and cheese.

- Marinate tofu in low-sugar barbecue sauce and cook it on the grill.

- Mash it with cottage cheese and seasonings to use as a spread on whole grain rye crackers.

- Use extra-firm tofu instead of beef in stews.

- For Asian stir-fry dishes, use extra-firm tofu with red bell pepper strips, carrot strips, and snow peas.

- Make a tofu salad with cubes of firm tofu stir-fried in canola oil. Add to Romaine lettuce, corn, sliced avocado, sliced tomatoes, and chopped cilantro. Top with roasted pumpkin seeds and squeeze lime juice on top.

- Create a tofu curry with stir-fried tofu, red bell pepper strips, chickpeas, vegetable oil, curry powder (it contains turmeric, a Magic spice), and sesame seeds. Serve over brown or converted rice.

Soy milk

- If you like soy milk, use it in place of regular milk in smoothies, on cereal, and in recipes. Buy the low-fat, unsweetened variety.

RELATED recipes

Asian Noodle Hot Pot *225*
Asian Peanut Dip *204*
Cherry-Almond Gratin *288*
Chocolate-Raspberry Cheesecake *284*
Mediterranean Salad with Edamame *215*
Pumpkin Custards *278*
Spring Vegetable Stir-Fry with Tofu *260*
Whole Wheat Noodles with Peanut Sauce and Chicken *214*

spinach AND OTHER DARK GREENS

GL VERY LOW

If everyone ate more spinach, we'd all have less diabetes, not to mention diseases like heart disease and cancer. No, spinach doesn't have any special power to lower your blood sugar, other than some soluble fiber and the fact that it's a vegetable, so that like almost all vegetables, it has little impact on your blood sugar. But the more fruits and vegetables you eat, the lower your risk of being overweight and of developing diabetes. It's that simple (remember secret number 3 of Magic eating, Eat More Fruits and Vegetables). Spinach is so all-around good for you, with so many nutrients and so few calories, it's a must for a Magic diet.

Despite what Popeye may have thought, spinach is not a very good source of iron. That's because the iron it contains isn't absorbed very well by the body. But it's loaded with other nutrients that can help stave off or treat just about every health concern, especially if you have diabetes or any of the risk factors for it.

Because spinach contains lots of potassium and magnesium, it (and other dark greens) can help keep blood pressure in check. Thanks to its store of carotenoids, it's one of the most antioxidant-rich vegetables on Earth. These antioxidants are powerful weapons against diabetes-related complications, including heart disease and nerve damage, not to mention cancer.

Speaking of antioxidants, spinach is a surprisingly good source of vitamin C. Two cups of raw leaves (enough for a nice-size salad) provides 28 percent of a day's allowance while dishing out only 14 calories. With such a small calorie count, spinach can help lower the overall calories of any dish you add it to.

Health Bonus

Popeye probably never got cancer. Several studies have found that people who eat a lot of green, leafy vegetables, including spinach, have a lower risk of developing cancer than people who eat little of the leafy stuff.

Researchers have identified at least a dozen antioxidant compounds in spinach that may have anti-cancer activity. Lutein and beta-carotene are two at the top of the list. Known as carotenoids, they've been linked time and again with a reduced risk of several kinds of cancer, including colon and prostate cancers, lower risk of heart disease, and better eye health.

Spinach for your eyes? That's right. Spinach and its kin—kale, collards, turnip greens, and Romaine lettuce—are some of the richest sources of lutein, which research shows may help protect against cataracts and age-related macular degeneration, two conditions most likely to rob you of your sight as you age.

Another fact to bone up on: A single serving of spinach offers a full day's supply of vitamin K, which

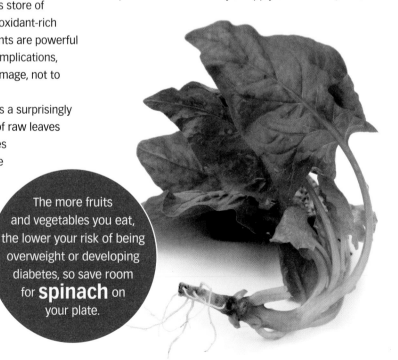

The more fruits and vegetables you eat, the lower your risk of being overweight or developing diabetes, so save room for **spinach** on your plate.

researchers now know is needed for a strong skeleton. Too many "senior moments"? Eat more spinach. Studies carried out by the USDA found that feeding middle-aged rats a spinach extract prevented some of the loss of long-term memory and learning ability that rats normally experience. Researchers chalk it up to the stash of antioxidant compounds in spinach.

Cooks Tips

Wash fresh spinach thoroughly with cold water—twice. In addition to washing off any bacteria that may be lurking in the leaves, you want to get rid of the dirt that can make spinach gritty. (It does, after all, grow on the ground, and it does best in sandy soil.) If you buy bagged greens to save time, it's still a good idea to rinse them well before eating. Remove the stems, at least the larger, thicker ones, before cooking.

Menu Magic

Look for any and every opportunity to "go green," from good old spinach salad to these ideas.

- For a super-nutritious side dish, sauté spinach (Swiss chard or kale works well, too) and sliced onions in olive oil. Sprinkle with sesame seeds, another Magic food.

- Stir steamed spinach into mashed potatoes so you get less potato and a lower GL with every bite. Top with sliced scallions.

- Top pizza with spinach.

- Steam spinach, then puree with parsley and lemon juice and use as a sauce for chicken or pasta.

- Make spinach pesto. Puree raw spinach with almonds, garlic, olive oil, and a bit of Parmesan cheese, then toss with whole grain pasta and chickpeas.

PERFECT portions: 1 cup raw

Because spinach shrinks so much, a serving of cooked spinach is 1/2 cup. These are official serving sizes, but when it comes to spinach, the more the better.

- "Beef" up lasagna with spinach instead of meat.

- Serve spinach with garlic and olive oil over pasta cooked al dente. Sprinkle with sesame seeds.

- For a quick soup, puree steamed spinach with garlic and low-fat plain yogurt.

RELATED recipes

Bean and Barley Soup 222
Cauliflower and Spinach Casserole 270
Dahl with Spinach 261
Greek Lentil Salad 217
Macaroni and Cheese with Spinach 255
Penne with Asparagus, Ricotta and Lemon 252
Quick Spinach and Sausage Lasagna 253
Salmon Sandwiches with Wasabi Mayonnaise 220
Sautéed Spinach with Ginger and Soy Sauce 275
Sole Florentine 247
Spinach and Goat Cheese Omelet 194
Spinach, Grapefruit and Avocado Salad with Poppy Seed Dressing 216
Spinach with Pine Nuts and Currants 274
Tuna and Cannellini Salad with Lemon 213
Turkey-Noodle Casserole with Spinach 239
Whole Wheat Pasta with Sausage, Beans and Greens 254

sweet potatoes

GL
MEDIUM

These sweet-tasting super-spuds hold a real surprise. Eat a baked sweet potato instead of a baked white potato, and your blood sugar will rise about 30 percent less! Compared to regular potatoes, a.k.a. blood sugar bombs, sweets rank relatively low on the GL scale. And the fact that they're packed with nutrients and disease-fighting fiber (almost 40 percent of which is soluble fiber, the kind that helps lower blood sugar and cholesterol) makes them a sweet deal indeed.

Sweet potatoes are extraordinarily rich in carotenoids, orange and yellow pigments that play a role in helping the body respond to insulin. And as unlikely as it may seem, coffee (another Magic food) and sweet potatoes have something in common: They're both rich in the natural plant compound chlorogenic acid, which may help reduce insulin resistance.

You may not think of vitamin C when you think of sweet potatoes, but they're actually an excellent source. That's important when you're battling high blood sugar, because the vitamin's antioxidant powers may help keep arteries from being damaged. Vitamin C may also help fight heart disease and complications of diabetes, such as nerve and eye damage.

Like so many other good-for-us foods, sweet potatoes are one of those staples that we like to gum up with gooey ingredients that essentially turn it into candy; think maple syrup, brown sugar, butter, and even marshmallows. If this is the only way you've ever enjoyed sweet potatoes, give some of our menu suggestions a try. Steer clear of canned sweets, which are usually packed in sugary syrup.

Health Bonus

A recent study found that among almost 2,000 men studied, those whose diets were richest in beta-carotene and vitamin C—two nutrients plentiful in

Yam I Am?

Is there a difference between sweet potatoes and yams? You bet. What you see in the super-market is most likely one of two popular varieties of sweet potato. One has orange flesh and is moist and sweet; the other is yellow fleshed, drier, and not as sweet. Unless you're shopping at a market that specializes in ethnic foods, you're unlikely to find yams, which are native to Central America. Considerably larger than sweet potatoes, they have ivory-colored flesh and aren't particularly sweet.

sweet potatoes—were more likely to survive prostate cancer than those whose diets contained little of the two nutrients.

The famous Nurses' Health Study at Harvard Medical School found that women who ate lots of foods rich in beta-carotene, such as sweet potatoes, reduced their risk of breast cancer by as much as 25 percent.

Eating sweet potatoes is a smart move for you if you have high blood pressure. That's because they're rich in potassium, a mineral known for bringing pressure down. You'll get more potassium from a sweet potato than you will from a banana!

Cooks Tips

Choose sweet potatoes that are heavy for their size, with intact peels (no decay). If you're going to cook them whole, buy potatoes that are similar in size so the cooking time will be the same. Peel or scrub thoroughly before cooking. They'll keep for a month if you keep them cool but not cold (don't put them in the fridge).

Menu Magic

Don't relegate sweet potatoes to candy-like dishes served only at Thanksgiving and Christmas. These spuds have a lot to offer all year round.

☺ Bake a sweet potato just as you would a white potato and serve alongside your favorite protein dish (beef, chicken, fish, pork, or lamb).

☺ If you're hooked on regular mashed potatoes, try using half regular potatoes and half sweets.

☺ For a Magic food trifecta, top mashed sweet potatoes with trans fat–free margarine, then season with cinnamon and sprinkle with chopped pecans.

☺ Grill sweet potato slices to serve with pork loin chops.

☺ Place sweet potato slices on top of your next casserole. Cover with foil to keep them moist and bake as usual.

☺ Add sweet potato cubes to soups and stews 30 to 45 minutes before the dish is done.

☺ Cube cooked sweet potatoes and use in stir-fries.

☺ Make roasted sweet potatoes seasoned with thyme for a savory side dish. Combine olive oil, minced garlic, thyme, salt, and coarsely ground black pepper in a bowl. Arrange peeled, sliced sweet potatoes in a single layer on a baking sheet and brush with the mixture. Bake at 425°F (220°C) until tender and slightly brown.

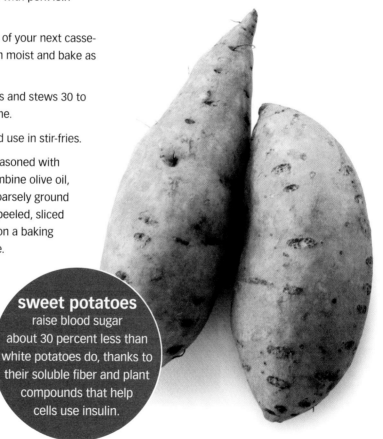

sweet potatoes raise blood sugar about 30 percent less than white potatoes do, thanks to their soluble fiber and plant compounds that help cells use insulin.

PERFECT portions: 1 medium

A medium sweet potato (5 ounces/140 g) is big enough to satisfy your appetite without tipping the blood sugar scales.

RELATED recipes

tea

GL VERY LOW

Fire up the kettle, because after reading this entry, you'll be ready for a nice hot cup of tea. Laboratory studies show that tea can boost insulin activity more than 15-fold! The research, carried out by the USDA, found that all types of tea—green, black, and oolong—have the ability to enhance insulin activity, which of course means lower blood sugar. Almost all of that power comes from the naturally occurring antioxidant compound EGCG (epigallocatechin gallate) in tea.

Skip the milk, though. Adding milk may decrease this insulin-activating power by as much as 90 percent. It's not that milk is bad for you, it's just that it binds with the EGCG, making it unavailable to the body.

Drinking tea could even benefit people already being treated for diabetes. In a Taiwanese study of 20 people with type 2 diabetes, all of whom were taking glucose-lowering medication, drinking a lot of oolong tea—about six 8-ounce (250-ml) glasses a day was linked with a 29 percent drop in blood sugar. Most of us won't want to drink that much (tea has a diuretic effect), but even a cup or two should benefit you.

Some research suggests that tea may even speed up the body's metabolism and help control weight, which by itself could help lower your risk of insulin resistance and type 2 diabetes. In a group of 10 healthy men, a green tea extract that provided the active compounds found in about 2 cups of green tea increased the number of calories burned in a 24-hour period by 4 percent as compared to when no extract was taken. Another study found that people who drank tea at

don't fall for it

Rumor has it that only green tea packs a big enough antioxidant punch to make a difference in your health. Not so. Tea is one of the most researched drinks around, and studies have found that while the exact types and amounts of antioxidant compounds vary from one tea type to the next, all types pack a healthy dose of these natural compounds.

PERFECT portions: unlimited

Tea has zero carbs and virtually no calories, so you can have several cups a day as long as you don't add sugar. If you're sensitive to caffeine, stick with one cup in the morning.

least once a week for more than 10 years had almost 20 percent lower body fat than people who seldom drank tea, even after taking into account other lifestyle factors such as diet and exercise.

Want to make tea even better for your blood sugar? Brew a cup of chai, which combines tea with spices such as cinnamon, another Magic food. Watch out for the chai lattes you get at baristas like Starbucks, though. They're usually made with premixed liquids that include milk and are generously sweetened. Ask for a chai tea bag instead, and don't add anything (or just one packet of sugar, if you must).

If you're used to sweetening your tea, try black teas—not herbal teas—that taste better plain, such as ginger-peach or mint tea. By the way, a cup of tea has about half the caffeine of a cup of coffee.

Health Bonus

Tea outranks even the best vegetables in terms of antioxidant wallop. Remember that antioxidants protect against everything from cancer to stroke to heart disease.

In a controlled study, 15 men and women who drank five 6-ounce (180-ml) cups of black tea a day for three weeks experienced an 11 percent drop in "bad" LDL cholesterol and a 6.5 percent drop in total cholesterol. Again, that's a lot of tea, but it's likely that drinking even a cup or two a day offers some benefits. In another study, more moderate tea drinkers had a 28 percent lower death rate after heart attacks than people who didn't drink tea.

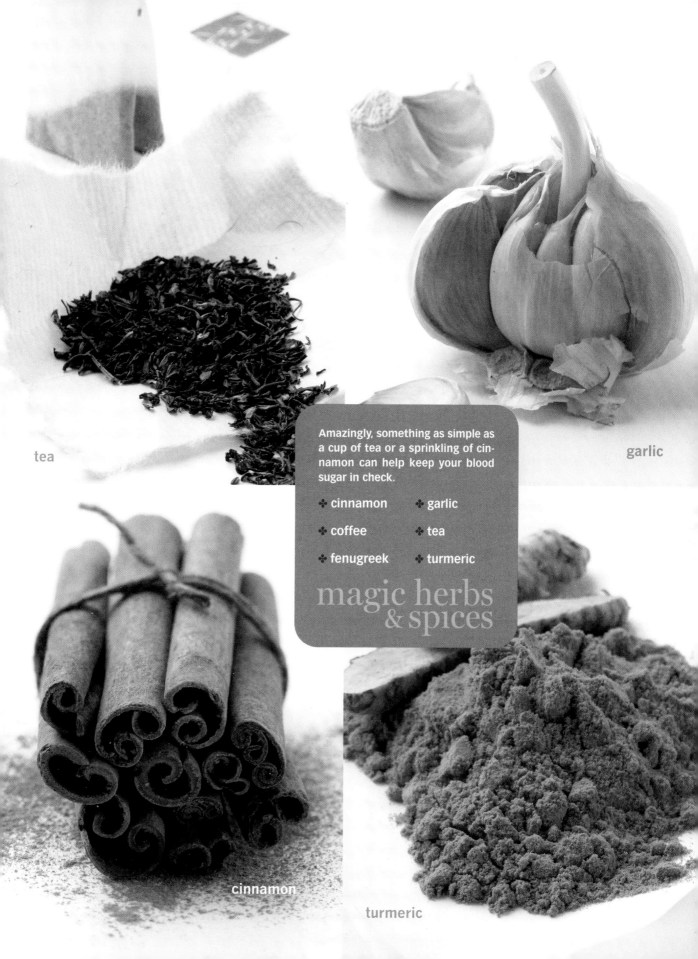

tea

garlic

Amazingly, something as simple as a cup of tea or a sprinkling of cinnamon can help keep your blood sugar in check.

✤ cinnamon   ✤ garlic

✤ coffee   ✤ tea

✤ fenugreek   ✤ turmeric

magic herbs & spices

cinnamon

turmeric

Cooks Tips

You'll need to store tea properly if you want to keep the same subtle flavors that helped you make it your choice in the first place. Always store tea, whether ground leaves or tea bags, in an airtight container away from light, moisture, and strong odors, which can be absorbed by the leaves.

Menu Magic

While drinking a cup of hot tea is the obvious way to consume this Magic food, tea is actually a more versatile plant than you might imagine.

✿ Grind oolong tea leaves in a pepper mill and blend them with freshly ground white pepper to sprinkle on chicken or pork.

✿ Tea also works wonders in a marinade; just add ground leaves to the mixture.

✿ Add tea leaves to chicken broth or stock for a dish with an Asian nuance.

RELATED recipes

Cantaloupe and Blueberry Compote with Green Tea and Lime *276*

Chai *208*

Peachy Iced Tea *209*

TEA glossary

True tea comes from the Camellia sinensis plant. Varieties are listed below. Herbal teas don't offer the same blood-sugar benefits.

White tea: It's picked and harvested before the leaf buds, which are covered with white fuzz, have opened. It's the least processed of the teas and has about half the amount of caffeine of black tea (about 15 milligrams per cup).

Green tea: The leaves are picked, then dried, steamed, or pan fried to keep enzymes in the tea from changing some of the antioxidant compounds and turning the tea dark.

Oolong tea: The leaves are dried for a longer time than for green tea, allowing the enzymes to work longer. Oolong is halfway between green and black tea in terms of processing.

Black tea: The leaves are processed longer to oxidize more of the compounds and produce a darker tea. Black tea contains the most caffeine (about 40 milligrams per cup).

Chai: This isn't a result of processing but rather is tea (usually black) that's combined with spices such as cardamom, cinnamon, cloves, and pepper.

tomatoes

GL VERY LOW

I say "tom-*ay*-to," you say "tom-*ah*-to," but what really matters is how many you eat. No matter how you slice it, tomatoes are terrific for your blood sugar. These juicy fruits are incredibly low in calories (just 22 per tomato) and carbs (less than 5 grams each). What's more, they're rich in vitamin C, which helps protect the body from blood sugar damage, and lycopene, a member of the carotenoid family along with beta-carotene.

Lycopene may have special power against diabetes. Researchers from the Centers for Disease Control and Prevention looked at 1,665 men and women with and without diabetes and found that those with impaired glucose tolerance (essentially, prediabetes) had blood levels of lycopene that were 6 percent lower than those of healthy people. Levels averaged 17 percent lower in people with newly diagnosed diabetes. Two other studies found similar connections.

Health Bonus

A Harvard study found that men who ate tomatoes and tomato products such as tomato sauce and tomato paste at least twice a week lowered their risk of prostate cancer by 24 to 36 percent.

Studies also suggest that eating tomatoes may reduce your risk of osteoporosis and asthma and may improve circulation and reduce inflammation.

Cooks Tips

Store tomatoes on the counter; never keep them in the fridge. It ruins the texture and flavor.

Menu Magic

The possibilities are virtually endless. Serve tomatoes raw, and you get the full vitamin C punch (heat destroys the vitamin); serve them cooked with a little oil, and you get the maximum lycopene dose (the oil helps the body absorb lycopene). Canned tomatoes, tomato sauce, and tomato paste all count, too. Ketchup isn't a good choice since it contains sugar, and while tomato juice is rich in lycopene, it's loaded with salt.

PERFECT portions: 1 medium

One juicy sliced tomato is a satisfying serving, but because tomatoes are so low in calories and carbs, feel free to have more.

- Include tomato wedges or grape tomatoes in green and pasta salads.
- Add tomato slices to your sandwiches.
- Whip up fresh tomato salsa using any recipe.
- Marinate peeled tomatoes in a mixture of olive oil, lemon juice, minced garlic, salt, pepper, and oregano and serve as an appetizer or side dish.
- Serve sliced tomatoes with low-fat mozzarella, balsamic vinegar, and olive oil as a snack or appetizer.
- Make a tomato pizza on a whole wheat pita. Brush the pita with olive oil and top with sliced tomatoes and onions. Sprinkle with basil and grated Parmesan cheese and bake.
- Come summertime, enjoy refreshing gazpacho.

RELATED recipes

Bean and Barley Soup *222*

Caponata *202*

Cherry Tomatoes Filled with Pesto Cream Cheese *200*

Dahl with Spinach *261*

Garden Pasta Salad *215*

Greek Pasta and Beef Casserole *230*

Lentil and Bean Chili *262*

Mediterranean Salad with Edamame *215*

Penne with Tomato and Eggplant Sauce *256*

Quick Spinach and Sausage Lasagna *253*

Seared Fish Steaks with Tomato-Olive Sauce *246*

Shrimp and Orzo Casserole *251*

Slow-Cooker Beef and Vegetable Stew *228*

Spiced Cauliflower with Peas *272*

Tuna and Cannellini Salad with Lemon *213*

Turkey and Bean Chili with Avocado Salsa *243*

Whole Wheat Pasta with Sausage, Beans and Greens *254*

turmeric

GL *VERY LOW*

Turmeric, the spice that gives mustard its bright yellow color and curried dishes their warm glow, may help tame wild blood sugar. That's because turmeric root, a relative of ginger, is one of Earth's most concentrated sources of curcumin, an antioxidant compound that's been shown to help prevent blood sugar surges, at least in diabetic animals. (Cumin is another source of curcumin.) While turmeric the spice has not been well studied, researchers have set their sights on extracts containing curcumin, the active ingredient. One study in lab rats, for example, found that 10 milligrams of a turmeric extract lowered blood sugar levels by 37 percent within 3 hours and by 55 percent after 6 hours.

Exactly how curcumin works isn't known, but researchers point to a number of different possibilities. The main one: It may act directly on the pancreas to stimulate the release of insulin.

Curcumin also has very powerful antioxidant effects that could help stave off heart disease as well as damage related to high blood sugar, including kidney disease, nerve damage, and retinopathy (eye damage).

Health Bonus

Turmeric has a long history as a folk medicine in India and other countries for treating stomach ailments, inflammation, arthritis, and sprains. It's also being studied as an anti-cancer spice. Population studies find dramatically reduced rates of colon cancer in people whose diets are rich in curcumin. And in test tube studies, curcumin has caused the death of cervical cancer cells and blocked harmful cell changes.

Most recently, researchers have begun to look at whether curcumin may help prevent Alzheimer's. In India, where turmeric is practically ubiquitous in food, there is a very low incidence of the disease. In animal studies, curcumin decreased the formation of amyloid, the stuff that makes up the brain deposits characteristic of people with Alzheimer's. While the findings are promising, curcumin has not yet been studied for the treatment or prevention of Alzheimer's in humans.

PERFECT portions: 1/8 to 1/4 teaspoon

Most of the studies with turmeric have used curcumin extracts derived from turmeric, so it's hard to know exactly how much is beneficial. The best advice? Use turmeric whenever you can. It adds deep color and richness to dishes you won't get from anything else.

Cooks Tips

Be careful to keep turmeric contained when you use it, because it will stain almost anything—your fingernails, plastic cups and utensils, and even some kitchen countertops.

Menu Magic

- Purchase bright yellow curry powder; it's likely to contain the most turmeric. Or add extra turmeric to your favorite brand of curry powder.

- Use yellow mustard on burgers and when cooking. Its color comes from turmeric.

- Add turmeric to rice instead of saffron in paella and Spanish rice.

- Include up to a teaspoon of turmeric in your favorite pea soup recipe.

- Add turmeric to stews and casseroles.

- A touch of turmeric works very well in lentil dishes.

RELATED recipes
Curried Butternut Squash Puree *269*
Spiced Cauliflower with Peas *272*

vinegar

GL
VERY LOW

Fans of folk medicine swear by vinegar to treat just about anything that could ail a person, from sunburns to stomachaches to dull hair. But there's one truly effective use for vinegar that most people don't know about. It turns out that simply adding a high-acid food like vinegar to your meals can reduce the blood sugar effect of the entire meal—by 19 to 55 percent!

In one small Italian study, when five people consumed 1 gram of acetic acid (the equivalent of 1 1/3 tablespoons of vinegar) and olive oil (sounds suspiciously like a vinaigrette salad dressing!), followed by 50 grams of carbohydrates from white bread (the amount in about four small slices), their blood sugar went up 31 percent less than when they ate just the bread.

In another study, this one from Arizona State University, when healthy people consumed about 4 teaspoons of cider vinegar before eating a high-GI meal (a bagel, butter, and orange juice), their blood sugar rose an average of 55 percent less after an hour than when they drank water sweetened with saccharin before the meal. And in another study by the same researchers, people with insulin resistance who consumed vinegar before a bagel meal had a 34 percent increase, on average, in insulin sensitivity—which of course translates to better blood sugar control.

Yet another study, this one from Japan, found that when vinegar was part of a meal, it reduced the glycemic index of white rice by an impressive 20 to 40 percent.

One reason for the dramatic findings: The acid in vinegar slows the rate at which food leaves your stomach, also slowing the transformation of a meal's carbohydrates into blood sugar. Animal studies also suggest the acid may help increase the storage of glycogen (the form in which blood sugar is stored for future energy needs) in the liver and skeletal muscles, getting it out of the bloodstream.

Health Bonus

Some of the same research that shows vinegar can lower blood sugar also shows that it can make you feel more satisfied after a meal—a boon to anyone trying to

PERFECT portions: 3 to 4 teaspoons

Research suggests that making this much vinegar part of a meal can significantly lower your blood sugar response to the meal.

lose weight. Vinegar also fights bacteria and fungi, which is why it's used in some homemade preparations for swimmer's ear.

Cooks Tips

Don't limit yourself to plain ol' distilled vinegar. Try red or white wine vinegar, rice vinegar, or apple cider vinegar. Or buy or make flavor-infused vinegars such as tarragon, raspberry, strawberry, and so on. See "Pump Up the Flavor" on page 160 to learn how to make your own flavored vinegar.

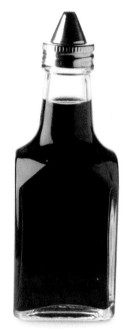

Menu Magic

- Start dinner with a spinach salad dressed with balsamic vinegar and oil.

- Add red wine vinegar to lentil soup.

- Mix up Asian coleslaw with shredded red cabbage and carrots, mung bean sprouts, chopped bok choy, olive oil, rice vinegar, sesame seed oil, chopped cilantro, and toasted sesame seeds.

- Marinate sliced beets in balsamic vinegar, rosemary, crushed garlic, and herbes de Provence for about 20 minutes. Place the beets and marinade in a foil packet, seal tightly, and grill until tender.

- Make a balsamic vinegar glaze for grilled salmon. In a saucepan, boil balsamic vinegar, red wine, and a bit of honey until thick. Serve over the salmon.

(continued)

vinegar continued

- Marinate chicken in cider vinegar and canola oil before baking or grilling.

- Serve soy-glazed chicken. In a skillet, sauté chopped garlic and shallots in olive oil, then add chopped tomato, distilled vinegar, soy sauce, honey, salt, and pepper. Stir well. Add cooked chicken breast and cook over medium-high heat, turning occasionally, until the vinegar mixture has thickened into a glaze.

- Pickle some carrots. In a medium saucepan, mix 1 cup distilled white vinegar, 2 tablespoons sugar, 1 teaspoon salt, pepper to taste, and 2/3 cup water. Bring to a boil, then remove from the heat and let cool slightly. Dice eight large carrots, place in sterile containers, and cover with the vinegar solution. Seal and refrigerate for 12 hours or overnight.

- For dessert, serve sliced strawberries splashed with balsamic vinegar and sprinkled with a few pinches of sugar.

RELATED recipes

Pump Up the Flavor

Here are basic instructions for making your own flavor-infused vinegar.

1. Use clean glass jars or bottles that are free of cracks or nicks and can be sealed with corks, screw-on caps, or two-piece canning lids.

2. Choose your flavoring and vinegar. White vinegar has a sharp, acidic taste and is good for delicately flavored herbs. Apple cider vinegar is milder and blends well with fruit. Wine and champagne vinegars work well with delicate herbs and lighter-flavored fruits. Red wine vinegar has a bolder flavor and complements spices and strong herbs like rosemary.

3. In a saucepan, heat the vinegar to just below the boiling point (at least 190° to 195°F/88° to 90°C).

4. Place three or four sprigs of fresh herbs, 3 tablespoons of dried herbs, 1 to 2 cups of fruits or vegetables, or the peel of one lemon or orange per pint of vinegar to be flavored into the jar. For some herbs, you may want to "bruise" the leaves or sprigs to release the flavors.

5. Pour the hot vinegar over the flavoring ingredient in the jar. Seal the jar and let stand undisturbed in a cool, dark place for three to four weeks.

6. Strain the vinegar through damp cheesecloth or a coffee filter until it's no longer cloudy, then pour it into a clean, dry glass jar.

Store all flavored vinegars in a cool, dark place in a tightly closed glass jar—not on your countertop in the sun. (If you keep it there for decoration, don't consume it.) Flavored vinegars will keep for three months in cool storage and for six to eight months in the fridge. Plain, unflavored distilled vinegar will keep indefinitely.

wheatberries

GL MEDIUM

In case you haven't noticed, we've been preaching the merits of whole grain foods in this book. (Remember secret number 2 of Magic eating, Make Three of Your Carb Servings Whole Grains?) Well, you can't get any more "whole grain" than wheatberries, which are, simply put, the entire grain (or "fruit") of the wheat plant, minus the hull. If you've read the bran and wheat germ entries, you know how good those are for your blood sugar and your health in general. Wheatberries offer both in one package.

As we said earlier, people who eat at least three daily servings of whole grain foods, like wheatberries, are much less likely to develop type 2 diabetes.

It's no wonder. According to a British study, eating wheatberries resulted in significantly lower levels of blood sugar and insulin than eating the same amount of carbs from flour. A Swedish study had similar results when healthy volunteers ate either white bread or coarse wheat bread made with wheatberries.

If you've shopped for prepared salads lately, you may have noticed some made with wheatberries. The berries have a nice, firm texture that requires some chewing, so they keep you from wolfing down your food. They're also more filling than other wheat products containing the same amount of carbohydrates, according to findings from Australia.

Health Bonus

Large-scale studies have shown that eating whole grain foods lowers the risk not only of diabetes but also of heart disease, stroke, and several types of cancer.

Wheatberries supply minerals and other compounds that are lost when the grains are milled into white flour. Their germ portion is a rich source of cholesterol-lowering sterols.

Cooks Tips

Since wheatberries take so long to cook (an hour or more, depending on whether you soak them first), you may want to cook extra, then store the surplus in a

covered container in the refrigerator for up to two days or in the freezer for up to six months. With cooked wheatberries on hand, it's easy to add them to salads, soups, pilafs, pancakes, muffins, and breads.

Menu Magic

Wheatberries are most often enjoyed in wheatberry salads featuring anything from cranberries and nuts to avocados and tomatoes. They can be served as side dishes or main dishes, warm or chilled. Here are a few other ideas for using cooked wheatberries.

- Combine wheatberries with avocado cubes and cherry tomatoes and toss with a vinaigrette.

- Mix them with grilled bell peppers, place on a bed of lettuce, and top with a vinaigrette.

- For a flavorful side dish, combine wheatberries with raisins, sliced almonds, chopped scallions, and curry powder.

- Use as a hot or cold breakfast cereal, plain or with milk or soy milk and topped with a bit of brown sugar and a dash of cinnamon.

- Fold wheatberries into bread dough or pancake batter.

- Combine them with cooked lentils and season to taste.

- Use them in Italian soups along with beans. They offer a nice textural contrast to the soft, creamy beans.

RELATED recipe

Wheatberry Salad with Dried Apricots and Mint *266*

wheat germ

GL
VERY LOW

You may wonder how any food whose name includes the word *germ* can be good for you, but don't let the name throw you. Wheat germ is another example of good things that come in small packages.

The germ (think of it as the grain's embryo) is the nutritional heart of the wheat kernel. Besides complex carbohydrates, it's packed with protein and sugar-stabilizing, hunger-fighting "good-for-you" fats as well as fiber, vitamins, and minerals, including zinc, selenium, and magnesium, which help the body manage blood sugar.

Magnesium is a potential diabetes fighter. Harvard researchers tallied the magnesium intakes of more than 127,000 men and women with no initial history of diabetes. After 18 years of follow-up in women and 12 years in men, they found that people whose diets provided the most magnesium were about 34 percent less likely to develop type 2 diabetes than those whose diets provided the least.

Health Bonus

Vitamin E is wheat germ's crowning glory. E is a powerful antioxidant that thwarts cell damage from free radicals, the rogue molecules that are suspected of playing a role in chronic conditions such as heart disease, cataracts, and Alzheimer's disease.

Like magnesium, diets rich in E may help stave off diabetes. As part of the Insulin Resistance and Atherosclerosis Study, University of South Carolina researchers measured the levels of E in the blood of nearly 900 people without diabetes for five years. They found that among people who didn't take vitamin E supplements, those with the highest blood levels of E were 88 percent less likely to develop type 2 diabetes than those with the lowest levels.

The "good" fat in wheat germ, along with its cholesterol-lowering plant sterols, can also help lower harmful (LDL) cholesterol.

PERFECT portions: 2 tablespoons

Wheat germ has a very low GL thanks to its fat and protein, but it does have calories (55 in 2 tablespoons), so portion size is important.

Cooks Tips

Buy plain toasted wheat germ and steer clear of sweetened varieties. Once the jar has been opened, store it in the refrigerator to prevent the wheat germ from going rancid.

Menu Magic

Wheat germ's crunchy texture and nutty flavor make it perfect for a variety of uses.

- Add nutty crunch to steamed vegetables and green salads with a sprinkling of wheat germ.
- Sprinkle it on oatmeal or cold cereal.
- Top low-fat yogurt with berries and wheat germ.
- When coating chicken or fish, skip the bread crumbs in favor of a mixture of wheat germ, grated Parmesan cheese, and dried parsley.
- Add wheat germ to smoothies made with low-fat plain yogurt and fruit.
- Substitute wheat germ for some of the meat in your favorite meat loaf or meatball recipe.
- Add wheat germ to muffins, pancakes, casseroles, pizza dough, and savory piecrusts.

RELATED recipes
Macaroni and Cheese with Spinach *255*
Multi-Grain Pancakes or Waffles *192*

whole wheat BREAD AND FLOUR

GL MEDIUM

Let's face it, bread isn't exactly a banner food for better blood sugar. So why eat it? If it's whole grain bread, here's all the reason you should need: People who eat more whole grains have a much lower risk of diabetes.

Whole grains also help improve the body's sensitivity to insulin, the hormone that manages blood sugar. In one study of 978 men and women, the higher their intake of whole grains, the greater their insulin sensitivity, which translates into better blood-sugar control.

There's another reason to eat whole grains: your heart. Countless studies have confirmed that people who eat a lot of whole grain foods cut their heart disease risk by anywhere from 15 to 30 percent compared with people who go "white" all the way (or avoid grains altogether). Chalk up whole wheat bread's heart benefits to its antioxidants, fiber, and cholesterol-reducing plant sterols.

Want to lose weight? Switch to whole wheat. The famous Nurses' Health Study from the Harvard School of Public Health looked at more than 74,000 women and found that those who ate the most whole grains were a whopping 49 percent less likely to gain weight over a 12-year period than those who ate the least. Why? Whole grains are filling, in large part because of their hefty fiber content (remember, fiber contains no calories, because it can't be digested). And of course, they're gentler on your blood sugar than their refined-grain counterparts. Steadier blood sugar means steadier weight.

Blood sugar aside, whole wheat bread has the edge over white bread in every other conceivable way. It contains the germ of wheat, where most of the nutrients are located (you may not know that whole wheat bread is a terrific source of antioxidants!). The germ is stripped out to make white bread, as is the bran, where most of the fiber is found. Just about all that's left in white bread is the starchy endosperm.

Want to make sure the good stuff is still in your bread? You'll have to become a label reader. See "The Whole Truth about Whole Wheat" on page 164 to learn exactly what to look for.

PERFECT portions: 1 slice

One small slice of whole wheat bread provides about 70 calories. But watch out: Some heftier slices have as many as 110 calories each.

Health Bonus

Whole grains have surprising power to prevent certain cancers, including breast cancer and other hormone-related cancers, such as uterine and ovarian cancers, and gastrointestinal cancers, such as stomach and colorectal cancers. In fact, according to various studies, you can cut your overall risk of cancer by as much as 40 percent by eating plenty of whole grains. According to the American Institute for Cancer Research, for instance, when data from 40 recent studies on whole grains and cancer risk were combined and analyzed, the risk of cancer was reduced by 34 percent on average in people who ate a lot of whole grains compared to those who ate very little.

How can whole grain bread help prevent cancer? That depends on the cancer, but the ingredients at work probably include fiber, flavonoids (special types of antioxidants), and lignans, estrogen-like compounds found in the bran and germ layers of the grain.

Probably thanks to their fiber, whole grains also help prevent constipation as well as an intestinal disorder called diverticulitis.

Cooks Tips

Since whole wheat flour contains more fat (it's the beneficial type) than white flour does, it's more perishable. Store it in an airtight container in the refrigerator or freezer.

You can usually replace up to half the white flour called for in recipes with whole wheat flour. But when making delicate baked goods like biscuits, opt for whole wheat pastry flour. It contains less gluten-forming protein than regular whole wheat flour and helps ensure a tender result.

(continued)

Menu Magic

✪ Use whole wheat bread instead of refined white bread for sandwiches (when you're not using rye, pumpernickel, or sourdough, which are all Magic foods, too).

✪ Look for whole wheat hamburger buns.

✪ Make your pizza with whole wheat dough (see our recipe on page 258).

✪ If you're using croutons for soups or salads, make them whole wheat. The same goes for bread crumbs in cooking and baking. To make croutons, cube two slices of whole wheat bread (2 cups) and toss with 2 teaspoons olive oil, then spread in a small baking pan and bake at 350°F (175°C) until crisp, 15 to 25 minutes.

✪ Use whole wheat pitas as the base for quick, healthy lunches. Stuff with carrots and tuna or other good-for-you fixin's, such as chickpeas, tomatoes, arugula, and so on, or top with grilled vegetables, tomato sauce, and a bit of cheese for a fast pizza.

✪ If you enjoy baking bread and would like to make loaves with 100 percent whole wheat flour, add wheat gluten (vital gluten, found in the bulk section of natural foods stores) at a ratio of 1 tablespoon gluten to 2 cups flour. This helps compensate for the additional bran and germ in the whole wheat, which does not contain gluten.

RELATED recipes

The Whole Truth about Whole Wheat

Buying whole wheat bread is trickier than it may seem. There are dozens of "wheat breads" on the shelves, but guess what? Most of them are white bread. You see, all flour comes from wheat, so any old bread can be called wheat bread, even if it's made with refined white flour. Some "wheat" breads may contain a bit of whole wheat flour, but usually not much.

The bottom line: It's not enough to look for the word *wheat* on *labels*. Instead, look for the word *whole*, preferably in the very first ingredient, to make sure the bread you buy is truly made from whole grain. That goes for any bread labeled "multigrain" as well—if the word *whole* isn't at the top of the list, pass it up.

You may have seen new breads on the market called whole grain white breads. Even though they're whole wheat, they look like white bread because they're made from a special variety of wheat (albino wheat) that's lighter in color, plus a host of "dough conditioners" that keep the bread soft like white bread. These breads are more processed than regular whole wheat breads because the whole grains are pulverized into tiny bits by special machinery to make the bread smooth. We don't know what effect this has on the bread's GL, but it certainly doesn't help it.

yogurt

GL
LOW

Like milk, yogurt has a naturally low GL (after all, yogurt is nothing more than fermented milk). The unidentified natural component in milk that experts think may help prevent insulin resistance is there in yogurt, too. Since it's fermented by bacteria, yogurt also contains acids, and you've already read that acids can help lower blood sugar.

You can drink your yogurt in a smoothie or eat it with fresh fruit. Another reason we like yogurt: It's a perfectly acceptable lower-fat substitute for some or all of the mayonnaise in creamy salads and the sour cream in baked goods, soups, and chip dips.

Compared to milk, yogurt is usually better tolerated by people who are lactose intolerant. Even though yogurt contains lactose, or milk sugar, the bacterial cultures used to make it produce the lactase enzyme required for proper digestion.

When it comes to yogurt types, low fat and fat free are of course your best choices. Skip "fruit on the bottom" brands, which are usually loaded with added sugar. You can always add your own fresh fruit.

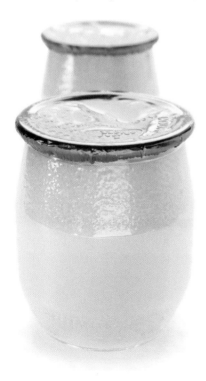

PERFECT portions: 1 cup plain

This amount will give you a low glycemic load and a good deal of calcium.

Health Bonus

You can count yogurt in as a calcium-rich bone builder. It provides the same 300 milligrams per 8 ounces (250 ml) as milk. And it counts as a dairy food in the famously healthy DASH diet, proven to help control high blood pressure.

Yogurt contains "good" bacteria, the kind that offer numerous health benefits, including boosting the immune system, alleviating diarrhea caused by some infections or treatment with antibiotics, relieving constipation, and even reducing the risk of developing colon cancer. Some people like to eat yogurt whenever they're taking antibiotics to replace the beneficial bacteria in the gut that the drugs obliterate.

As far as yogurt's immune benefits go, more than 70 percent of the body's natural immune defenses are located in the digestive tract. Building up the population of good bacteria there may help boost production of important immune system compounds, making you more resistant to viruses.

There's also evidence that women who regularly eat yogurt with live *Lactobacillus acidophilus* cultures get fewer yeast infections.

(continued)

don't fall for it

Frozen yogurt may seem like the next best thing to regular yogurt, but it's not. First, almost all frozen yogurt is sweetened and flavored. While there are several low-fat and fat-free options, they're typically high in sugar. In addition, levels of beneficial bacteria vary greatly. Some brands are heat treated after the bacterial cultures are added, rendering the bacteria useless to your health. In others, the bacteria are added to an ice cream–like mixture after the fact.

Only yogurts labeled "contains live, active cultures" have bacteria that are still active (unless they were pasteurized after the bacterial cultures were added, which destroys the bacteria; these yogurts should be labeled "heat-treated after culturing").

Cooks Tips

To get the most bacterial benefit from yogurt, use it by the expiration date on the carton. The "friendly" bacteria begin dying when the yogurt is no longer fresh. Cooking destroys the beneficial bacteria, but even cooked yogurt is a low-GL food.

Cooking with yogurt on top of the stove can be tricky since it usually curdles when boiled. When adding it to hot dishes, stabilize it first by mixing in 1 teaspoon of cornstarch per cup of yogurt. Add it toward the end of the cooking time.

Menu Magic

- ❖ Substitute yogurt for sour cream in baked goods.

- ❖ Make your favorite chip or vegetable dip using low-fat plain yogurt instead of sour cream.

- ❖ Replace half the mayonnaise in creamy salad dressings with yogurt.

- ❖ Use yogurt as a restaurant-worthy garnish for pureed vegetable soups, such as a squash or carrot soup. First, thin the yogurt with low-fat milk to make it the same consistency as the soup. Drop dollops of the mixture into the soup, then draw the tip of a knife or toothpick through it to create swirls.

- ❖ Use a dollop on chili instead of sour cream.

- ❖ Make cool, creamy fruit soup with low-fat plain yogurt, sliced peaches, strawberries, orange juice, and honey. Process in the blender, then garnish with fresh mint leaves.

- ❖ Serve a cucumber salad made with grated cucumbers and carrots, diced onion, chopped dill, low-fat plain yogurt, and salt and pepper to taste.

- ❖ Top sliced fruit with yogurt or create a beautiful breakfast parfait. In a tall, chilled parfait glass, layer low-fat plain yogurt with fresh blueberries and oat and nut granola.

- ❖ Dip Granny Smith apples into yogurt for a refreshing snack.

- ❖ Make a refreshing yogurt cooler (*ayran,* a traditional Turkish beverage) by combining equal parts yogurt and cold water and a pinch of salt in a blender. Serve over crushed ice.

- ❖ To make yogurt creamier and richer tasting, make yogurt "cheese." Spoon yogurt into a cheesecloth-lined sieve, set over a bowl, and refrigerate for at least 6 hours or overnight. Discard the liquid (whey) that has accumulated in the bowl. Use the "cheese" as a substitute for cream cheese or sour cream. Stir in chopped fresh herbs, scallions, and garlic to make a delicious low-fat herbed cheese spread.

RELATED recipes

Meal Makeovers

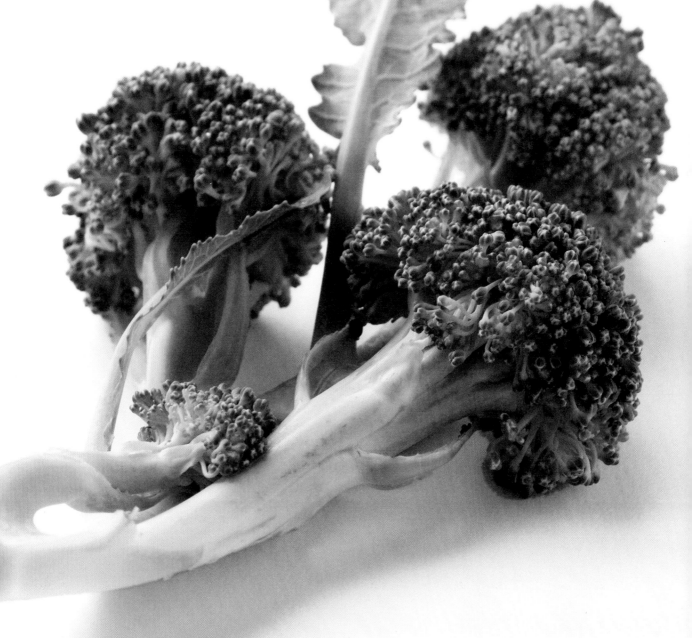

BREAKFAST makeovers

If your idea of breakfast is a bagel, a bowl of cornflakes, or a pile of pancakes or waffles, help is here.

Nothing sabotages your daily efforts to follow the Magic eating plan like a high-GL breakfast—the kind most of us eat. Breakfast is usually the most carbohydrate-filled meal of the day and thus the one that raises your blood sugar the most dramatically. That doesn't mean you should cut out the carbs, though. Just switching to "slower-acting" carbs, and eating less of them, will do the trick. You'll also want to find ways to add some protein to your plate.

Our top five BREAKFAST GUIDELINES:

1 Limit carbohydrates to one serving. Have one slice of bread instead of two, eat half a bagel (or a mini-bagel) instead of a whole one, and pour only 3/4 to 1 cup cold cereal instead of a huge bowlful (stick to 1/2 to 3/4 cup for hot cereal).

2 Choose lower-GL cereals. These usually include whole grain cereals with at least 5 grams of fiber per serving (see "How Cereals Rate" in the bran entry on page 85). Bran cereals such as All Bran, Bran Buds, and 100% Bran are good choices, along with high-fiber, high-protein cereals such as Kashi GoLean and oat cereals such as Barbara's Shredded Oats.

3 Totally avoid "white" carbs. This means no Pop-Tarts, white toast with jelly, or muffins made with white flour.

4 Replace some carbohydrate calories with fruit and a high-protein food. Have some orange slices with your eggs, sprinkle nuts and berries on cereal, or enjoy grapefruit along with a bagel or toast spread with peanut butter. This will not only make the meal more filling, it will also lower its effect on your blood sugar.

5 Use small glasses for juice. Fruit juice is fine for you—in moderation. Drink too much, and it quickly becomes a high-GL (and high-calorie) food.

In many ways, breakfast really is the most important meal of the day. If you start the day with a Magic breakfast, you're more likely to stay off the blood sugar rollercoaster—and eat less—all day long.

Typical Breakfast

3 4-inch (10-cm) white flour waffles with
3 tablespoons maple syrup

2 slices regular bacon

8 ounces (250 ml) orange juice

1 cup coffee

Total GL: 105
Total calories: 597

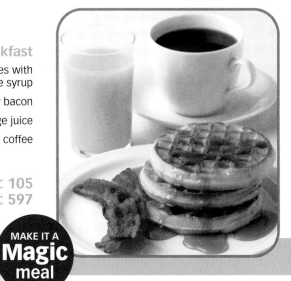

MAKE IT A
Magic
meal

Magic BREAKFAST

1 4-inch (10-cm) Multigrain Waffle
(recipe on page 192) with 1 tablespoon maple syrup

2 large eggs, scrambled

2 slices Canadian back bacon

1/2 medium grapefruit

1 cup coffee or tea

THE FIXES

- Substituted fiber-rich whole grain waffles for the white flour waffles to lower the GL.

- Decreased the number of waffles from three to one.

- Added protein-rich eggs to replace the waffle calories.

- Decreased the amount of maple syrup for fewer calories and a lower GL.

- Substituted Canadian back bacon for regular bacon. It's much lower in saturated fat—which, you'll recall, contributes to insulin resistance.

- Replaced the orange juice with half a grapefruit. Remember, whole fruit has more fiber and a lower GL than fruit juice.

Total GL: 15
Total calories: 337

BETTER still: Substitute a slice of rye toast for the waffle.

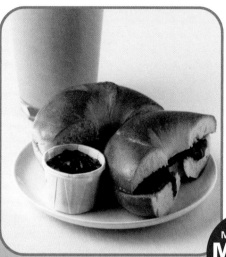

Typical Breakfast

1 toasted large plain bagel with 2 tablespoons jam or jelly

12 ounces (341 ml) French vanilla coffee beverage

Total GL: 46
Total calories: 612

MAKE IT A
Magic
meal

Magic BREAKFAST

1/2 toasted large whole wheat bagel with 1 tablespoon peanut butter

1 medium apple

1 cup coffee or tea

THE FIXES

- Substituted a whole grain bagel for the white flour bagel for more fiber and a lower GL.

- Cut the bagel portion in half to limit carbs.

- Added peanut butter as a filling source of protein and "good" fat to add back calories without increasing the GL.

- Replaced the high-calorie, high-GL coffee beverage with plain coffee or tea.

Total GL: 17
Total calories: 275

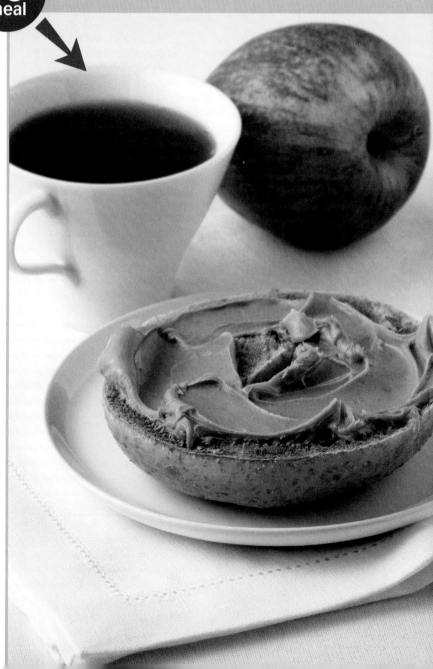

Typical Breakfast

2 cups cornflakes with 1 cup 2% milk

1 cup coffee or tea

Total GL: 49
Total calories: 321

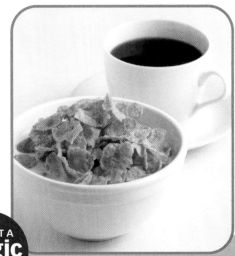

MAKE IT A
Magic
meal

Magic BREAKFAST

3/4 cup Grape-Nuts Flakes with:
    1/2 cup fat-free milk
    1/2 cup strawberries
    1/2 ounce (14 g) slivered almonds

1 cup coffee or tea

THE FIXES

- Switched the high-GL cereal for a lower-GL cereal.

- Decreased the cereal serving to further cut the GL.

- Cut calories and fat by switching from 2% milk to fat-free milk.

- Added fruit and nuts to the cereal to make up for the smaller portion. The fruit provides extra vitamins and phytochemicals, and the nuts, with their healthy fats, slow the digestion of the meal for a slower rise in blood sugar.

Total GL: 19
Total calories: 258

BETTER still: Go for All Bran cereal instead of Grape-Nuts Flakes.

LUNCH**makeovers**

Lunch can be a tough meal because we often grab it on the go, and healthy fare can be harder to find when you're not at home. Regardless of where you eat lunch, though, you can make choices that will be gentler on your blood sugar.

Our top six LUNCH GUIDELINES:

1 Make your lunch at home. You'll have all the control you need over what you eat. If you do have to grab something from a fast-food place, we give some examples of smarter ordering.

2 Switch your sandwich bread to whole grain. Choose rye or pumpernickel for the lowest possible GL. Whole wheat is also a good choice. If you do choose white bread, make it sourdough; its acids make its GL lower than that of other white breads.

3 Ask for mustard instead of mayo. Mustard might as well be a Magic food because of its vinegar and turmeric content. Mayonnaise...well, it isn't.

4 Favor fruit. Lunch is a great time to get one or more of your fruit servings for the day.

5 Select a smart salad. Make sure it contains plenty of protein in the form of eggs, chicken, tuna, beans, tofu, or low-fat cheese. And choose a Magic vinegar-based dressing, not a creamy one.

6 Skip the soda. It has a sky-high GL unless you order diet soda or stick to 8 ounces (250 ml)—less than one can. Opt for mineral water or unsweetened iced tea instead. If you prefer juice, look for one that's 100% juice and unsweetened (most are anything but, crammed with sugar in the form of high-fructose corn syrup), and either stick to 6 ounces (180 ml) or less or dilute it with seltzer.

Finally, don't forget to have a snack between lunch and dinner to keep your blood sugar on an even keel. See our snack makeovers starting page 178.

Typical Lunch

2 slices white bread with 2 slices roasted turkey,
2 slices processed cheese, 1 tablespoon mayonnaise

1 medium banana

3 or 4 graham crackers

16 ounces (495 ml) apple juice

Total GL: 59
Total calories: 891

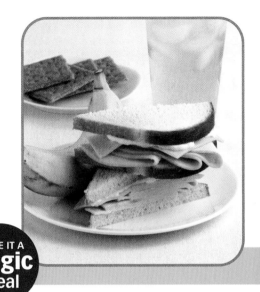

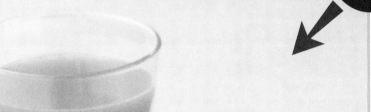

LUNCH MAKEOVERS **LUNCH** MAKEOVERS

**MAKE IT A
Magic
meal**

Magic LUNCH

2 slices whole grain bread with:
  2 slices roasted turkey
  1 slice processed cheese
  Lettuce
  2 slices tomato
  1 tablespoon mustard

12 sweet cherries

1 ounce (30 g) dark chocolate–
  covered almonds

6 ounces (180 ml) unsweetened
  grapefruit juice

THE FIXES

- Swapped white bread for whole grain to boost fiber and lower the GL.

- Cut approximately 60 calories by switching from mayo to mustard.

- Exchanged the apple juice for grapefruit juice, which has a lower GL, and cut the quantity to reduce calories and further lower the GL.

- Switched the banana for cherries. All stone fruits have lower GLs than bananas do.

- Included dark chocolate–covered almonds instead of graham crackers. The almonds offer protein, "good" fats, vitamins, and fiber, while the crackers don't provide much nutrition and add significantly to the meal's GL.

**Total GL: 17
Total calories: 452**

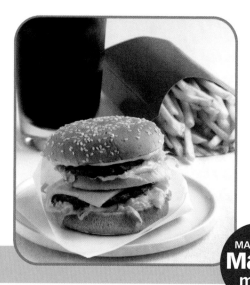

Typical Lunch

McDonald's Big Mac

Large order of French fries

32 ounces (730 ml) soda

Total GL: 109
Total calories: 1,427

Magic LUNCH

McDonald's Quarter Pounder

6 ounces (180 ml) Berries and Yogurt
or Yogurt Parfait

Bottled water

THE FIXES

- Switched to the Quarter Pounder, which has less bread and more meat than the Big Mac. Ordered it without cheese to keep calories in check.

- Avoided French fries, a.k.a. blood sugar bombs, and ordered Berries and Yogurt (or Yogurt Parfait) instead for fewer calories, less fat, and more nutrition.

Total GL: 10
Total calories: 550

BETTER still: A single hamburger and a side salad with vinaigrette dressing.

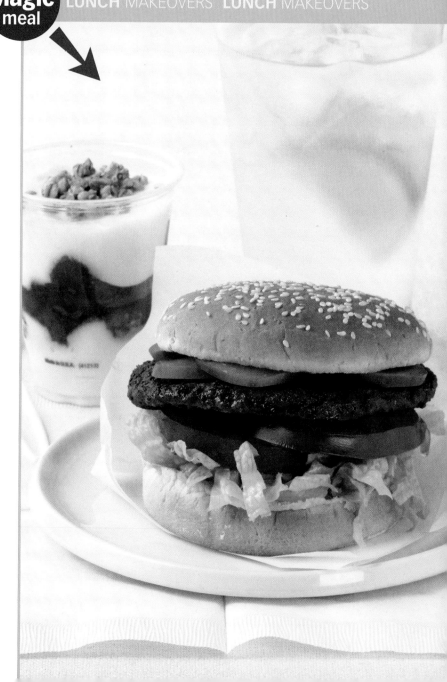

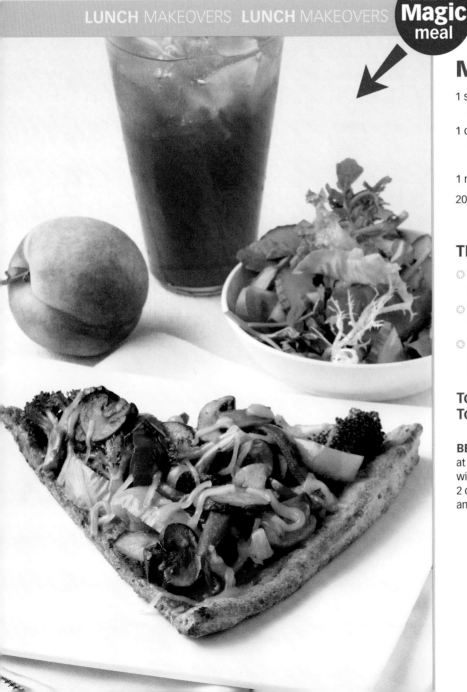

Typical Lunch

2 slices regular cheese pizza

32 ounces (730 ml) soda

Total GL: 86
Total calories: 580

MAKE IT A
Magic meal

Magic LUNCH

1 slice whole wheat pizza with cheese
and vegetables

1 cup side salad with:
Lettuce, tomato, and cucumber
1 tablespoon oil and vinegar dressing

1 medium peach

20 ounces (495 ml) unsweetened
iced tea

THE FIXES

- Cut carbs, fat, and calories by limiting pizza to one slice.

- Boosted fiber by switching to whole wheat crust and adding vegetables.

- Made up for the slice you're not eating by adding a salad and a piece of fruit, both nutritious, low-GL foods.

Total GL: 14
Total calories: 333

BETTER still: Make your own pizza at home by topping a whole grain pita with 2 tablespoons tomato sauce, 2 ounces (60 g) part-skim mozzarella, and plenty of veggies.

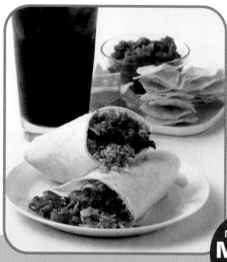

Typical Lunch

1 large burrito made with a 13-inch (33-cm) white flour tortilla and 1 cup white rice, 2 ounces (60 g) beef filling 1 ounce (30 g) cheddar cheese, 2 tablespoons salsa

1.5 ounces (45 g) tortilla chips

1/4 cup salsa

32 ounces (730 ml) soda

Total GL: 120
Total calories: 1,422

MAKE IT A
Magic meal

Magic LUNCH

1 small burrito made with a 6-inch
(15-cm) whole wheat tortilla and:
  1/2 cup black beans
  1.5 ounces (42 g) roasted chicken
  Plenty of lettuce, tomato, and salsa
  1/2 ounce (15 g) cheddar cheese

1/2 mango

Bottled water

THE FIXES

○ Cut carbs and lowered the GL by switching from an overgrown white flour tortilla to a more reasonably sized whole wheat tortilla.

○ Lowered the GL significantly and added fiber by eliminating the white rice and including black beans instead.

○ Added fruit instead of tortilla chips. Chips are an "empty-calorie" food, whereas fruit is packed with fiber and vitamins, not to mention having a low GL.

Total GL: 22
Total calories: 519

BETTER still: A grilled chicken or steak salad, if it's on the menu (no taco shell). If it's not, ask for a "naked burrito"— burrito filling without the tortilla.

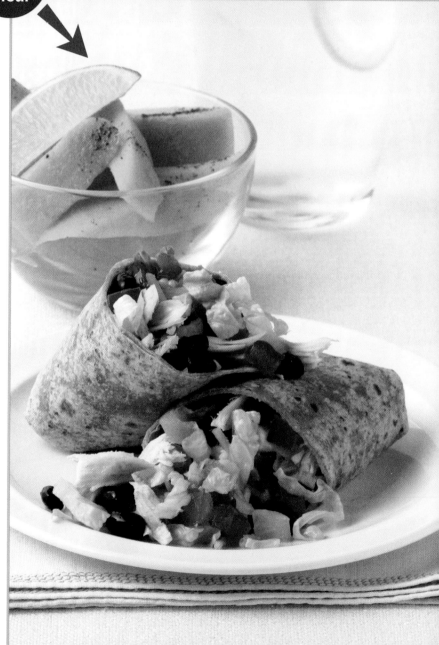

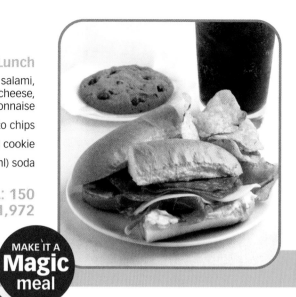

Typical Lunch

1 large white sub roll with 4 slices salami, 4 slices prosciutto, 2 slices provolone cheese, 1 tablespoon mayonnaise

2-ounce (60-g) bag potato chips

1 large chocolate chip cookie

32 ounces (730 ml) soda

Total GL: 150
Total calories: 1,972

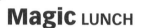

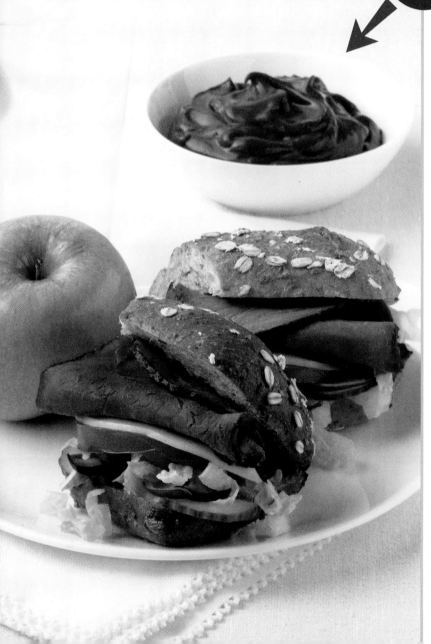

MAKE IT A
Magic
meal

Magic LUNCH

1/2 whole grain sub roll with:
   2 slices lean roast beef
   1 slice provolone cheese
   Oil and vinegar
   Lettuce, tomato, cucumber,
    onion, and olives

1 medium apple

4 ounces (125 ml) "light" chocolate
   pudding

Mineral water with lemon

THE FIXES

○ Switched to a whole grain roll, which has more fiber, and cut it in half to cut carbs.

○ Substituted leaner meat for meats high in saturated fat, reduced the quantity of meat, and "beefed up" the sandwich with a generous helping of veggies.

○ Replaced the chips with fruit for much less fat and more nutrients.

○ Cut saturated fat and calories by replacing the cookie with light pudding, which also provides some calcium.

Total GL: 38
Total calories: 588

BETTER still: Enjoy a chef's salad with rolled cold cuts, cheese, and veggies.

SNACK**makeovers**

It's 3:00 p.m., and your energy is dipping, as are your eyelids. You're thinking about raiding the vending machine, and your resolve is weakening. The good news: Snacking is good for you because going too long without eating sets you up for a huge blood sugar dip that could wreck your Magic eating for the rest of the day. The bad news: Most of the snacks in the vending machine are rotten choices.

Our top three SNACKING GUIDELINES:

1 Pack your snack with your lunch. It's easy enough to grab some carrot or celery sticks, some grapes or grape tomatoes, a container of yogurt, or some nuts and stick them in your "lunchbox."

2 Stay away from chips and go easy on pretzels, which are not much more than white flour, with barely any protein to balance it out.

3 Seek out protein. Peanut butter, nuts, yogurt, and even a hard-boiled egg are good snack sources.

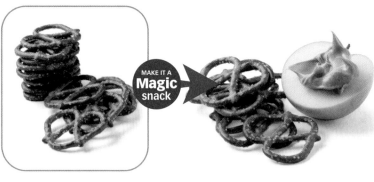

2 ounces (60 g)
pretzels

Total GL: 33
Total calories: 216

3/4 ounce (20 g) pretzels
1/2 green apple with 1 tablespoon peanut butter

Total GL: 14
Total calories: 208

THE FIXES

○ Decreased the number of pretzels by more than half to limit refined carbs.

○ Beefed up the snack with a filling piece of fruit and some peanut butter for blood sugar "staying power." This snack will help you stay full longer than if you ate just the pretzels.

1 berry cereal bar

Total GL: 26
Total calories: 140

14 ounces (125 ml) low-fat mixed-berry yogurt
topped with 2 tablespoons All Bran cereal

Total GL: 9
Total calories: 148

THE FIXES

○ Substituted yogurt for the cereal bar to slash the GL. Because these bars contain cereal, we often assume they're good for us, but they're often lower in fiber and higher in sugar than their cereal counterparts.

○ Added All Bran cereal on top for crunch and a bit of whole grain.

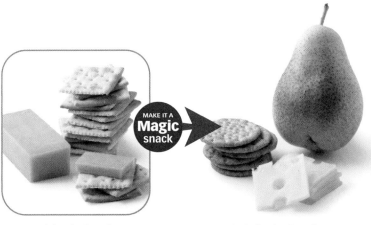

15 plain salted crackers
3 ounces (85 g) cheddar cheese

Total GL: 22
Total calories: 624

6 whole wheat crackers
1 ounce (30 g) Swiss cheese, 1 small pear

Total GL: 13
Total calories: 299

THE FIXES

- Switched to whole wheat crackers and cut the portion by more than half to decrease the GL.

- Limited the cheese to decrease saturated fat. Cheese is indeed a Magic food, but you need to eat it in moderation.

- Added a piece of fruit to add back some calories. Because of its fiber and water, the pear will fill you up more than the crackers.

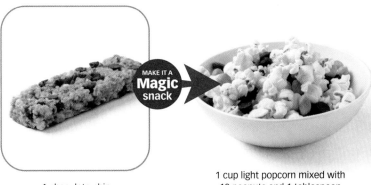

1 chocolate chip
granola bar

Total GL: 14
Total calories: 163

1 cup light popcorn mixed with
10 peanuts and 1 tablespoon
semisweet chocolate chips

Total GL: 8
Total calories: 160

THE FIXES

- Swapped the granola bar, filled with added sugar, for popcorn (a whole grain, high-fiber food) to lower the GL.

- Added peanuts for a sugar-stabilizing dose of protein and "good" fats that will help you stay fuller longer.

- Threw in some chocolate chips to satisfy your sweet tooth.

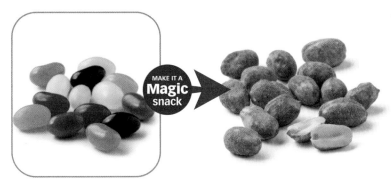

14 jelly beans

Total GL: 27
Total calories: 150

15 dry-roasted peanuts

Total GL: 1
Total calories: 84

THE FIX

- Slashed the GL to almost nothing by substituting peanuts, which are satisfying and full of protein, fiber, and healthy fat, for jelly beans, full of nothing but blood sugar–raising sugar.

DINNER**makeovers**

The most chaotic time in most households is dinnertime. You're tired, the family is hungry, and you just want to get something on the table fast. The good news is that you can make your dinner more Magic without spending any extra time making the meal.

Our top five DINNER GUIDELINES:

1 Limit yourself to one or two servings of carbohydrates. One serving would be 1/2 cup of pasta, potatoes, rice, or stuffing; two servings would be 1 cup.

2 Fill the hole on your plate with veggies. Here's your best shot at meeting your vegetable quota for the day. Even if you're having a salad on the side, put at least 1/2 cup of veggies, such as sautéed carrots or green beans, on your plate. Rely on frozen veggies and prewashed, bagged salad greens if you're short on time.

3 Leave the bread at the store. Bread isn't bad for you, but if you had a sandwich for lunch, that's probably all the bread you need for the day. Adding bread to dinner means you may not eat other, healthier foods; almost always adds butter to your meal; and certainly increases the GL.

4 Keep your protein lean. Think turkey meatballs instead of beef, flank steak instead of ground beef, and chicken without the skin instead of fried chicken. Tofu, beans, fish, and shrimp are also good protein sources.

5 Stick with water as your beverage of choice. Or, if you like milk, have a glass of fat-free. Wine is fine occasionally if your doctor okays it, but soda and juice add calories and GL without adding much (or any) nutrition. Most of us don't drink enough water throughout the day and come home feeling wilted. Drink a cold glassful at dinner to rehydrate.

Dish the food onto plates instead of placing a serving dish on the table for everyone to dig into. You're likely to eat less. A final tip: After dinner (or dessert, if you have it), close up the kitchen. For many people, late-night eating is a prime reason for eating too many calories in a day.

Typical Dinner

7 ounces (200 g) grilled "select" sirloin steak

1 medium baked potato with 1 tablespoon butter

1 cup salad with 1 tablespoon ranch dressing

1 slice French bread with 1 tablespoon butter

4 ounces (125 ml) red wine

Total GL: 64
Total calories: 1,003

MAKE IT A
Magic
meal

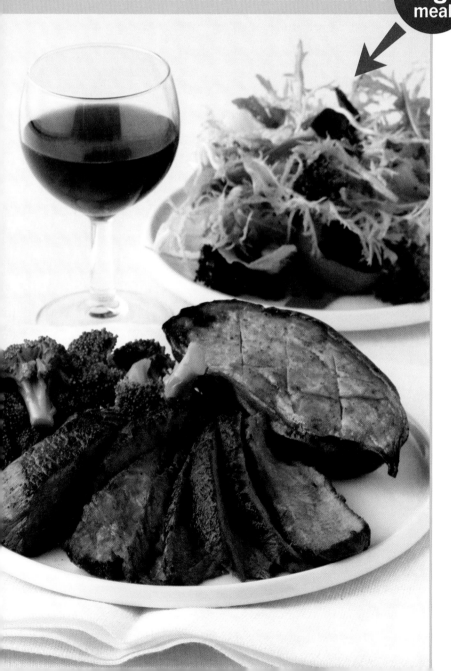

Magic DINNER

7 ounces (200 g) grilled "select" sirloin steak

1/2 baked medium sweet potato with:
   1/2 tablespoon good-for-you margarine
   Cinnamon
   Nutmeg

1/2 cup steamed broccoli

2 cups mixed greens salad with:
   Roasted red and yellow bell peppers
   2 tablespoons oil and vinegar dressing

4 ounces (125 ml) red wine

THE FIXES

- Replaced the white potato with half a sweet potato to dramatically decrease the GL. Eat the skin for added fiber.

- Doubled the salad size. Salad is filling and full of low-GL nutrition.

- Changed the ranch dressing to oil and vinegar to decrease unhealthy saturated fat and provide extra acidity, which lowers the meal's GL.

- Replaced the bread with broccoli to add vitamins and fiber and lower the GL.

Total GL: 12
Total calories: 481

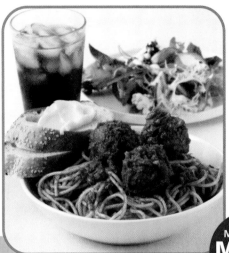

2 cups cooked regular spaghetti with
1 cup tomato sauce, 3.5 ounces (100 g) beef meatballs

2 small slices Italian bread with 1 tablespoon butter

1 cup salad with
Cucumber, tomato, 1 tablespoon blue cheese dressing

8 ounces (250 ml) soda

Total GL: 62
Total calories: 1,170

MAKE IT A
Magic
meal DINNER MAKEOVERS DINNER MAKEOVERS

Magic DINNER

1 cup cooked whole wheat spaghetti
with:
　1/2 cup tomato sauce
　3.5 ounces (100 g) turkey meatballs
　　(made with 90% fat-free
　　ground turkey)

2 cups salad with:
　Tomato, cucumber, olives,
　　and red onion
　2 tablespoons oil and vinegar dressing

8 ounces (250 ml) unsweetened iced tea

THE FIXES

◦ Cut the spaghetti portion in half and
switched to whole wheat spaghetti
to add fiber and lower the GL.

◦ Eliminated the bread and doubled
the size of the salad (just as filling as
bread), thus swapping empty calories
for fiber and vitamins and lowering
the GL.

◦ Topped the salad with oil and vinegar
dressing instead of blue cheese to cut
saturated fat and add a dose of sugar-
lowering acid from the vinegar.

Total GL: 14
Total calories: 550

BETTER still: Choose a pasta like
Barilla Plus, which contains extra protein,
fiber, and omega-3 fatty acids.

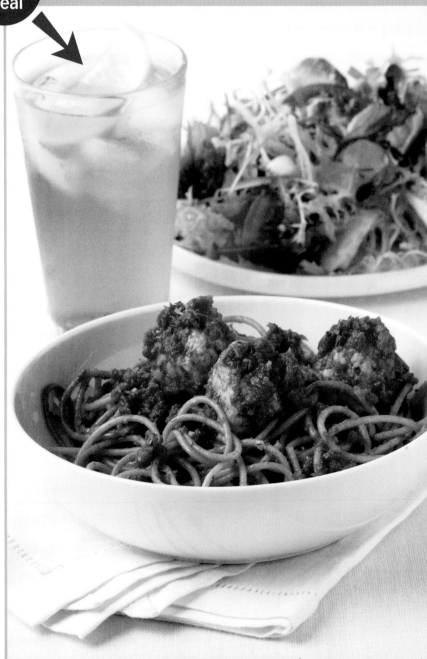

Typical Dinner

1 4-ounce (125-g) pork chop

1 1/2 cups cooked fettucine with
1 tablespoon butter, 1 tablespoon
Parmesan cheese, 1 tablespoon parsley

1 white dinner roll with 1 tablespoon butter

12 ounces (341 ml) beer

Total GL: 33
Total calories: 627

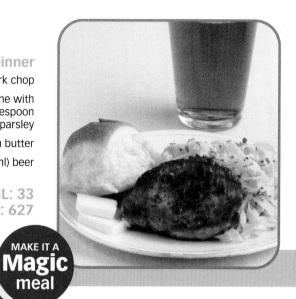

MAKE IT A
Magic
meal

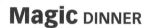

Magic DINNER

1 4-ounce (125-g) pork chop

1/2 cup Bulgur with Ginger and Orange
(recipe on page 264)

Sautéed Spinach with Ginger and Soy
Sauce (recipe on page 275)

12 ounces (341 ml) light beer

THE FIXES

- Swapped the fettucine for a better carbohydrate choice, bulgur. Pasta's not bad for you, but bulgur has more fiber and a lower GL.

- Eliminated the white roll, which adds nothing but GL to the meal.

- Added sautéed spinach to replace the roll. Spinach is loaded with fiber and nutrients and has a very low GL (and far fewer calories).

- Changed the regular beer to light beer to reduce carbs and calories.

Total GL: 17
Total calories: 665

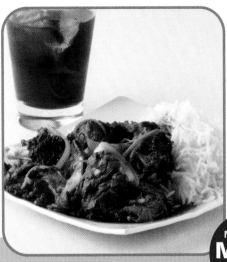

1 1/2 cups takeout beef and broccoli stir-fry

1 cup white rice

8 ounces (250 ml) soda

Total GL: 49
Total calories: 1,223

MAKE IT A
Magic
meal

DINNER MAKEOVERS DINNER MAKEOVERS

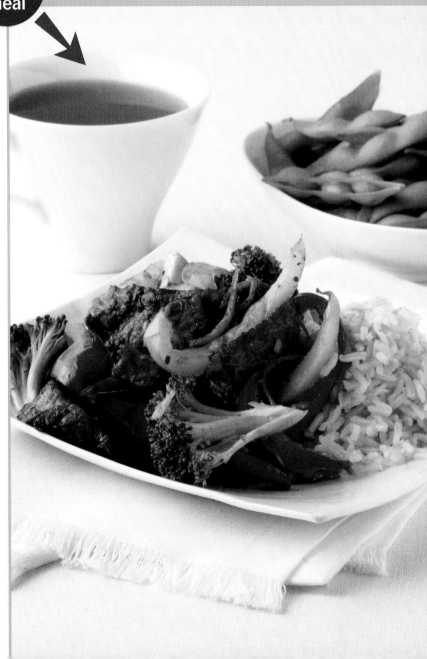

Magic DINNER

1 cup unshelled edamame

1 1/2 cups Orange Beef Stir-Fry with
Broccoli and Red Pepper
(recipe on page 226)

1/2 cup brown rice

Black or green tea

THE FIXES

⬡ Made the stir-fry at home using leaner
beef, less oil, and more vegetables.
The result: fewer calories and less
saturated fat, which clogs arteries
and hampers insulin sensitivity.

⬡ Substituted brown rice for white and
cut the portion in half to dramatically
decrease the meal's GL.

⬡ Started the meal with edamame
(steamed green soybeans) to fill you
up on a low-GL, fiber- and protein-rich
food so you won't miss the rest of the
rice. Edamame also slows eating
because it takes time to get the beans
out of their shells.

⬡ Replaced high-GL soda with no-GL
green tea.

Total GL: 14
Total calories: 612

Typical Dinner

1 roasted chicken breast with skin

1 cup mashed potatoes

1/2 cup gravy

1 cup stuffing

Mineral water with lemon

Total GL: 51
Total calories: 1,053

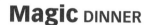

MAKE IT A
Magic
meal

Magic DINNER

1 roasted chicken breast without skin

1/3 cup gravy

1 cup apple-walnut stuffing

3/4 cup Moroccan Spiced Carrots
(recipe on page 274)

Mineral water with lemon

THE FIXES

- Eliminated the chicken skin, a significant source of saturated fat (which hampers insulin sensitivity) and calories.

- Cut out the un-Magic mashed potatoes and replaced them with carrots to increase fiber and vitamins and substantially lower the GL of the meal.

- Added apples and walnuts to the stuffing to decrease the GL (more apples and walnuts mean less bread) and add some "good" fat from the nuts to further lower the GL.

Total GL: 28
Total calories: 760

DESSERT**makeovers**

Everyone likes dessert—but nowhere else do the evils of white flour, sugar, and saturated fat converge in such a perfect storm, making your blood sugar surge. In terms of glycemic load and extra calories, most desserts are the last thing you need. But that doesn't mean dessert in general is off-limits. When the cake comes around, don't say no; instead, say, "I'll take half a piece please, with lots of berries on top."

Our top four DESSERT GUIDELINES:

(1) Think fruit, fruit, fruit. It's sweet and refreshing and easily transformed into an almost endless variety of attractive, easy-to-make desserts (for proof, check out the dessert recipes in Part 4).

(2) Watch portion sizes. The truth is, you can eat whatever you like if the portion is small enough. Use a small plate, such as a saucer, or a child-size cereal bowl for ice cream to help make smaller portions look more substantial. Or, to make your dessert fill up a big plate or bowl, add fruit such as pineapple, blueberries, or banana.

(3) Hunt for whole grains. Most baked goods are made with white flour, but they don't have to be. In fact, many of our dessert recipes in Part 4 cut down the amount of white flour in favor of blood sugar–friendly oats, whole wheat flour, and so on.

(4) Go low fat. Whether it's the ice cream you buy or the cream cheese you put in your cheesecake, make it reduced fat to avoid the nasty saturated fats that hamper your body's ability to handle blood sugar.

Finally, think of dessert as a treat—not a daily habit. Indulge twice a week to keep your sweet tooth happy. The rest of the week, top off dinner with an evening stroll instead.

Typical Dessert

1 slice apple pie
with 1/2 cup ice cream

Total GL: 29
Total calories: 363

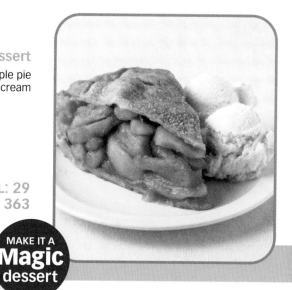

DESSERT MAKEOVERS   DESSERT MAKEOVERS

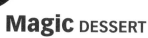

MAKE IT A
Magic
dessert

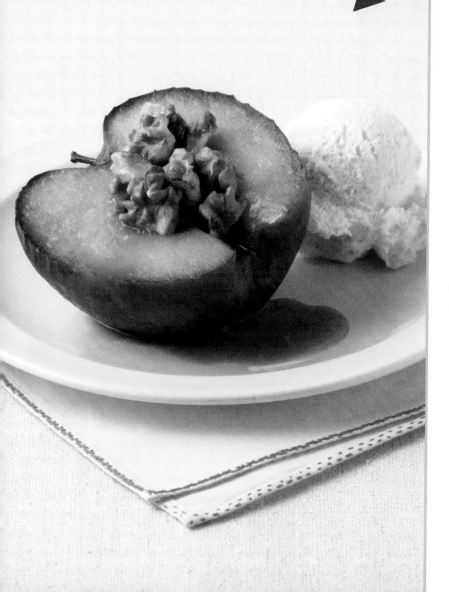

Magic DESSERT

1 Maple-Walnut Roasted Apple
  with ice cream (recipe on page 282)

THE FIXES

◌ Kept the apple but got rid of the piecrust and the extra sugar used for the filling. Both of these ingredients are responsible for increasing the GL of this dessert (plus, the piecrust is high in calories and full of saturated fat).

◌ Added walnuts for protein and "good" fat to help fill you up and further lower the dessert's GL.

◌ Cut the ice cream down to one small scoop and switched to reduced-fat ice cream to lower the saturated fat.

Total GL: 17
Total calories: 207

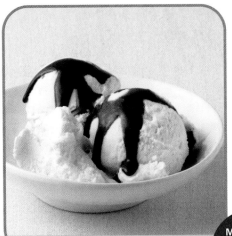

1 cup vanilla ice cream with
1/3 cup hot fudge sauce

Total GL: 39
Total calories: 329

MAKE IT A
Magic
dessert

DESSERT MAKEOVERS   DESSERT MAKEOVERS

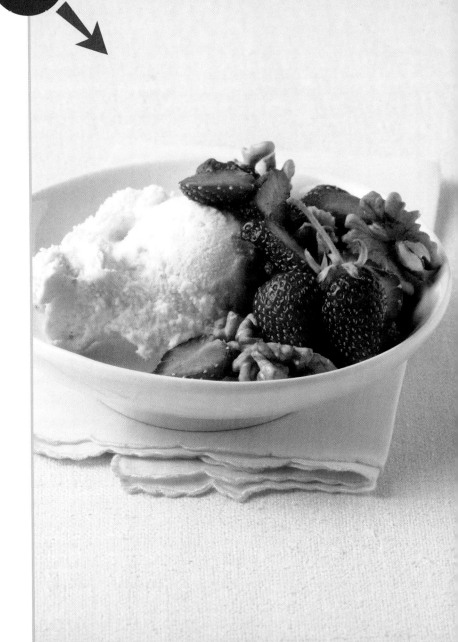

Magic DESSERT

1/2 cup vanilla ice cream with:
　1/2 cup strawberries
　5 toasted walnut halves

THE FIXES

○ Decreased the portion of ice cream
　since it has a lot of sugar and a high
　GL, not to mention saturated fat,
　which hampers insulin sensitivity.

○ Scrapped the sugar-laden hot fudge,
　along with its glycemic load.

○ Added walnuts and strawberries
　to fill up the bowl and provide fiber,
　nutrients, and healthy fats (from
　the walnuts) to help improve insulin
　sensitivity.

Total GL: 12
Total calories: 224

Typical Dessert

1 large piece chocolate cake
with frosting

Total GL: 23
Total calories: 439

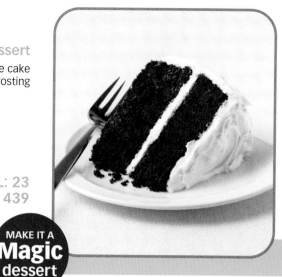

MAKE IT A
Magic
dessert

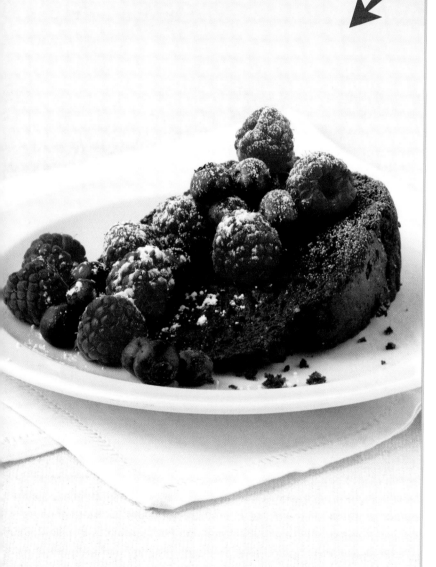

Magic DESSERT

1 small piece unfrosted chocolate cake
dusted with confectioner's sugar

1/2 cup mixed blueberries and
raspberries

THE FIXES

- Decreased the portion size of the
cake to cut refined carbohydrates
and therefore the GL.

- Eliminated the frosting, which has
a high GL.

- Added berries to increase the
nutritional value of the dessert
and make the smaller portion of
cake more satisfying.

**Total GL: 12
Total calories: 309**

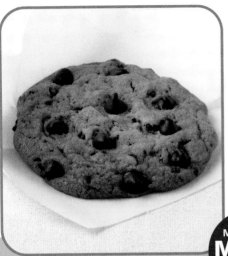

Typical Dessert
1 large chocolate chip cookie

Total GL: 19
Total calories: 196

Magic DESSERT

1 Oatmeal–Peanut Butter Trail Bar
   (recipe on page 207)

THE FIX

○ Swapped the cookie, made with the triple evils of sugar, butter, and white flour, for an even more delicious trail bar made with whole grains (full of fiber) and peanut butter (full of protein and "good" fat) to lower the GL and keep you fuller longer. The bar also provides extra nutrition from dried fruit.

Total GL: 13
Total calories: 175

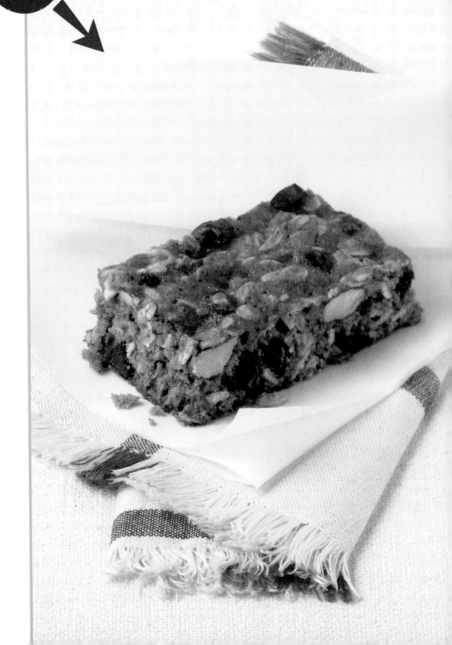

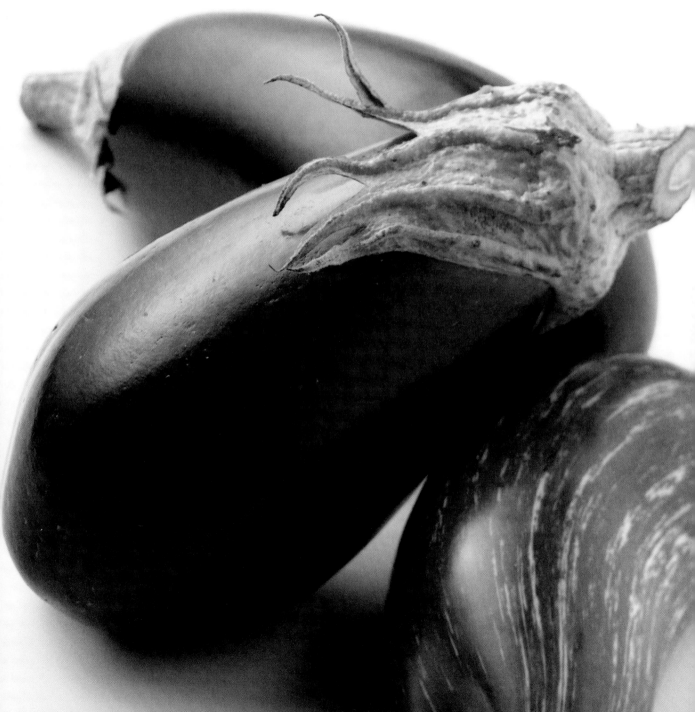

part 4

Magic Recipes
and meal plans

BREAKFASTS

Multi-Grain Pancakes or Waffles

8 Serves | Preparation time: 20 minutes
Cooking time: 15 to 20 minutes

Most pancakes are anything but Magic, but here the weekend treats have been entirely re-imagined. We've slashed the white flour and added whole wheat flour and oats, plus an unexpected dash of sugar-lowering cinnamon. Wheat germ provides healthy fats, extra fiber, and deliciously nutty flavor. *See photo on page 195.*

2 cups low-fat buttermilk (see Tip, page 198)

1/2 cup old-fashioned rolled **oats**

2/3 cup **whole wheat flour**

2/3 cup all-purpose flour

1/4 cup toasted **wheat germ**

1 1/2 teaspoons baking powder

1/2 teaspoon baking soda

1/4 teaspoon salt

1 teaspoon **cinnamon**

2 large **eggs**

1/4 cup firmly packed brown sugar

1 tablespoon canola oil

2 teaspoons vanilla extract

1 cup maple syrup, warmed

1 1/2 cups sliced **strawberries** or **blueberries**

1. Mix the buttermilk and oats in a small bowl. Let stand for 15 minutes.

2. Whisk the whole wheat flour, all-purpose flour, wheat germ, baking powder, baking soda, salt, and cinnamon in a large bowl.

3. Whisk the eggs, sugar, oil, and vanilla in a medium bowl. Add the buttermilk mixture. Add this mixture to the flour mixture and mix with a rubber spatula just until flour mixture is moistened.

4. To cook the pancakes: Coat a large nonstick skillet with cooking spray. Heat over medium heat. Spoon about 1/4 cup batter for each pancake into the skillet and cook until bottoms are golden and small bubbles start to form on top, about 3 minutes. Flip the pancakes and cook until browned and cooked through, 1 to 2 minutes. (Adjust the heat as necessary for even browning.) Keep the pancakes warm in a 200°F (90°C) oven while you finish cooking the remaining batter.

To cook the waffles: Coat a waffle iron with cooking spray. Heat the iron. Spoon in enough of the batter to cover three-quarters of the surface, close the iron, and cook until the waffles are crisp and golden brown, 4 to 5 minutes. Keep the waffles warm in a 200°F (90°C) oven while you finish cooking the remaining batter.

5. Top with maple syrup and strawberries (or blueberries). One serving is 2 pancakes or waffles. Wrap any leftover pancakes or waffles individually in plastic wrap and refrigerate for up to 2 days or freeze for up to 1 month. Reheat in a toaster or toaster oven.

Per serving: 292 calories, 8 g protein, 60 g carbohydrates, 3 g fiber, 3 g total fat, 1 g saturated fat, 56 mg cholesterol, 331 mg sodium.

Oatmeal with Apple and Flaxseeds

4
Serves

Preparation time: 5 minutes

Cooking time: 10 minutes

What better way to start your day than with a comforting bowl of steaming oatmeal? This simple breakfast packs not one or two but *six* Magic foods to steady your blood sugar and keep you full till lunch.

2 cups low-fat (1%) **milk** or vanilla **soy milk**

3/4 cup old-fashioned rolled **oats** (*not* quick oats)

1 medium **apple,** peeled, cored and chopped

1/3 cup dried cranberries or raisins

1/2 teaspoon **cinnamon**

1/4 cup whole **flaxseeds,** ground (see Tip, page 197) or 1/3 cup flaxseed meal

1/4 cup nonfat plain or vanilla **yogurt**

1/4 cup maple syrup, warmed, or 2 tablespoons brown sugar

1. Combine the milk, rolled oats, apple, dried cranberries (or raisins), and cinnamon in a heavy medium saucepan. Bring to a simmer over medium-high heat, stirring almost constantly.

2. Reduce the heat to medium-low and cook, stirring often, until creamy and thickened, 3 to 5 minutes.

3. Stir in the flaxseeds. Spoon the cereal into individual bowls and top each serving with a dollop of yogurt and a drizzle of maple syrup. One serving is 2/3 cup. Leftovers will keep, covered, in the refrigerator for up to 2 days. Reheat in the microwave.

Per serving: 282 calories, 10 g protein, 47 g carbohydrates, 6 g fiber, 7 g total fat, 1 g saturated fat, 8 mg cholesterol, 84 mg sodium.

Zucchini-Basil Frittata

2
Serves

Preparation time: 15 minutes

Cooking time: 8 to 12 minutes

Eggs are one of our favorite Magic foods because they're an inexpensive and remarkably complete source of protein, which doesn't budge blood sugar a bit. This frittata (an Italian-style flat omelet) includes zucchini to help you get more veggies into your diet.

1 tablespoon **olive oil,** divided

1/2 cup thinly sliced **onion** (1 small)

1 1/2 cups shredded **zucchini** (1 small)

2 **garlic** cloves, minced

4 large **eggs**

1/2 teaspoon hot red pepper sauce, such as Tabasco

1/8 teaspoon salt, or to taste

Freshly ground black pepper to taste

1/2 cup grated Parmesan **cheese**

1/3 cup chopped fresh basil

1. Heat 2 teaspoons oil in a 10-inch (25-centimeter) nonstick broiler-proof skillet over medium heat. Add onion and cook, stirring often, until softened, 1 1/2 to 2 minutes. Add zucchini and garlic; cook, stirring often, until zucchini is tender and most of the moisture has evaporated, 2 to 3 minutes. Transfer to a plate and let cool slightly. Rinse and dry the skillet.

2. Blend the eggs, hot sauce, salt, and pepper briskly with a fork in a medium bowl. Stir in the zucchini mixture, Parmesan, and basil.

3. Preheat the broiler. Brush the remaining 1 teaspoon oil over the skillet. Heat over medium-low heat. Pour in the egg mixture. Cook, lifting edges with a heat-resistant rubber spatula and tilting the skillet to allow the uncooked egg to flow underneath from time to time, until the bottom is golden, 3 to 4 minutes.

4. Place the skillet under the broiler and cook until the top is firm to touch and set, 2 to 4 minutes. Slide the frittata onto a plate and cut into wedges.

Per serving: 219 calories, 17 g protein, 9 g carbohydrates, 2 g fiber, 13 g total fat, 4 g saturated fat, 18 mg cholesterol, 580 mg sodium.

Spinach and Goat Cheese Omelet

1
Serves | Preparation time: 10 minutes
| Cooking time: 2 minutes

A French-style, folded omelet is one of the fastest protein-rich meals you can make. It is also an excellent strategy for healthy solo dining. Omelet filling options are limitless. Try the variations below or improvise with leftover cooked vegetables or ingredients at hand. *See photo on next page.*

2 cups baby **spinach,** rinsed

2 tablespoons crumbled goat **cheese** or feta cheese

1 tablespoon chopped **scallion**

1 large **egg**

2 large **egg** whites

1/4 teaspoon hot red pepper sauce, such as Tabasco

Pinch of salt

Pinch of freshly ground black pepper

1 teaspoon **olive oil**

1. Bring about 1 inch (2.5 centimeters) of water to a boil in a large saucepan. Drop in spinach and cook just until wilted, about 30 seconds. Drain, press out liquid and chop coarsely. (Alternatively, place spinach in a microwave-safe bowl, cover with vented plastic wrap, and microwave on high for 1 to 2 minutes.) Place the spinach in a small bowl. Stir in the cheese and scallion.

2. Blend egg, egg whites, hot sauce, salt, and pepper briskly with a fork in a medium bowl. Heat oil in a 7- to 10-inch (18- to 25-centimeter) nonstick skillet over medium-high heat until hot. Tilt the skillet to swirl oil over surface. Pour in egg mixture. Immediately stir egg mixture with heat-resistant rubber spatula or fork for a few seconds. Then use spatula to push cooked portions at edges toward the center, tilting the skillet to allow uncooked egg mixture to fill in areas around edges. Sprinkle spinach mixture over the omelet. Continue to cook until almost set, and the bottom is golden. The entire cooking process should take about 1 minute.

3. Use a spatula to fold one-third of the omelet over the filling. Tip the skillet and, using spatula as a guide, slide the omelet onto a plate so that it lands, folded in thirds, seam-side down.

Per serving: 235 calories, 20 g protein, 4 g carbohydrates, 1 g fiber, 15 g total fat, 6 g saturated fat, 228 mg cholesterol, 471 mg sodium.

VARIATIONS
Mushroom Omelet

Omit the spinach, goat cheese, and scallion. In Step 1, heat 1 teaspoon oil in a medium nonstick skillet over medium-high heat. Add 1/2 cup sliced mushrooms. Cook, stirring often, until browned, 3 to 4 minutes. Stir in 1 tablespoon parsley and a pinch of salt and pepper. In Step 2, sprinkle the mushroom mixture over the omelet.

Broccoli and Cheese Omelet

Substitute 2 tablespoons chopped cooked broccoli and 2 tablespoons shredded Swiss or cheddar cheese for the spinach, goat cheese, and scallion in the filling.

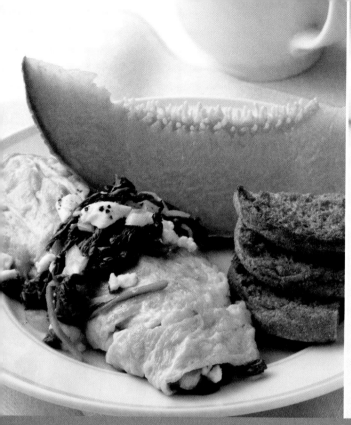

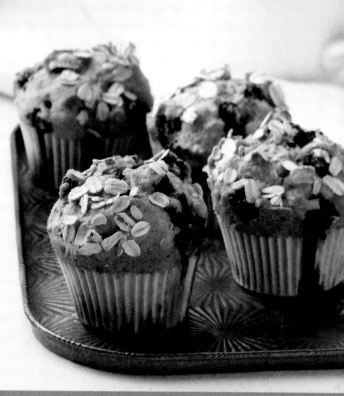

Spinach and Goat Cheese Omelet *page 194*
spinach • cheese • scallion • egg • olive oil

Whole Wheat Flaxseed Bread *page 196*
whole wheat flour • flaxseed • milk • olive oil

Blueberry-Oatmeal Muffins *page 198*
**whole wheat flour • cinnamon • oats • egg
• berries**

Multi-Grain Pancakes or Waffles *page 192*
**oats • whole wheat flour • wheat germ • cinnamon
• egg • berries**

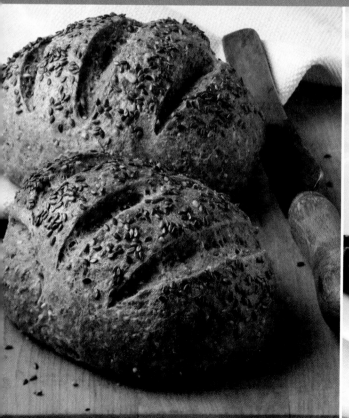

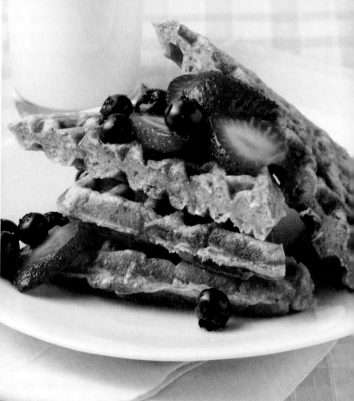

BREADS AND MUFFINS

Whole Wheat Flaxseed Bread

1
Loaf

| **Preparation time: 20 minutes**
| **Rising/baking time (for food processor method): about 3 hours**

Many of the healthy-sounding multi-grain and wheat breads on the shelves actually contain only a tiny proportion of whole grain. An enjoyable way to make sure you're getting at least 50 percent whole wheat flour in a loaf is to make your own. Flaxseed is a Magic addition to this bread; it increases the amount of blood sugar–lowering soluble fiber and contributes a delightful nutty taste. Note: Since bread machines come in both a 1-pound/450-gram (2 cup) and a 1 1/2-pound/700-gram (3-cup) capacity, we offer proportions to suit either. *See photo on page 195.*

1-POUND (450-GRAM) LOAF (8 SLICES)

1 1/3 cups whole wheat flour

2/3 cup bread flour or all-purpose flour

3 tablespoons whole flaxseed, ground (see Tip, opposite page), or 1/4 cup flaxseed meal

2 tablespoons nonfat dry milk

1 1/2 teaspoons bread machine yeast

3/4 teaspoon salt

3/4 cup water, at room temperature

1 tablespoon molasses or honey

1 tablespoon olive oil

1 1/2-POUND (700-GRAM) LOAF (12 SLICES)

2 cups whole wheat flour

1 cup bread flour or all-purpose flour

1/4 cup whole flaxseed, ground (see Tip, opposite page), or 1/3 cup flaxseed meal

3 tablespoons nonfat dry milk

2 teaspoons bread machine yeast

1 teaspoon salt

1 cup plus 2 tablespoons water, at room temperature

2 tablespoons molasses or honey

1 tablespoon olive oil

TOPPING FOR FOOD PROCESSOR/OVEN METHOD

1 egg white, lightly beaten with 1 tablespoon water

1 tablespoon whole flaxseed

To mix the dough and bake the bread in a bread machine: Place all of the ingredients in a bread machine pan in the order recommended by the manufacturer (do not place the yeast in direct contact with the liquids and salt). Select the whole wheat or basic cycle and medium crust, then press start. Once the dough is mixed, check the consistency; it should be smooth yet soft to the touch. Adjust if necessary by adding flour 1 tablespoon at a time or water 1 teaspoon at a time. When the bread has finished the baking cycle, transfer it to a rack to cool.

To mix the dough in a food processor and bake the bread in the oven:

1. In a food processor fitted with a metal chopping blade, combine the whole wheat flour, bread (or all-purpose) flour, ground flaxseed (or flaxseed meal), dry milk, yeast, and salt and pulse several times to blend. In a measuring cup, stir together the water, molasses (or honey), and oil until the molasses is fully dissolved; set aside. With the motor running, slowly pour enough of the liquid through the feeder tube to make a smooth dough that pulls away from the sides of

the workbowl. The consistency should be smooth yet soft to the touch; adjust if necessary by adding flour 1 tablespoon at a time or water 1 teaspoon at a time. Process for 1 minute to knead. Transfer the dough to a bowl coated with cooking spray and turn to coat. Cover with plastic wrap and let rise at room temperature until doubled in bulk, 1 1/2 to 1 3/4 hours.

2. Coat a baking sheet with cooking spray. When the dough has doubled, turn it out onto a lightly floured surface. Punch it down and shape into a round or oval loaf (or make 2 small loaves). Place the loaf on the baking sheet. Coat a sheet of plastic wrap with cooking spray and cover the loaf with it. Let rise until almost doubled in bulk, about 1 hour.

3. Meanwhile, place a small metal baking pan on the bottom oven rack. Preheat the oven to 400°F (200°C).

4. When the loaf has risen, brush it with the egg white mixture and sprinkle with the whole flaxseed. Pour 1 cup water into the baking pan in the oven to create steam. Use a serrated knife to score four 1/4-inch (5-millimeter)-deep slashes in the loaf. Bake until the bread is golden and sounds hollow when tapped, 20 to 30 minutes. Transfer to a wire rack to cool. One serving is 1 slice.

Per serving: 155 calories, 5 g protein, 27 g carbohydrates, 3 g fiber, 4 g total fat, 1 g saturated fat, 0 mg cholesterol, 229 mg sodium.

Tip: To grind flaxseeds, use a spice mill (such as a clean coffee grinder) or a blender to grind it into coarse meal. Flaxseeds must be ground in order for your body to reap the nutritional benefits.

Apple-Bran Muffins

12 muffins

| Preparation time: 20 minutes |
| Baking time: 20 minutes |

Bran muffins never tasted so good or boasted so many Magic ingredients. Applesauce keeps these low-fat, fiber-rich treats moist and tender. If you bake a batch on the weekend, you can wrap the leftovers individually in plastic wrap and freeze them so you can enjoy wholesome, homemade muffins on busy weekday mornings.

2 large eggs

1/2 cup packed light brown sugar

1 cup unsweetened applesauce

3/4 cup low-fat buttermilk (see Tip, next page)

1 cup unprocessed wheat bran

3 tablespoons canola oil

1 teaspoon vanilla extract

1 cup whole wheat flour

3/4 cup all-purpose flour

1 1/2 teaspoons baking powder

1/2 teaspoon baking soda

1/4 teaspoon salt

2 teaspoons ground cinnamon

1/4 teaspoon ground nutmeg

1 cup chopped peeled apple (1 medium)

1/3 cup chopped walnuts

1. Preheat the oven to 400°F (200°C). Coat 12 standard-size muffin cups (2 3/4 x 1 1/4-inch/ 7 x 3-centimeter) with cooking spray.

2. In a medium bowl, whisk the eggs and brown sugar until smooth. Add the applesauce, buttermilk, bran, oil, and vanilla and whisk until blended.

3. In a large bowl, whisk together the whole wheat flour, all-purpose flour, baking powder, baking soda, salt, cinnamon, and nutmeg. Add the egg mixture and mix with a rubber spatula

just until the dry ingredients are moistened. Fold in the apple. Spoon the batter into the muffin cups and sprinkle with the walnuts.

4. Bake until the tops of the muffins spring back when touched lightly, 18 to 22 minutes. Let cool in the pan on a rack for 5 minutes, then loosen the edges of the muffins and turn out onto a wire rack. Let cool slightly before serving. One serving is 1 muffin.

Per serving: 194 calories, 5 g protein, 31 g carbohydrates, 4 g fiber, 7 g total fat, 1 g saturated fat, 36 mg cholesterol, 194 mg sodium.

Tip: To thaw a frozen muffin, remove the plastic wrap, wrap in a paper towel, and microwave on defrost (20% power) for 1 to 2 minutes. To thaw in the oven, wrap in foil and bake at 300°F (150°C) for 25 to 35 minutes.

Blueberry-Oatmeal Muffins

12 muffins | **Preparation time: 25 minutes**

Baking time: 20 minutes

Pairing rolled oats—filled with blood sugar–lowering soluble fiber—with antioxidant-rich blueberries makes for a Magic breakfast, especially when you add cinnamon, as we have. Maple syrup provides subtle sweetness; it complements the blueberries and lets the fruity flavor shine through—and it has a lower GL than table sugar. *See photo on page 195.*

3/4 cup plus 2 tablespoons whole wheat flour

3/4 cup all-purpose flour

1 1/2 teaspoons baking powder

1/2 teaspoon baking soda

1/4 teaspoon salt

1 teaspoon ground cinnamon

1 cup plus 2 tablespoons old-fashioned rolled oats

1 large egg

2 large egg whites

1/2 cup maple syrup

3/4 cup low-fat buttermilk (see Tip)

3 tablespoons canola oil

2 teaspoons grated orange zest

1 tablespoon orange juice

1 teaspoon vanilla extract

1 1/2 cups fresh blueberries, rinsed and patted dry

1. Preheat the oven to 400°F (200°C). Coat 12 standard-size (2 3/4 x 1 1/4-inch/7 x 3-centimeter) muffin cups with cooking spray or insert paper liners.

2. In a large bowl, whisk together the whole wheat flour, all-purpose flour, baking powder, baking soda, salt, and cinnamon. Stir in 1 cup rolled oats.

3. In a medium bowl, whisk the egg, egg white, and syrup until smooth. Add the buttermilk, oil, orange zest, orange juice, and vanilla and whisk until blended. Add to the flour mixture and mix with a rubber spatula just until the dry ingredients are moistened. Fold in the blueberries. Spoon the batter into the muffin cups, filling them almost to the top. Sprinkle the tops with the remaining 2 tablespoons rolled oats.

4. Bake until the muffins are lightly browned and the tops spring back when touched lightly, 18 to 22 minutes. Loosen the edges of the muffins, turn out onto a wire rack, and let cool slightly before serving. One serving is 1 muffin.

Per serving: 180 calories, 5 g protein, 30 g carbohydrates, 3 g fiber, 5 g total fat, 0 g saturated fat, 18 mg cholesterol, 190 mg sodium.

Tip: If you don't have buttermilk on hand, make your own "sour milk" by mixing 1 tablespoon lemon juice or vinegar with enough low-fat milk or plain soy milk to measure 1 cup. Alternatively, blend equal proportions of fat-free plain yogurt and low-fat milk. Shelf-stable buttermilk powder is another option; substitute according to package directions, but for added calcium and body, replace liquid with low-fat milk instead of water.

Upside-Down Nectarine Muffins

12 muffins
Preparation time: 25 minutes

Baking time: 20 minutes

There is nothing ordinary about these muffins. A bit like individual upside-down cakes, they boast an irresistible caramelized fruit topping. They're tasty treats indeed—with the Magic benefits of whole grains, stone fruit, nuts, and cinnamon.

TOPPING

2 tablespoons packed light brown sugar

1/4 cup **walnuts,** chopped

12 ounces (340 grams) **nectarines** (about 3 medium), pitted and cut into 1/4-inch (5-millimeter)-thick wedges

MUFFINS

1 cup **whole wheat flour**

1 cup all-purpose flour

1 1/2 teaspoons baking powder

1/2 teaspoon baking soda

1/4 teaspoon salt

1 1/2 teaspoons ground **cinnamon**

1/2 teaspoon ground nutmeg

2 large **eggs**

1/2 cup packed light brown sugar

1 cup low-fat buttermilk (see Tip, page 198)

3 tablespoons canola oil

1 teaspoon vanilla extract

1. Preheat the oven to 400°F (200°C). Coat 12 standard-size (2 3/4 x 1 1/4-inch/7 x 3-centimeter) muffin cups with cooking spray.

2. **To make the topping:** Sprinkle about 1/2 teaspoon brown sugar into each muffin cup and pat into an even layer, then sprinkle about 1 teaspoon walnuts into each cup. Arrange 3 or 4 nectarine slices, slightly overlapping, over the walnuts and brown sugar. Cover and set aside. Coarsely chop the remaining nectarines (you should have about 3/4 cup); set aside.

3. **To make the muffins:** In a large bowl, whisk together the whole wheat flour, all-purpose flour, baking powder, baking soda, salt, cinnamon, and nutmeg.

4. In a medium bowl, whisk the eggs and brown sugar until smooth. Whisk in the buttermilk, oil, and vanilla. Add to the flour mixture and mix with a rubber spatula just until the dry ingredients are moistened, then fold in the reserved nectarines. Spoon the batter into the muffin cups (they will seem quite full; the nectarine wedges will collapse during baking).

5. Bake until the muffins are lightly browned and the tops spring back when touched lightly, 18 to 22 minutes. Immediately loosen the edges and carefully turn the muffins out onto a wire rack. Replace any stray nectarine slices and spoon on any walnut pieces remaining in the muffin cups. Let cool slightly before serving. One serving is 1 muffin.

Per serving: 202 calories, 5 g protein, 32 g carbohydrates, 2 g fiber, 6 g total fat, 1 g saturated fat, 41 g cholesterol, 153 mg sodium.

VARIATION

Substitute 12 ounces (340 grams) plums or apricots for the nectarines.

SNACKS, APPETIZERS, AND BEVERAGES

Cherry Tomatoes Filled with Pesto Cream Cheese

16 Serves | Preparation time: 35 minutes
Cooking time: 0 minutes

Pesto and tomatoes are one of those time-honored combinations that taste better every time you try it. In this recipe, pesto is thickened with low-fat cream cheese to make a filling that bursts with the flavor of summer. Stuffed into cherry tomatoes, it makes an exceptionally attractive appetizer that is not at all hard to prepare. You can make the pesto cream cheese filling ahead of time (refrigerate it, covered, for up to 2 days), but wait until shortly before serving to stuff the tomatoes. *See photo on page 201.*

3 cups fresh basil leaves, washed and dried

1/3 cup plus 2 tablespoons pine **nuts,** toasted (see Tip)

2 medium **garlic** cloves, minced

1/2 teaspoon salt, or to taste

Freshly ground pepper to taste

1 tablespoon extra-virgin **olive oil**

1 package (8 ounces/250 grams) reduced-fat cream **cheese** (Neufchâtel), cut into chunks

2 pints (4 cups) cherry **tomatoes,** washed and dried

1. Combine the basil, 1/3 cup pine nuts, garlic, salt, and pepper in a food processor. Process until pine nuts are ground. With motor running, drizzle in olive oil. Add cream cheese and pulse until smooth and creamy.

2. Shortly before serving, make an X on the rounded side (opposite stem) of each cherry tomato with a serrated or sharp paring knife. Scoop out the seeds with a grapefruit spoon or your fingertips, taking care to keep the tomatoes intact.

3. Scrape the cream cheese filling into a pastry bag fitted with a star tip or small plastic food bag with a 1/2-inch (1-centimeter) hole snipped in one corner. Pipe a rosette of filling into each cherry tomato cavity. Garnish the cherry tomatoes with the remaining pine nuts. One serving equals 3 filled cherry tomatoes.

Per serving: 70 calories, 2 g protein, 2 g carbohydrates, 0 g fiber, 6 g total fat, 2 g saturated fat, 8 mg cholesterol, 116 mg sodium.

Tip: Toast pine nuts in a small dry skillet over medium-low heat, stirring constantly, until light golden and fragrant, 2 to 3 minutes. Transfer to a small bowl and let cool.

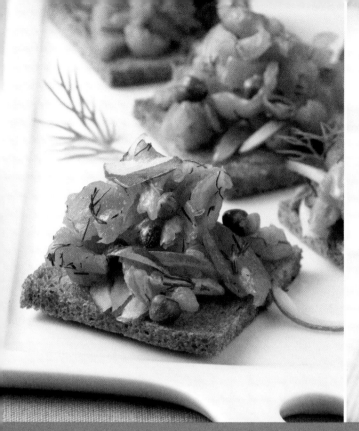

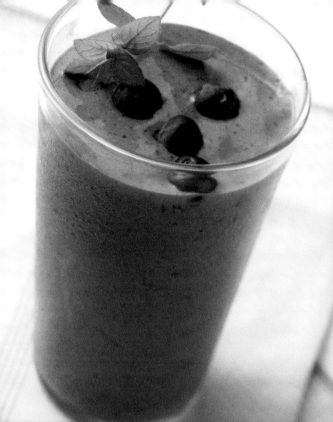

Smoked Salmon Canapés *page 203*
rye bread • lemon • tea • olive oil • salmon • onion

Warm Artichoke and Bean Dip *page 204*
beans • garlic • cheese

Berry-Flaxseed Smoothie *page 208*
flaxseed • yogurt • berries

Cherry Tomatoes Filled with Pesto Cream Cheese *page 200*
nuts • garlic • olive oil • cheese • tomato

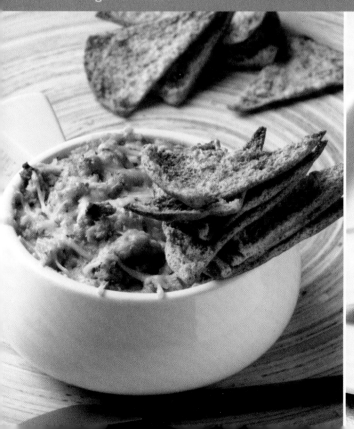

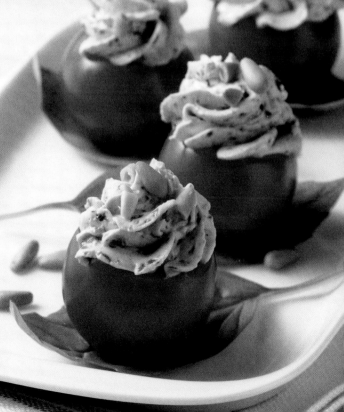

Caponata

12 Serves
Preparation time: 25 minutes

Cooking time: 30 to 35 minutes

Caponata is terrific for entertaining because you can make it ahead of time. In fact, it gets better as it sits. Serve it in an attractive bowl, surrounded by whole grain crackers or toasted whole wheat baguette slices. You can also use it to perk up a sandwich filling or enliven a tomato-based pasta sauce. Made with plenty of vegetables and well flavored with olive oil—a "good fat" that may help reverse insulin resistance—this is a Magic way to begin a meal.

3 tablespoons **olive oil**

1 pound (450 grams) **eggplant,** cut into 1/2-inch (1 centimeter) cubes (6 cups)

1 cup chopped **onion** (1 small)

1 cup finely diced celery (4 stalks)

4 **garlic** cloves, minced

1/8 teaspoon crushed red pepper

1 can (14 1/2 ounces/398 milliliters) diced **tomatoes** (undrained)

1/4 cup sun-dried **tomatoes** (*not* oil-packed), finely chopped

3 tablespoons red-wine **vinegar**

8 cracked green **olives,** pitted and chopped (1/3 cup)

2 tablespoons drained capers, rinsed

1 tablespoon sugar

3 tablespoons currants

1/4 cup pine **nuts,** toasted (see Tip, page 256)

3 tablespoons chopped fresh parsley

1. Heat 1 tablespoon of oil in large nonstick skillet over medium-high heat. Add half of the eggplant and cook, stirring and turning eggplant, until browned and tender, 4 to 6 minutes. Transfer to a plate and set aside. Add 1 tablespoon oil to the skillet and repeat with the remaining eggplant. Set aside.

2. Add the remaining 1 tablespoon oil to the skillet. Add the onion and celery. Cook, stirring often until softened, 3 to 5 minutes. Add the garlic and red pepper. Cook, stirring, for 30 seconds. Add the diced tomatoes, sun-dried tomatoes, vinegar, olives, capers, sugar, and reserved eggplant. Bring to a simmer. Reduce heat to medium-low, cover skillet, and cook, stirring occasionally, until mixture has a chunky jam-like consistency, about 15 minutes. Add the currants and cook, covered, for 1 minute. Remove from heat. Stir in pine nuts and parsley. Let cool before serving. One serving is 2 1/2 tablespoons.

Per serving: 96 calories, 2 g protein, 10 g carbohydrates, 3 g fiber, 6 g total fat, 1 g saturated fat, 0 mg cholesterol, 182 mg sodium.

Marinated Olives

8 Serves
Preparation time: 5 minutes

Cooking time: 2 minutes

Full of "good fats," these highly savory nuggets are a perfect appetizer for better blood sugar.

2 teaspoons **olive oil**

2 **garlic** cloves

4 (2 x 1/2-inch/5 x 1-centimeter) strips orange peel

1 1/2 teaspoons fennel seeds

2 cups rinsed kalamata **olives**

2 tablespoons orange juice

1. Heat olive oil in medium skillet over low heat until warm. Add garlic, orange peel and fennel seeds. Cook, stirring, until fragrant, 30 to 60 seconds. Add olives. Cook, stirring, until warmed through but not hot, about 1 minute.

2. Remove from heat. Stir in the orange juice. Cover and let stand at room temperature for 1 hour. Serve at room temperature. One serving is 2 tablespoons. Refrigerate leftovers.

Per serving: 93 calories, 1 g protein, 3 g carbohydrates, 0 g fiber, 9 g total fat, 1 g saturated fat, 0 mg cholesterol, 509 mg sodium.

Smoked Salmon Canapés

12 Serves | Preparation time: 15 minutes | Baking time: 15 minutes

Party fare doesn't have to be a minefield of fatty foods and fast-acting carbohydrates. These elegant hors d'oeuvres offer a delectable bite of smoked salmon (a good source of protein and omega-3s), moistened with a light, lemony vinaigrette. Low-GL rye bread toasts make an excellent platform for the smoked salmon topping. Both the topping and toasts can be made early in the day. Refrigerate the topping, covered, for up to 8 hours. Store the toasts in an airtight container at room temperature. *See photo on page 201.*

24 slices cocktail **rye bread**

2 tablespoons **lemon** juice

2 tablespoons brewed black **tea** or vodka

1 tablespoon extra-virgin **olive oil**

2 teaspoons Dijon mustard

Freshly ground pepper to taste

8 ounces (250 grams) sliced smoked **salmon,** finely chopped (1 1/3 cups)

1/4 cup finely diced red **onion**

3 tablespoons chopped fresh dill, plus sprigs for garnish

2 tablespoons drained capers, rinsed and coarsely chopped

1. Preheat the oven to 325°F (160°C). Coat a baking sheet with nonstick spray. Arrange the cocktail rye bread slices in a single layer on the baking sheet. Spray the tops of slices lightly with nonstick spray. Bake the slices just until crisp, 12 to 15 minutes.

2. Whisk the lemon juice, tea (or vodka), oil, mustard, and pepper in a medium bowl. Add the smoked salmon, onion, dill, and capers. Toss to mix well.

3. Shortly before serving, mound about 1 tablespoon of topping on each slice of toast. Garnish each with a dill sprig. One serving is 2 canapés.

Per serving: 84 calories, 5 g protein, 9 g carbohydrates, 1 g fiber, 3 g total fat, 0 g saturated fat, 4 mg cholesterol, 311 mg sodium.

Spiced Almonds

8 Serves | Preparation time: 5 minutes | Cooking time: 25 to 30 minutes

Warm spices turn plain almonds into irresistible nibbles. And thanks to almonds' protein and "good fat," these are blood sugar–smart.

1 cup unpeeled whole **almonds**

1 teaspoon **olive oil**

3/4 teaspoon ground cumin

1/4 teaspoon salt

1/8 teaspoon cayenne pepper

1. Toss the almonds with olive oil, cumin, salt, and cayenne in a pie plate or shallow baking dish.

2. Bake at 350°F (180°C), stirring occasionally, until fragrant, 25 to 30 minutes. Let cool. One serving is 2 tablespoons. Almonds will keep, enclosed in an airtight container, for up to 1 week.

Per serving: 112 calories, 4 g protein, 4 g carbohydrates, 2 g fiber, 10 g total fat, 1 g saturated fat, 0 mg cholesterol, 73 mg sodium.

Warm Artichoke and Bean Dip

8
Serves

| Preparation time: 10 minutes |
| Baking time: 20 to 25 minutes |

Beans are the Magic ingredient in this lower-fat, higher-fiber version of a classic cheesy artichoke dip. It makes an appealing holiday appetizer and is an excellent choice for year-round entertaining as well. Try it with Whole Wheat Pita Crisps (page 207) or low-fat, whole grain crackers, such as Wasa, Kavli, or Ryvita. *See photo on page 201.*

1 can (19 or 15 ounces/540 or 398 milliliters) cannellini (white kidney) **beans,** drained and rinsed

1 can (14 ounces/398 milliliters) artichoke hearts, drained and rinsed

3 **garlic** cloves, minced

1 tablespoon reduced-fat mayonnaise

Pinch of cayenne pepper

Freshly ground pepper to taste

2/3 cup plus 2 tablespoons grated Parmesan **cheese**

1/4 cup chopped fresh parsley

1 teaspoon freshly grated lemon zest

1. Preheat the oven to 400°F (200°C). Coat a 2- to 3-cup baking dish with nonstick spray.

2. Place the beans, artichoke hearts, garlic, mayonnaise, cayenne, and black pepper in a food processor. Process until almost smooth, stopping to scrape down the sides of the workbowl once or twice. Transfer to a medium bowl. Stir in 2/3 cup of the Parmesan, parsley, and lemon zest. Scrape into the baking dish and smooth with a spatula. Sprinkle with the remaining 2 tablespoons Parmesan.

3. Bake the dip, uncovered, until heated through, 20 to 25 minutes. One serving is 1/4 cup.

Per serving: 116 calories, 7 g protein, 16 g carbohydrates, 5 g fiber, 3 g total fat, 2 g saturated fat, 7 mg cholesterol, 517 mg sodium.

Tip: Canned beans are high in sodium, but you can reduce the sodium by about 40 percent just by draining them. A 30-second rinse reduces sodium by another 3 percent. In our nutrition analyses we've assumed you've drained and rinsed the beans.

Asian Peanut Dip

8
Serves

| Preparation time: 10 minutes |
| Cooking time: 0 minutes |

Tofu stretches the peanut butter in this spicy dip, reducing calories and giving it a velvety consistency. Serve with crudités or as a spread for grown-up peanut butter sandwiches, made with whole wheat bread, grated carrots, sliced cucumbers, and lettuce. The dip also can be used as a dressing for an Asian noodle salad.

1/2 cup natural-style **peanut butter**

1/3 cup low-fat, firm silken **tofu**

3 tablespoons firmly packed light brown sugar

2 tablespoons reduced-sodium soy sauce

2 tablespoons **lime** juice

1/2 to 3/4 teaspoon crushed red pepper

2 **garlic** cloves, crushed

Place all of the ingredients in a food processor and process until smooth and creamy, stopping once or twice to scrape down sides of the workbowl. One serving is 2 tablespoons. The dip will keep, covered, in the refrigerator for up to 2 days.

Per serving: 120 calories, 5 g protein, 10 g carbohydrates, 1 g fiber, 7 g total fat, 2 g saturated fat, 0 mg cholesterol, 216 mg sodium.

Mediterranean Split Pea Spread

16 Serves
Preparation time: 10 minutes
Cooking time: 50 minutes

This Greek appetizer illustrates how the traditional Mediterranean diet can be healthy, and at the same time, delicious. The base of the spread is simply yellow split peas—boasting slow-acting complex carbohydrates. When seasoned with cumin, garlic, lemon juice, and fruity olive oil, they are transformed into a mouth-watering appetizer. Enjoy this spread as an opener to a leisurely meal, accompanied by Whole Wheat Pita Crisps (see page 207), whole grain crackers, olives, and feta cheese. It also makes a delicious sandwich filling.

2 1/4 cups water

3/4 cup dried yellow split peas or chana dahl, sorted and rinsed

6 garlic cloves, crushed

1/8 teaspoon crushed red pepper

3 tablespoons lemon juice

3 tablespoons extra-virgin olive oil, divided

1 1/2 teaspoons ground cumin

3/4 teaspoon salt, or to taste

2 tablespoons finely diced red onion

2 tablespoons coarsely chopped fresh dill

1. Combine the water, split peas (or chana dahl), garlic, and red pepper in a heavy medium saucepan. Bring to a boil. Reduce the heat to low, partially cover, and simmer, stirring occasionally, until the split peas are tender and most of the liquid has been absorbed, 40 to 50 minutes. (Add more water during cooking, if necessary. If the mixture seems too soupy at the end of cooking, simmer, uncovered, stirring constantly, for a few minutes, or until mixture has consistency of *very* thick split pea soup.) Let cool slightly.

2. Transfer the split pea mixture to a food processor. Add the lemon juice, 2 tablespoons of the olive oil, cumin, and salt. Process until smooth. To serve, spread the puree in a shallow serving dish. Drizzle with the remaining 1 tablespoon oil. Sprinkle with the red onion and dill. One serving is 2 tablespoons. The spread will keep, covered, in the refrigerator for up to 4 days.

Per serving: 58 calories, 2 g protein, 7 g carbohydrates, 1 g fiber, 3 g total fat, 0 g saturated fat, 0 mg cholesterol, 112 mg sodium.

White Bean Spread with Italian Flavors

12 Serves
Preparation time: 10 minutes
Cooking time: 0 minutes

A snap to make and wonderfully flavorful, this could be the perfect spread.

1 can (19 or 15 ounces/540 or 398 milliliters) cannellini beans, drained and rinsed

2 tablespoons extra-virgin olive oil

2 tablespoons lemon juice

1 garlic clove, minced

Pinch of cayenne pepper

Pinch of salt

Freshly ground pepper

1 1/2 teaspoons chopped fresh rosemary

1. Combine cannellini beans, olive oil, lemon juice, garlic, cayenne pepper, salt, and ground pepper to taste in a food processor. Pulse into a chunky puree. Transfer to a medium bowl and stir in rosemary. One serving is 2 tablespoons.

Per serving: 55 calories, 2 g protein, 6 g carbohydrates, 2 g fiber, 3 g total fat, 0 g saturated fat, 0 mg cholesterol, 66 mg sodium.

Chickpea Spread with Indian Flavors

12 Serves | Preparation time: 10 minutes

Cooking time: 1 minute

This spread has a bit of a kick, offset nicely by the cool yogurt.

2 tablespoons canola oil

2 jalapeño peppers, seeded and minced

1 tablespoon minced fresh ginger

2 garlic cloves, minced

2 teaspoons ground cumin

1 teaspoon ground coriander

1 can (19 or 15 ounces/540 or 398 milliliters) chickpeas, drained and rinsed

1/3 cup nonfat plain yogurt

2 tablespoons lime juice

1/8 teaspoon salt

Freshly ground pepper to taste

2 tablespoons chopped fresh cilantro (or parsley)

1. Heat canola oil in a small skillet over medium-high heat. Add jalapeño peppers, ginger and garlic. Cook, stirring, until fragrant, about 30 seconds. Stir in cumin and coriander. Remove from heat and transfer to a food processor.

2. Add chickpeas, yogurt, lime juice, salt, and pepper to taste. Process until smooth. Transfer to a medium bowl and stir in cilantro (or parsley). One serving is 2 1/3 tablespoons.

Per serving: 65 calories, 2 g protein, 7 g carbohydrates, 2 g fiber, 3 g total fat, 0 g saturated fat, 0 mg cholesterol, 108 mg sodium.

Black Bean Spread with Mexican Flavors

12 Serves | Preparation time: 10 minutes

Cooking time: 0 minutes

Fiber-rich canned beans provide the base for an easy spread that makes a satisfying snack to serve with crudités, whole grain crackers, Whole Wheat Pita Crisps (recipe next page) or Baked Tortilla Chips (recipe next page). It can also be used as a sandwich filling—spread on sourdough or whole wheat bread and top with grated carrots, sliced cucumber, tomatoes, and lettuce.

1 can (19 or 15 ounces/540 or 398 milliliters) black beans, drained and rinsed

2 tablespoons lime juice

1 tablespoon extra-virgin olive oil

1 garlic clove, minced

1 teaspoon ground cumin

1/4 teaspoon hot red pepper sauce, such as Tabasco

Pinch of salt

Freshly ground pepper to taste

2 tablespoons chopped fresh cilantro or parsley

1. Combine the black beans, lime juice, oil, garlic, cumin, hot sauce, salt, and pepper in a food processor. Process until smooth, stopping to scrape down the sides of the workbowl once or twice. Transfer to a medium bowl and stir in cilantro (or parsley). One serving is 2 tablespoons. The spread will keep, covered, in the refrigerator for up to 4 days.

Per serving: 36 calories, 2 g protein, 7 g carbohydrates, 2 g fiber, 2 g total fat, 0 g saturated fat, 0 mg cholesterol, 162 mg sodium

Baked Tortilla Crisps

8
Serves

Preparation time: 2 minutes

Cooking time: 10 to 15 minutes

These are a smart alternative to store-bought corn chips, which are much higher in fat and sodium.

1 package (9 ounces/297 grams) white corn tortillas (12 tortillas)

1/4 teaspoon salt

1. Stack tortillas and cut into 4 wedges. Spread wedges in a single layer on 2 baking sheets. Spray lightly with nonstick spray. Sprinkle with salt. Bake at 400°F (200°C) until light golden and crisp, 10 to 15 minutes. One serving is 6 crisps.

Per serving: 98 calories, 3 g protein, 20 g carbohydrates, 4 g fiber, 1 g total fat, 0 g saturated fat, 0 mg cholesterol, 411 mg sodium.

Whole Wheat Pita Crisps

8
Serves

Preparation time: 3 minutes

Cooking time: 8 to 10 minutes

Here is a healthy whole grain dipper for any of the spreads here.

4 whole wheat pita breads

1. Cut each pita bread into 4 triangles. Separate each triangle into 2 halves at the fold. Arrange, rough side up, on a baking sheet. Spritz lightly with olive oil nonstick spray. Bake at 425°F (220°C) until crisp, 8 to 10 minutes. One serving is 4 crisps.

Per serving: 60 calories, 2 g protein, 12 g carbohydrates, 2 g fiber, 1 g total fat, 0 g saturated fat, 0 mg cholesterol, 120 mg sodium.

Oatmeal-Peanut Butter Trail Bars

24
Bars

Preparation time: 25 minutes

Baking time: 20 to 25 minutes

When you bake your own "energy" bars, you can be assured that they include whole grains like rolled oats and whole wheat flour and healthy fats like canola oil, peanut butter, and walnuts. Peanut butter stands in for butter in these treats, reducing the saturated fat and boosting protein. These bars make ideal snacks—tuck one into your pocket when you head out the door.

1/2 cup **whole wheat flour**

1 teaspoon **cinnamon**

1/2 teaspoon baking soda

1/8 teaspoon salt

1/2 cup natural-style smooth **peanut butter** (see Ingredient Note, next page)

1/2 cup firmly packed brown sugar

1/3 cup honey

1 large **egg**

2 large **egg** whites (see Tip, next page)

2 tablespoons canola oil

2 teaspoons vanilla extract

2 cups old-fashioned rolled **oats**

1 cup dried cranberries (or raisins)

1/2 cup coarsely chopped **walnuts** or **almonds** (2 ounces/60 grams)

1/2 cup bittersweet or semisweet chocolate chips

1. Preheat the oven to 350°F (180°C). Coat a 9 x 13-inch (23 x 33-centimeter) baking pan with nonstick spray.

2. Whisk the flour, cinnamon, baking soda, and salt in a medium bowl. Beat the peanut butter, sugar, and honey in a large mixing bowl with an electric mixer until blended. Blend egg and egg whites with a fork in a small bowl. Add to the peanut butter mixture, along with oil and vanilla.

Beat until smooth. Add reserved flour mixture and mix with a rubber spatula. Mix in oats, dried cranberries (or raisins), walnuts (or almonds), and chocolate chips. Scrape batter into the prepared baking dish. Use a piece of plastic wrap to spread batter into an even layer.

3. Bake the bars until lightly browned and firm to the touch, 20 to 25 minutes. Let cool completely in the pan on a rack before cutting into 24 bars. One serving is one 2 x 2-inch (5 x 5-centimeter) bar.

Per serving: 175 calories, 4 g protein, 24 g carbohydrates, 2 g fiber, 8 g total fat, 1 g saturated fat, 9 mg cholesterol, 68 mg sodium.

Ingredient Note: If you must avoid peanut butter because of an allergy, you can substitute soy nut butter or sunflower seed butter (for tips on adapting recipes to sunflower seed butter, visit www.sunbutter.com). You can replace the nuts with unsalted roasted pepitas (pumpkin seeds) and/or sunflower seeds (look for unsalted seeds in the bulk bins of natural foods stores).

Tip: To avoid wasting the egg yolks, use reconstituted dried egg whites, such as Just Whites, which are available in the baking or natural foods sections of large supermarkets.

Chai

2	Preparation time: 2 minutes
Serves	Cooking time: 10 minutes

Chai, a milky spiced tea beverage that originated in India, is suddenly everywhere. It's easy to brew your own blend of this warming drink, and it's a good way to get some milk into your diet. This homemade version has a fraction of the calories and fat grams of coffee bar varieties—and it's much easier on your wallet.

1 1/2 cups water

1/4 teaspoon cinnamon

1/4 teaspoon ground cloves

1/4 teaspoon ground ginger

3 black tea bags

2/3 cup low-fat (1%) milk or vanilla soy milk

2 teaspoons honey, divided, or to taste

1. Combine the water, cinnamon, cloves, and ginger in a small saucepan. Bring to a simmer. Reduce heat to low, cover, and simmer for 5 minutes. Add the milk (or soy milk) and heat until steaming but not boiling. Remove from heat. Add the tea bags, cover, and let steep for 3 to 4 minutes. Pour the chai into 2 mugs and sweeten with honey, if desired. One serving is 1 cup.

Per serving: 63 calories, 3 g protein, 11 g carbohydrates, 0 g fiber, 1 g total fat, 1 g saturated fat, 3 mg cholesterol, 49 mg sodium.

Berry-Flaxseed Smoothie

2	Preparation time: 5 minutes
Serves	Cooking time: 0 minutes

A smoothie is a smart way to start your day, especially when it includes this tasty mix of Magic foods. Flaxseeds may seem like an unusual addition, but they blend in seamlessly and make this breakfast drink an excellent source of fiber. *See photo on page 201.*

2 tablespoons whole flaxseeds

1/2 cup orange juice

1/2 cup nonfat vanilla yogurt

1 cup unsweetened frozen mixed berries or blueberries

1 small banana, sliced

1. Place the flaxseeds in dry blender, cover, and blend until ground into a fine powder. Add the orange juice, yogurt, mixed berries (or blueberries), and banana. Cover and blend until smooth and creamy. One serving is 1 cup.

Per serving: 200 calories, 5 g protein, 36 g carbohydrates, 7 g fiber, 5 g total fat, 0 g saturated fat, 1 mg cholesterol, 33 mg sodium.

Peachy Iced Tea

8
Serves

| Preparation time: 5 minutes |
| Cooking time: 2 minutes |

To help wean you off soft drinks and sugary juice drinks made with high-fructose corn syrup, we've invented this delightfully refreshing iced tea enhanced with the sweet perfume of peach nectar. When buying the peach nectar or juice, look for a no-sugar-added variety, usually available in the natural foods section of supermarkets.

7 black or green **tea** bags

6 cups boiling water

2 cups no-sugar-added peach nectar or juice

2 cups sliced **peaches** (2 medium)

Ice cubes

Mint sprigs (optional)

1. Steep the tea bags in boiling water for 5 minutes. Remove the tea bags. Combine the brewed tea and nectar in a large pitcher. Stir in the peaches. Refrigerate until chilled, at least 3 hours or overnight. Serve over ice and garnish with mint sprigs, if desired. One serving is 1 cup.

Per serving: 52 calories, 0 g protein, 13 g carbohydrates, 1 g fiber, 0 g total fat, 0 g saturated fat, 0 mg cholesterol, 9 mg sodium.

VARIATION Berry Iced Tea

Substitute blackberry or blueberry juice for the peach nectar and fresh blackberries for the peaches.

Iced Coffee Frappé

1
Serves

| Preparation time: 5 minutes |
| Cooking time: 0 minutes |

Coffee bar drinks may seem innocent enough, but they are often outrageously high in calories, especially if you opt for the typical oversize portion. It is very easy to make your own frothy coffee-flavored drink. Our recipe has less than half the calories of a Starbucks Frappuccino.

2 teaspoons instant **coffee**

1 teaspoon sugar, or to taste

2 ice cubes

1/4 cup cold water

1/3 cup chilled vanilla **soy milk** or low-fat (1%) **milk**

Pinch of **cinnamon**

1. Combine the instant coffee, sugar, ice cubes, and water in a cocktail shaker or wide-mouth jar with tight-fitting lid (about 24-ounce/700-milliliter capacity). Secure lid and shake vigorously until frothy, about 30 seconds. Pour into a tall glass. Add the soy milk (or milk) and stir to mix. Sprinkle with cinnamon and serve with a straw. One serving is 2/3 cup.

Per serving: 70 calories, 3 g protein, 12 g carbohydrates, 0 g fiber, 1 g total fat, 0 g saturated fat, 0 mg cholesterol, 47 mg sodium.

SALADS, SANDWICHES, AND SOUPS

Grilled Chicken Salad with Oranges

4
Serves

| Preparation time: 25 minutes |
| Marinating time: 20 minutes |
| Cooking time: 10 to 15 minutes |

Slices of grilled chicken transform a fruity, Mediterranean salad into a satisfying hot-weather dinner that's packed with flavor—and Magic foods. Note: When marinating meat, fish, and poultry, remember to set aside a few tablespoons of the marinade for basting. Do not contaminate cooked food with marinade that has been in contact with raw meat. *See photo on page 218.*

1/3 cup orange juice

2 tablespoons lemon juice

3 tablespoons extra-virgin olive oil

1 tablespoon Dijon mustard

2 garlic cloves, minced

1/4 teaspoon salt, or to taste

Freshly ground pepper to taste

1 pound (450 grams) boneless skinless chicken breasts, trimmed

1/4 cup pistachios, or slivered almonds toasted

8 cups (5 ounces/140 grams) mesclun salad mix, rinsed and dried

1/2 cup thinly sliced red onion

2 medium oranges, peeled, quartered, and sliced

1. Place the orange juice, lemon juice, oil, mustard, garlic, salt, and pepper in a small bowl or jar with a tight-fitting lid; whisk or shake to blend. Reserve 1/3 cup of this dressing for the salad and 3 tablespoons for basting.

2. Place the remaining dressing in a shallow glass dish or a resealable plastic bag. Add the chicken and turn to coat. Cover or seal and marinate in the refrigerator for at least 20 minutes or up to 2 hours.

3. Preheat the grill to medium. Lightly oil grill rack by rubbing it with a piece of crumpled, oil-soaked paper towel (use tongs to hold paper towel). Remove chicken from marinade and discard marinade. Grill the chicken 4 to 6 inches (10 to 15 centimeters) from the heat source, basting the cooked sides with dressing reserved for basting, until no longer pink in the center and an instant-read thermometer inserted in the thickest part registers 170°F (75°C), 4 to 6 minutes per side. Transfer to a cutting board and let stand for 5 minutes.

4. Meanwhile, toast the almonds (or pistachios) in a small dry skillet over medium-low heat, stirring constantly, until light golden, 2 to 3 minutes. Transfer to a bowl and let cool.

5. Place the salad mix and onion in a large bowl. Toss with the dressing reserved for the salad. Divide the salad among 4 plates. Slice the chicken and distribute over the salads. Scatter orange slices over top and sprinkle with pistachios (or almonds).

Per serving: 331 calories, 30 g protein, 18 g carbohydrates, 5 g fiber, 16 g total fat, 3 g saturated fat, 68 mg cholesterol, 290 mg sodium.

Barley Salad with Snow Peas and Lemon Dressing

8
Serves

Preparation time: 30 minutes

Cooking time: 40 to 45 minutes

As this delightful, colorful salad attests, sugar-lowering barley isn't just for soups. Peas add even more sugar-busting, cholesterol-bashing soluble fiber. What's more, the refreshing lemon dressing helps slow down your body's conversion of carbohydrates into blood sugar. To turn this into a main-course salad, just add some diced cooked chicken, salmon, or firm baked tofu.

DRESSING

2 teaspoons freshly grated lemon zest

1/4 cup fresh **lemon** juice

1/4 cup finely chopped **shallot**

1 **garlic** clove, minced

1/2 teaspoon salt, or to taste

Freshly ground pepper to taste

1/3 cup extra-virgin **olive oil**

SALAD

1 cup pearled **barley,** rinsed (see Tip)

2 1/2 cups water

1/4 teaspoon salt, or to taste

1 1/2 cups (6 ounces/170 grams) snow **peas** or sugar snap peas

1 medium red bell pepper, seeded and diced

1 cup grated **carrots** (3–4 medium)

1/4 cup chopped fresh parsley

1/4 cup snipped fresh chives

1. **To make the dressing:** Whisk the lemon zest, lemon juice, shallot, garlic, 1/2 teaspoon salt, and pepper in a medium bowl. Gradually whisk in the oil.

2. **To make the salad:** Place the barley, water, and 1/4 teaspoon salt in a large saucepan and bring to a simmer over medium-high heat. Reduce the heat to low and cook, covered, until the barley is tender and most of the liquid has been absorbed, 40 to 45 minutes. Transfer to a large bowl and let cool, fluffing with a fork occasionally to prevent sticking.

3. Meanwhile, remove the stem ends and strings from peas. Cut in half on the diagonal. Cook the peas in a large saucepan of lightly salted water or steam them until just tender, about 2 minutes. Drain and rinse with cold running water.

4. Add the peas, bell pepper, carrots, parsley, and chives to the barley. Drizzle the dressing over the salad and toss to coat well. One serving is 3/4 cup. To make ahead, prepare the dressing and salad and refrigerate in separate covered containers for up to 1 day. Toss the salad with dressing shortly before serving.

Per serving: 202 calories, 4 g protein, 25 g carbohydrates, 5 g fiber, 10 g total fat, 1 g saturated fat, 0 mg cholesterol, 234 mg sodium.

Tip: To save time, you can substitute quick-cooking barley. In Step 2, use 1 1/2 cups quick-cooking barley, 2 1/2 cups water, and 1/4 teaspoon salt. Bring to a simmer and cook, covered, for 10 to 12 minutes.

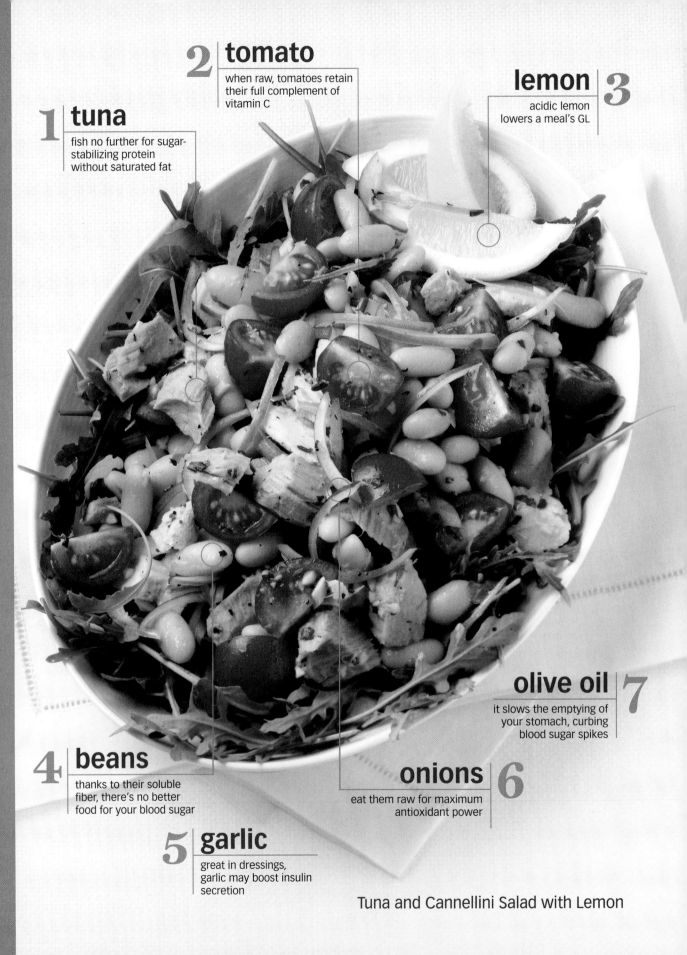

2 tomato
when raw, tomatoes retain their full complement of vitamin C

1 tuna
fish no further for sugar-stabilizing protein without saturated fat

lemon 3
acidic lemon lowers a meal's GL

olive oil 7
it slows the emptying of your stomach, curbing blood sugar spikes

4 beans
thanks to their soluble fiber, there's no better food for your blood sugar

onions 6
eat them raw for maximum antioxidant power

5 garlic
great in dressings, garlic may boost insulin secretion

Tuna and Cannellini Salad with Lemon

Tuna and Cannellini Salad with Lemon

4 Serves

Preparation time: 25 minutes
Cooking time: 0 minutes

Tuna and beans are a classic combo as well as a practical and nutritious one. If you keep canned tuna and canned beans on hand, you can put this recipe together from pantry staples—just add fresh greens and cherry tomatoes. This version is distinguished by a seasoning of lemon zest and rosemary. It is perfect for a special lunch, picnic, or dinner on a steamy evening.

LEMON-GARLIC DRESSING

3 tablespoons lemon juice

1 garlic clove, minced

1/4 teaspoon salt, or to taste

1/8 teaspoon crushed red pepper

1/4 cup extra-virgin olive oil

Freshly ground pepper to taste

SALAD

1 can (19 or 15 ounces/540 or 398 milliliters) cannellini beans, drained and rinsed

1 can (6 ounces/170 grams) water-packed chunk light tuna, drained and flaked

1/3 cup finely diced red onion

2 teaspoons chopped fresh rosemary

1 1/2 teaspoons freshly grated lemon zest

6 cups arugula, washed, dried, and torn into bite-size pieces

1 cup cherry tomatoes, quartered

1. **To make the dressing:** Combine the lemon juice, garlic, salt, and crushed red pepper in a small bowl. Gradually whisk in the oil. Season with pepper.

2. **To make the salad:** Combine the beans, tuna, onion, rosemary, and lemon zest in a medium bowl. Add 1/4 cup of the lemon-garlic dressing (save remaining dressing for the arugula). Toss to coat well. (The tuna-bean salad will keep, covered, in the refrigerator for up to 1 day.)

3. Just before serving, place the arugula in a large bowl. Add the reserved lemon-garlic dressing and toss to coat well. Divide the arugula mixture among 4 plates. Top with tuna-bean salad and garnish with cherry tomatoes. One serving is 2/3 cup tuna-bean salad and 1 1/2 cups arugula.

Per serving: 305 calories, 18 g protein, 25 g carbohydrates, 7 g fiber, 15 g total fat, 2 g saturated fat, 26 mg cholesterol, 500 mg sodium.

Black Bean and Barley Salad

6 Serves

Preparation time: 25 minutes
Cooking time: 10 minutes

With an all-star Magic foods lineup of barley, beans, vinegar, and citrus, this hearty salad is a real winner. It's great for picnics and barbecues and is an excellent accompaniment for grilled chicken, pork, or fish. *See photo on page 219.*

1 1/4 cups reduced-sodium chicken broth or vegetable broth

3/4 cup quick-cooking barley

1/4 cup cider vinegar

1/4 cup orange juice

1/4 cup extra-virgin olive oil

1 1/2 teaspoons ground cumin

1 teaspoon dried oregano

1 garlic clove, minced

1/4 teaspoon salt, or to taste

Freshly ground pepper to taste

1 can (15 1/2 or 19 ounces/398 or 540 milliliters) black beans, drained and rinsed

1 large red or yellow bell pepper, seeded and diced

2/3 cup chopped scallions, trimmed (1 bunch)

1/2 cup coarsely chopped fresh cilantro

Lime wedges

1. Combine the broth and barley in a medium saucepan and bring to a simmer. Cover and reduce heat to low. Simmer until the barley is tender and most of the liquid has been absorbed, about 10 minutes. Transfer the barley to a large bowl. Fluff with a fork and let cool.

2. Meanwhile, combine the vinegar, orange juice, oil, cumin, oregano, garlic, salt, and pepper in a jar with tight-fitting lid or small bowl. Shake or whisk to blend.

3. Add the beans, bell pepper, scallions, and cilantro to the barley. Drizzle with the dressing and toss to coat well. Garnish with lime wedges. One serving is 3/4 cup. The salad will keep, covered, in the refrigerator for up to 1 day.

Per serving: 230 calories, 7 g protein, 29 g carbohydrates, 7 g fiber, 11 g total fat, 2 g saturated fat, 0 mg cholesterol, 410 mg sodium.

Whole Wheat Noodles with Peanut Sauce and Chicken

8
Serves

Preparation time: 35 minutes

Cooking time: 8 to 10 minutes

This dish will be a big hit at your next potluck. Nutty-tasting whole wheat spaghetti complements the peanut sauce. Tofu stretches the peanut butter in the recipe, helping to keep calories in check and giving the sauce a velvety consistency. For a vegetarian version, substitute diced, baked, seasoned tofu for the chicken. If you are making the salad ahead, it is best to prepare all the components and toss the salad with the dressing shortly before serving.

DRESSING

1/2 cup natural-style peanut butter

1/3 cup low-fat firm silken tofu

1/4 cup reduced-sodium soy sauce

3 tablespoons lime juice

3 garlic cloves, minced

2 tablespoons firmly packed light brown sugar

3/4 teaspoon crushed red pepper

SALAD

12 ounces (340 grams) whole wheat spaghetti

2 teaspoons toasted sesame oil

2 1/2 cups shredded cooked skinless chicken breast

1 cup grated carrots (2–4 medium)

1 cup finely diced red bell pepper (1 small)

3/4 cup grated seedless (English) cucumber (1/4 medium)

1/3 cup coarsely chopped fresh cilantro leaves

1/4 cup chopped scallions

3 tablespoons unsalted dry-roasted peanuts, chopped

Lime wedges

1. Bring a large pot of lightly salted water to a boil for cooking the spaghetti.

2. To make the dressing: Combine all of the dressing ingredients in a food processor. Process until smooth and creamy, stopping once or twice to scrape down sides of workbowl. Set aside.

3. To make the salad: Cook the spaghetti in the boiling water, stirring often, until al dente (just tender), 6 to 9 minutes, or according to package directions. Drain and rinse with cold running water. Transfer to a large bowl. Drizzle with the oil and toss to coat.

4. Add the chicken, carrots, and bell pepper to the spaghetti. Add the peanut dressing and toss to coat. Sprinkle with the cucumber, cilantro, scallions, and peanuts. Serve with the lime wedges. One serving is 1 1/4 cups.

Per serving: 364 calories, 22 g protein, 43 g carbohydrates, 8 g fiber, 13 g total fat, 2 g saturated fat, 28 g cholesterol, 560 mg sodium.

Mediterranean Salad with Edamame

8
Serves

Preparation time: 25 minutes

Cooking time: 4 minutes

Torn leaves of fragrant herbs and delicate, protein-rich edamame beans distinguish this variation of a classic Greek salad. Edamame are immature soybeans. You can find them in the freezer section or the natural foods section of supermarkets or in natural foods stores. *See photo on page 218.*

1 cup frozen shelled **edamame** beans

1/3 cup extra-virgin **olive oil**

3 tablespoons **lemon** juice

2 **garlic** cloves, minced

1/4 teaspoon salt, or to taste

1/4 teaspoon sugar

Freshly ground pepper to taste

2 cups shredded romaine lettuce (1/2 small head)

2 cups cherry **tomatoes,** halved, or 2 medium tomatoes, cored, cut into 2- by 1-inch (5- by 2.5-centimeter) wedges

1 cup sliced English cucumber

2/3 cup chopped **scallions**

1/2 cup pitted kalamata **olives,** halved

1/2 cup fresh mint leaves, washed, dried, and torn into 1/2-inch (1-centimeter) pieces

1/2 cup fresh flat-leaf parsley leaves, washed, dried, and torn into 1/2-inch (1-centimeter) pieces

1 cup crumbled feta **cheese**

1. Bring a large saucepan of lightly salted water to a boil. Add the edamame beans and cook, covered, over medium heat until tender, 3 to 4 minutes. Drain and rinse with cold running water.

2. Combine the oil, lemon juice, garlic, salt, sugar, and pepper in a screw-top jar with a tight-fitting lid. Shake to blend.

3. Combine the lettuce, tomatoes, cucumber, scallions, olives, mint, parsley, and cooked edamame beans in a large bowl. Just before serving, drizzle the lemon dressing over salad and toss to coat well. Sprinkle each serving with feta. One serving is 1 1/4 cups.

Per serving: 220 calories, 7 g protein, 10 g carbohydrates, 3 g fiber, 17 g total fat, 5 g saturated fat, 15 mg cholesterol, 500 mg sodium.

Garden Pasta Salad

6
Serves

Preparation time: 30 minutes

Cooking time: 8 to 10 minutes

Pasta salads are perfect for potlucks, picnics, and backyard barbecues. This version has been upgraded with whole wheat pasta and a generous quantity of colorful vegetables. Reduced-fat mayonnaise, blended with low-fat yogurt, makes a creamy dressing that has a fraction of the saturated fat and calories of typical mayonnaise dressings. If you'd like to make this salad more substantial, toss in canned tuna, cooked chicken, or chickpeas. *See photo on page 218.*

2 cups (6 ounces/170 grams) whole wheat rotini or fusilli **pasta**

1/3 cup reduced-fat mayonnaise

1/3 cup low-fat plain **yogurt**

2 tablespoons extra-virgin **olive oil**

1 tablespoon red-wine **vinegar** or **lemon juice**

1 **garlic** clove, minced

1/8 teaspoon salt, or to taste

Freshly ground pepper to taste

1 cup cherry or grape **tomatoes,** halved

1 cup diced yellow or red bell pepper (1 small)

1 cup grated **carrots** (2–4 medium)

1/2 cup chopped **scallions** (4 medium)

1/2 cup chopped pitted kalamata **olives**

1/3 cup slivered fresh basil

1. Bring a large pot of lightly salted water to a boil. Cook pasta, stirring often, until firm-tender, 8 to 10 minutes, or according to package directions. Drain and refresh under cold running water.

2. Whisk mayonnaise, yogurt, oil, vinegar, garlic, salt, and pepper in a large bowl until smooth. Add the pasta and toss to coat. Add the tomatoes, bell pepper, carrots, scallions, olives, and basil. Toss to coat well. One serving size is 1 cup. The salad will keep, covered, in the refrigerator for up to 1 day.

Per serving: 205 calories, 6 g protein, 29 g carbohydrates, 4 g fiber, 9 g total fat, 2 g saturated fat, 1 mg cholesterol, 291 mg sodium.

No-Mayonnaise Creamy Coleslaw

6
Serves | **Preparation time: 20 minutes**
| **Cooking time: 0 minutes**

You can't have a picnic without coleslaw, but the traditional version is drowned in a fatty, overly sweet dressing. Our version uses yogurt enriched with olive oil (a good fat) instead of mayonnaise. If you have red cabbage on hand, use a mix of red and green cabbage for extra color and to take advantage of the red variety's anthocyanins, pigments that may help boost insulin production and lower blood sugar. To save time, you can use 5 cups packaged coleslaw mix. *See photo on page 219.*

1/3 cup nonfat plain **yogurt**

4 teaspoons Dijon mustard

4 teaspoons apple cider **vinegar**

4 teaspoons extra-virgin **olive oil**

1 1/2 teaspoons sugar

1/2 teaspoon caraway **seeds** or celery seeds

1/4 teaspoon salt

1/4 teaspoon freshly ground pepper

4 cups shredded green **cabbage** (1/2 medium)

1 cup grated **carrots** (2–4 medium)

1. Whisk the yogurt, mustard, vinegar, oil, sugar, caraway seeds, salt, and pepper in a small bowl until smooth.

2. Combine the cabbage and carrots in a large bowl. Add the dressing and toss to coat well. One serving is 3/4 cup. The coleslaw will keep, covered, in the refrigerator for up to 1 day.

Per serving: 63 calories, 2 g protein, 7 g carbohydrates, 2 g fiber, 4 g total fat, 1 g saturated fat, 0 mg cholesterol, 141 mg sodium.

Spinach, Grapefruit, and Avocado Salad with Poppy Seed Dressing

4
Serves | **Preparation time: 30 minutes**
| **Cooking time: 0 minutes**

Consider this salad a trifecta of Magic foods. Juicy, tart grapefruit makes a delicious contrast to buttery avocado and crisp spinach. Serve it as an impressive starter salad or add cooked shrimp and/or scallops and enjoy it as a refreshing warm-weather main dish. You can prepare recipe through Step 2 up to 2 days ahead. Cover and refrigerate the grapefruit segments and dressing separately.

2 pink **grapefruit**

1 tablespoon white-wine **vinegar** or rice vinegar

1/4 cup finely chopped **shallot** (1 large)

2 teaspoons poppy **seeds**

1 teaspoon honey

1 teaspoon Dijon mustard

3 tablespoons extra-virgin **olive oil**

1/2 teaspoon salt, or to taste

Freshly ground pepper to taste

8 cups (6 ounces/170 grams) baby **spinach,** rinsed and dried

1 cup sliced radishes (1 bunch)

2 Haas **avocados,** peeled, pitted, and sliced

1. Place a sieve over a medium bowl. Using a sharp knife, remove the skin and white pith from the grapefruit. Working over the sieve, cut the grapefruit segments from their surrounding membrane, letting the segments collect in the sieve and the juices collect in the bowl. When you have removed all of the segments, squeeze the membrane to extract as much juice as possible.

2. Place 1/4 cup of the grapefruit juice (reserve the remainder for another use) in a small bowl or a jar with a tight-fitting lid. Add the vinegar, shallot, poppy seeds, honey, mustard, oil, salt, and pepper. Whisk or shake to blend.

3. Just before serving, place the spinach and radishes in a large bowl. Toss with half of the grapefruit juice dressing. Divide the salad among 4 plates. Strew the avocado slices and grapefruit segments over salads and drizzle with the remaining dressing. One serving is 2 cups.

Per serving: 326 calories, 4 g protein, 29 g carbohydrates, 10 g fiber, 25 g total fat, 3 g saturated fat, 0 mg cholesterol, 416 mg sodium.

Greek Lentil Salad

6
Serves

Preparation time: 20 minutes

Cooking time: 25 to 30 minutes

Prized for their vegetable protein, soluble fiber, and high folate content, lentils are an essential Magic Foods pantry staple. And there is no need to wait for chilly soup weather to prepare lentils. They are also delicious in summer salads like this one. Feel free to substitute two cans (15 ounces/398 milliliters) of lentils (drained and rinsed) for the dried lentils.

1 cup dried green or brown lentils
    (see Ingredient Note), rinsed

1 teaspoon salt, divided

3 tablespoons lemon juice

2 tablespoons extra-virgin olive oil

1 garlic clove, minced

Freshly ground pepper to taste

1 cup chopped scallions (1 bunch)

1 cup (12 ounces) roasted red peppers from a jar,
    rinsed and diced

1/2 cup (2 ounces/60 grams) crumbled feta cheese

1/3 cup chopped fresh dill

6 cups trimmed arugula or watercress,
    washed, dried, and torn

1. Place the lentils in a large saucepan and cover with water. Bring to simmer. Reduce heat to medium-low, partially cover, and simmer for 15 minutes. Add 1/2 teaspoon of salt and cook until lentils are tender but not broken down, 10 to 15 minutes longer. Drain and let cool slightly.

2. Whisk the lemon juice, oil, garlic, the remaining 1/2 teaspoon salt, and the pepper in a large bowl. Add the warm lentils and toss gently to mix. Add the scallions, roasted red peppers, feta, and dill. Toss again. To serve, mound lentil mixture on a bed of arugula. One serving is 3/4 cup.

Per serving: 160 calories, 10 g protein, 13 g carbohydrates, 10 g fiber, 7 g total fat, 2 g saturated fat, 5 mg cholesterol, 700 mg sodium.

Ingredient Note: Common brown lentils are fine for this recipe, but small green lentils from France (often known as Le Puy lentils) are preferred for salads because they retain their shape and have an appealing chewy texture. Total cooking time is about 20 minutes for green lentils and 25 to 30 minutes for brown lentils.

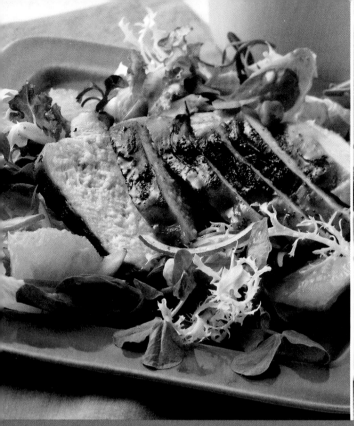

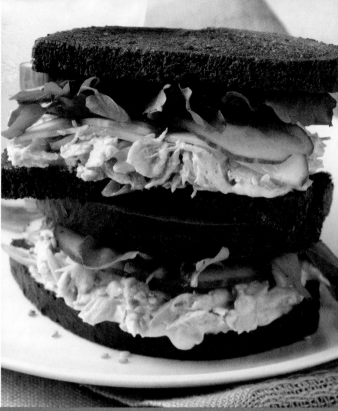

Grilled Chicken Salad with Oranges *page 210*
lemon • olive oil • garlic • chicken • pistachios
• onion • orange

Salmon Sandwiches with Wasabi Mayonnaise *page 220*
vinegar • salmon • scallion • seeds
• pumpernickel bread

Garden Pasta Salad *page 215*
pasta • yogurt • olive oil • vinegar • garlic
• tomato • carrot • scallion • olives

Mediterranean Salad with Edamame *page 215*
edamame • olive oil • lemon • garlic • tomato
• scallion • olives • cheese

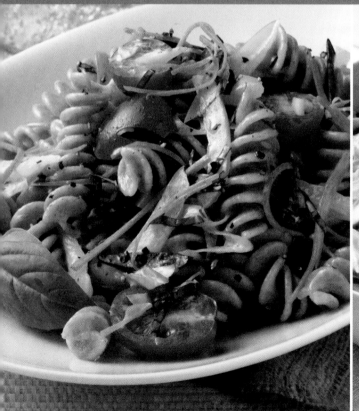

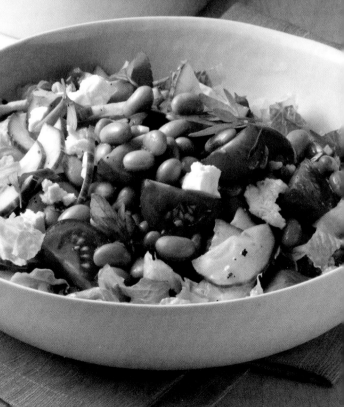

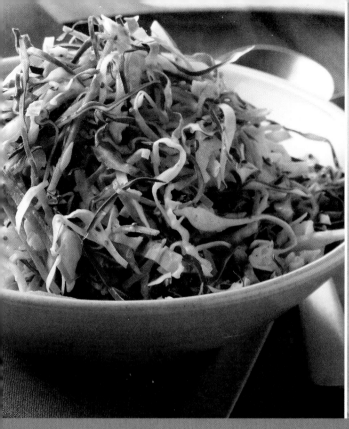

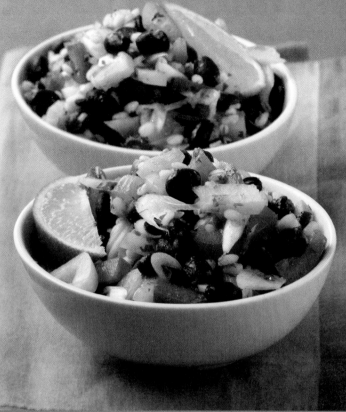

No-Mayonnaise Creamy Coleslaw *page 216*
yogurt • vinegar • olive oil • seeds • cabbage
• carrot

Black Bean and Barley Salad *page 213*
barley • vinegar • olive oil • garlic • beans
• scallion • lime

Tuna and Carrot Sandwich on Rye *page 222*
carrot • lemon • olive oil • scallion
• tuna • rye or pumpernickel bread

Curried Red Lentil Soup *page 224*
onions • garlic • lentils • tomato • cinnamon
• lemon • yogurt • scallion

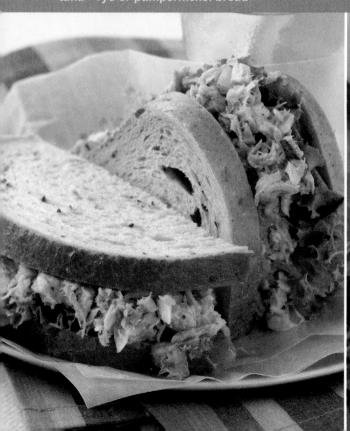

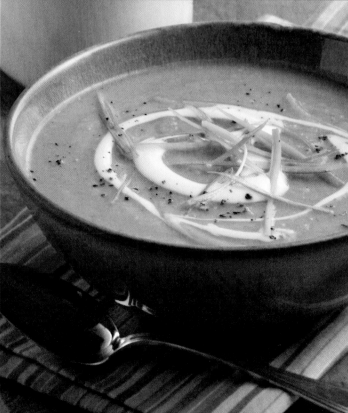

Salmon Sandwiches with Wasabi Mayonnaise

4	Preparation time: 20 minutes
Serves	Cooking time: 0 minutes

When you get tired of tuna sandwiches, try this recipe, which takes its inspiration from the sushi bar. Canned salmon is an essential pantry staple and a great way to get the benefits of wild salmon without paying the premium prices for fresh wild salmon. *See photo on page 218.*

6 tablespoons reduced-fat mayonnaise, divided

2 tablespoons rice vinegar

1 tablespoon grated fresh ginger

1 1/2 teaspoons wasabi powder
   (see Ingredient Note)

1 teaspoon mirin (see Ingredient Note)

1 can (7.5 ounces/213 grams) salmon,
   drained and flaked

2 tablespoons chopped scallions

1 tablespoon sesame seeds, toasted (see Tip)

8 slices pumpernickel bread

1 cup thinly sliced cucumber

1 cup trimmed watercress sprigs,
   rinsed and dried

1. Whisk 3 tablespoons of the mayonnaise, the rice vinegar, ginger, wasabi powder, and mirin in a medium bowl. Add the salmon, scallions, and sesame seeds. Mix well.

2. Spread the remaining 3 tablespoons mayonnaise over 1 side of each bread slice. Divide the salmon mixture among 4 of the bread slices, spreading evenly. Top with cucumber and watercress. Set the remaining bread slices on top. Cut the sandwiches in half. One serving is 2 sandwich halves.

Per serving: 314 calories, 18 g protein, 36 g carbohydrates, 5 g fiber, 12 g total fat, 2 g saturated fat, 34 mg cholesterol, 860 mg sodium.

Tip: Toast the sesame seeds in a small dry skillet, stirring constantly, until light golden and fragrant, 2 to 3 minutes.

Ingredient Notes:

• Wasabi, the pungent sushi condiment, is made from the stem of a semi-aquatic member of the cabbage family. Add water to the powder to make the paste that accompanies sushi. Large supermarkets stock wasabi powder in the Asian foods section or with the sushi.

• Also known as rice wine, mirin is a sweet wine made from glutinous rice. It has a low alcohol content, and you can find it in the Asian foods section of most supermarkets.

Grilled Eggplant Sandwiches with Red Pepper-Walnut Sauce

4	Preparation time: 30 minutes
Serves	Cooking time: 0 minutes

When it comes to sandwiches, think beyond the deli counter. This sophisticated and delicious combination pairs beautifully with low-GL sourdough breads and makes a special picnic sandwich. If you toast the bread and serve it right away, the sandwich makes a refreshing hot-weather supper. For panini (Italian-style grilled sandwiches), spritz the outside of the bread with non-stick spray and grill the sandwiches in a panini grill or contact grill.

3/4 cup Red Pepper-Walnut Sauce (recipe on
   opposite page)

2 medium-large baby eggplants, cut crosswise
   into 3/8-inch (1-centimeter)-thick slices

1/4 teaspoon salt, or to taste

Freshly ground pepper to taste

8 small slices **sourdough bread,**
  toasted, if desired

4 ounces (125 grams) creamy goat **cheese,**
  cut into 3/8-inch (1-centimeter)-thick slices

3/4 cup arugula leaves, washed and dried

1. Make the Red Pepper-Walnut Sauce.

2. Preheat the grill or broiler.

3. Spritz both sides of the eggplant slices with the cooking spray and season with salt and pepper. Lightly oil the grill or broiler rack by rubbing it with a piece of oil-soaked paper towel (use tongs to hold the paper towel when working over a hot grill). Grill or broil the eggplant until very tender and browned, 4 to 6 minutes per side.

4. Spread about 1 1/2 tablespoons of the Red Pepper-Walnut sauce over one side of each bread slice. Layer the eggplant slices and goat cheese slices on four slices of bread. Top with the arugula. Set the remaining bread slices on the sandwiches. Cut the sandwiches in half. One serving is 2 sandwich halves. The sandwiches will keep, wrapped in plastic wrap or foil, in the refrigerator or a cooler packed with ice packs for up to 2 days.

Per serving: 349 calories, 14 g protein, 44 g carbohydrates, 6 g fiber, 13 g total fat, 5 g saturated fat, 13 mg cholesterol, 910 mg sodium.

Tip: Place a fine-meshed vegetable grill rack over the grill grate to prevent the eggplant slices from falling through.

Red Pepper-Walnut Sauce

 4
Serves

| Preparation time: 10 minutes |
| Cooking time: 0 minutes |

In addition to perking up sandwich fillings, this intensely flavored sauce also makes an excellent appetizer spread to serve with whole grain crackers or toasted Whole Wheat Pita Crisps (page 207).

1/4 cup **walnuts**

1 tablespoon fine dry unseasoned bread crumbs

1 **garlic** clove, minced (1/2 teaspoon)

1 teaspoon ground cumin

1/8 teaspoon crushed red pepper

1/8 teaspoon salt, or to taste

1 jar (7 ounces/200 milliliters) roasted red peppers,
  drained and rinsed

1 tablespoon **lemon** juice

1. Combine the walnuts, bread crumbs, garlic, cumin, crushed red pepper and salt in a food processor; process until the walnuts are ground. Add the roasted red peppers and lemon juice; process until smooth. One serving is 3 tablespoons. The spread will keep, covered, in the refrigerator for up to 4 days. Makes 3/4 cup.

Per serving: 76 calories, 2 g protein, 6 g carbohydrates, 1 g fiber, 5 g total fat, 1 g saturated fat, 0 mg cholesterol, 268 mg sodium.

Tuna and Carrot Sandwich on Rye

2 Serves | **Preparation time: 15 minutes**
Cooking time: 0 minutes

Adding more omega-3–rich seafood to your diet can be as simple as packing a tuna sandwich for lunch. This one is boosted by a lemony grated carrot salad, adding crunch and appeal while squeezing some vegetable into your sandwich. We've put it on rye bread, which can actually help *lower* your blood sugar. *See photo on page 219.*

2/3 cup shredded carrot (1 medium)

2 teaspoons lemon juice

2 teaspoons extra-virgin olive oil

1 tablespoon chopped scallion

1 tablespoon chopped fresh dill or parsley

1/8 teaspoon salt, or to taste

1 can (3 ounces/85 grams) water-packed chunk light tuna, drained and flaked

1/4 cup finely chopped celery

2 tablespoons reduced-fat mayonnaise, divided

4 slices rye or pumpernickel bread

4 lettuce leaves, rinsed and dried

1. Combine the carrot, lemon juice, oil, scallion, dill (or parsley), and salt in a small bowl. Toss with a fork to mix.

2. Mix the tuna, celery, and 1 tablespoon of the mayonnaise in a small bowl. Spread the remaining 1 tablespoon mayonnaise over the bread slices. Spread half of the tuna mixture over two of the bread slices. Top with the carrot salad and lettuce. Set remaining bread slices over filling. Cut each sandwich in half. One serving equals 2 sandwich halves. The sandwiches will keep, well wrapped, in the refrigerator or a cooler packed with ice packs for up to 1 day.

Per serving: 303 calories, 17 g protein, 38 g carbohydrates, 5 g fiber, 9 g total fat, 2 g saturated fat, 13 mg cholesterol, 758 mg sodium.

Bean and Barley Soup

8 Serves | **Preparation time: 30 minutes**
Cooking time: 40 minutes

A soothing soup is one of the most nourishing and practical meals possible. And a chunky soup like this one that focuses on low-GL carbohydrates, such as barley and beans, and Magic veggies like carrots and spinach, provides maximum satisfaction for just a few calories. Infusing canned low-sodium broth with garlic and herbs freshens the flavor and makes it taste as good as homemade.

7 cups reduced-sodium chicken broth or vegetable broth

6 garlic cloves, peeled and crushed

2 sprigs fresh rosemary (4 1/2 inches/ 10 centimeters long)

1/4 teaspoon crushed red pepper

1 can (19 or 15 ounces/540 or 398 milliliters) dark red kidney beans, drained and rinsed

2 teaspoons olive oil

1 cup chopped onion (1 medium)

1 cup diced peeled carrots (3–4 medium)

1/4 cup diced celery (1 stalk)

1 can (14 1/2 ounces/398 milliliters) diced tomatoes

1 cup quick-cooking barley

10 cups baby spinach, washed

Freshly ground black pepper to taste

1/2 cup grated Parmesan cheese

1. Bring the broth to a boil in a large saucepan. Add the garlic, rosemary, and crushed red pepper. Partially cover the saucepan and simmer over medium-low heat for 15 minutes to intensify flavor. Strain the broth through a sieve into a large bowl. Discard the solids.

2. Mash 1 cup of the kidney beans in a small bowl with a fork. Set the whole and mashed

beans aside. Heat the oil in a 4- to 6-quart (4- to 6-liter) soup pot over medium heat. Add the onion, carrots, and celery. Cook, stirring often, until softened, 3 to 4 minutes. Pour in the infused broth. Add the tomatoes, barley, and reserved mashed and whole beans. Bring to a simmer, stirring occasionally. Reduce heat to medium-low, cover, and cook at a lively simmer until the barley is almost tender, about 15 minutes.

3. Stir in the spinach. Cover and cook until the spinach has wilted and the barley is tender, 3 to 5 minutes. Season with ground pepper. Top each serving with 1 tablespoon Parmesan cheese. One serving is 1 1/3 cups. The soup will keep, covered, in the refrigerator for up to 2 days.

Per serving: 197 calories, 12 g protein, 30 g carbohydrates, 7 g fiber, 4 g total fat, 1 g saturated fat, 4 mg cholesterol, 757 mg sodium.

Hearty Split Pea Soup with Rye Croutons

4
Serves

Preparation time: 15 minutes
Cooking time: 1 hour

An old-fashioned split pea soup is back on the menu for Magic eating. Split peas, which are a good source of plant protein and fiber, are amazingly filling. This soup is wonderful for a supper and handy to tote to the office for lunch—it will easily sustain you until your afternoon snack. The rye bread croutons are a cinch to make and give the soup a final flourish. They're a far healthier alternative to store-bought croutons, which are typically made with white flour and often contain trans fat.

4 teaspoons olive oil, divided

1/2 cup diced Canadian back bacon, diced (2 ounces/60 grams or 4 slices)

1 cup chopped onion (1 medium)

1 cup chopped carrots (2–4 medium)

5 1/4 cups reduced-sodium chicken broth

1 cup green split peas, sorted and rinsed

1 teaspoon dried summer savory or thyme

1/8 teaspoon cayenne pepper

1 bay leaf

1 1/2 cups cubed rye bread (2 slices)

1. Heat 2 teaspoons of the oil in a 4- to 6-cup soup pot over medium heat. Add the bacon, onion, and carrots. Cook, stirring often, until softened and lightly browned, 3 to 5 minutes. Add the broth, split peas, savory (or thyme), cayenne, and bay leaf. Bring to a simmer. Reduce the heat to medium-low, cover, and cook until the split peas have broken down and thickened the soup, about 1 hour.

2. Meanwhile, preheat the oven to 350°F (180°C). Toss the bread cubes with the remaining 2 teaspoons oil in a medium bowl. Spread in a small baking pan and bake until crisp, 15 to 20 minutes.

3. When the soup is ready, discard the bay leaf. Garnish each serving with rye croutons. One serving is 1 cup. The soup will keep, covered, in the refrigerator, for up to 2 days

Per serving: 298 calories, 18 g protein, 44 g carbohydrates, 2 g fiber, 6 g total fat, 1 g saturated fat, 7 mg cholesterol, 298 mg sodium.

Curried Red Lentil Soup

8 **Preparation time: 15 minutes**
Serves | **Cooking time: 25 minutes**

You may think of lentils as something to store in the back of your pantry until a day when you have lots of time to wait for them to cook. But lentils, especially the red variety (sold in natural foods stores), are surprisingly convenient. They require no presoaking and cook up quickly—red lentils in just 20 minutes and brown lentils in about 30 minutes. *See photo on page 219.*

2 teaspoons canola oil

2 cups chopped onions (2 medium)

4 garlic cloves, minced

4–5 teaspoons curry powder

1 1/2 cups red lentils, rinsed and picked over

6 cups reduced-sodium chicken broth or vegetable broth

3/4 cup water

2 tablespoons tomato paste

1/4 teaspoon cinnamon

2 tablespoons lemon juice

1/4 teaspoon salt, or to taste

Freshly ground pepper to taste

1/2 cup nonfat plain yogurt

1/4 cup chopped scallion greens

1. Heat the oil in a 4- to 6-quart (4- to 6-liter) soup pot over medium heat. Add the onion and cook, stirring frequently, until softened, 2 to 3 minutes. Add the garlic and curry powder. Cook, stirring, for 30 seconds. Add the lentils and stir to coat. Add the broth, water, tomato paste, and cinnamon. Bring to a simmer, reduce heat to low, cover, and simmer until the lentils are very tender, about 20 minutes.

2. In batches, transfer the soup to a food processor or blender and puree. (Use caution when blending hot liquids.) Return the puree to the soup pot and heat through. Season with lemon juice, salt, and pepper. Garnish each serving with a dollop of yogurt and a sprinkling of scallion greens. One serving is 1 cup. The soup will keep, covered, in the refrigerator for up to 2 days.

Per serving: 187 calories, 14 g protein, 29 g carbohydrates, 12 g fiber, 2 g total fat, 1 g saturated fat, 4 mg cholesterol, 199 mg sodium.

Peanut Chicken Soup

8 **Preparation time: 20 minutes**
Serves | **Cooking time: 25 minutes**

If you think peanut butter is just for sandwiches, think again. The secret ingredient in this soup (based on a traditional African recipe), it contributes exceptionally rich flavor and body—without saturated fat. It also boosts the protein content of this simple but surprising recipe.

2 teaspoons canola oil

1 cup chopped onion (1 medium)

3 garlic cloves, minced

1 tablespoon curry powder

2 cans (14 ounces/398 milliliters each) reduced-sodium chicken broth

1 can (14 ounces/398 milliliters) diced tomatoes

1 small sweet potato, peeled and cut into 1/2-inch (1-centimeter) pieces (2 cups)

1 pound (450 grams) boneless skinless chicken breasts, trimmed and cut into 1/2-inch (1-centimeter) pieces

1/3 cup natural-style peanut butter

1/3 cup chopped fresh cilantro

2 tablespoons lime juice

Dash of hot pepper sauce, such as Tabasco

1. Heat the oil in a 4- to 6-quart (4- to 6-liter) Dutch oven or soup pot over medium-high heat. Add the onion and cook, stirring often, until softened, 2 to 3 minutes. Add the garlic and curry powder; cook, stirring, until fragrant, about 20 seconds. Add the broth, tomatoes, and sweet potato and bring to a simmer. Reduce heat to medium-low, cover, and simmer for 10 minutes.

2. Add the chicken, cover, and simmer until the sweet potatoes are tender and the chicken is cooked through, about 10 minutes. Add the peanut butter and stir until blended into the soup. Stir in the cilantro, lime juice, and hot sauce. One serving is 1 cup. The soup will keep, covered, in the refrigerator for up to 2 days.

Per serving: 175 calories, 14 g protein, 14 g carbohydrates, 3 g fiber, 7 g total fat, 1 g saturated fat, 21 mg cholesterol, 406 mg sodium.

Asian Noodle Hot Pot

4
Serves

Preparation time: 15 minutes

Cooking time: 30 minutes

Serving noodles in a fragrant, spicy broth is a good way to ensure an appropriate portion size. Canned broth is the base, but this soup is infused with ginger and garlic to give it a characteristic Asian flavor. Rounding out the broth and noodles are several key Magic foods: cabbage, carrots, tofu, and vinegar. You can substitute diced cooked chicken for the tofu, if you prefer.

5 1/4 cups reduced-sodium chicken broth or vegetable broth

3 slices (1/4 inch/5 millimeters thick) peeled fresh ginger

2 **garlic** cloves, crushed and peeled

1/4 teaspoon crushed red pepper

2 teaspoons canola oil

4 ounces (125 grams) fresh shiitake mushrooms, stems removed, wiped clean, and sliced

3 cups sliced napa **cabbage** (1/2 medium) or green cabbage (1/2 medium) (see Ingredient Note)

8 ounces (225 grams) firm regular **tofu,** drained, patted dry, cut into 3/4-inch (2.5-centimeter) cubes

1 cup shredded **carrots** (2–4 medium)

2 teaspoons reduced-sodium soy sauce

2 teaspoons rice **vinegar**

1 teaspoon toasted sesame oil

4 ounces (125 grams) **whole wheat linguine** or spaghetti

1/4 cup chopped **scallions** (2 medium)

1. Bring a large pot of lightly salted water to a boil.

2. Bring the broth to a simmer in a large saucepan. Add the ginger, garlic, and red pepper. Partially cover and simmer over medium-low heat for 15 minutes to intensify flavor. Strain the broth through a sieve into another large saucepan and discard the solids.

3. Heat the oil in large nonstick skillet over medium-high heat. Add the mushrooms and cook, stirring often, until tender, 3 to 5 minutes. Add the cabbage and cook, stirring often, until almost tender, 2 to 3 minutes. Add to the infused broth in the saucepan. Simmer, partially covered, over medium-low heat until cabbage is tender, about 5 minutes. Add the tofu and carrots and heat through. Stir in the soy sauce, vinegar, and sesame oil.

4. Meanwhile, cook the linguine (or spaghetti) in the boiling water until al dente (just tender), 6 to 9 minutes, or according to package directions. Drain the linguine and divide among 4 large soup bowls. Ladle the soup over the noodles and garnish each serving with scallions. One serving is 1 1/2 cups.

Per serving: 246 calories, 16 g protein, 32 g carbohydrates, 6 g fiber, 8 g total fat, 1 g saturated fat, 0 mg cholesterol, 917 mg sodium.

Ingredient Note: Napa, also known as Chinese cabbage, is a pale green, long, oval-shaped cabbage. Its flavor is more delicate than that of regular green cabbage.

BEEF, LAMB, AND PORK

Orange Beef Stir-Fry with Broccoli and Red Pepper

4 Serves | Preparation time: 30 minutes
| Cooking time: 8 minutes

Recipes for beef and broccoli stir-fries may be commonplace, but this one stands out. Stir-frying orange zest with fresh ginger gives the sauce extraordinary fragrance and satisfying flavor. This dish provides a generous quantity of vegetables balanced with lean protein, providing excellent nutritional value for the calories. For convenience, you can substitute 4 cups frozen broccoli florets for fresh and 2 1/2 cups frozen pepper stir-fry mix for the fresh bell pepper and onion. *See photo on opposite page.*

1/2 cup orange juice

2 tablespoons reduced-sodium soy sauce

1 tablespoon oyster-flavored sauce

1 tablespoon rice **vinegar**

1 1/2 teaspoons chile-garlic sauce or hot red pepper sauce

1 1/2 teaspoons cornstarch

1 tablespoon vegetable oil

12 ounces (340 grams) flank **steak,** trimmed, halved lengthwise, and cut into 1/4-inch (5-millimeter)-thick slices

1 tablespoon minced fresh ginger

2 teaspoons freshly grated orange zest (see Tip)

3 **garlic** cloves, minced

1 cup sliced **onion** (1 medium)

1 pound (450 grams) **broccoli** crowns, cut into 1-inch (2.5-centimeter) florets (4 cups)

1 red or yellow bell pepper, cut into 2- x 1/4-inch (5-centimeter x 5-millimeter) slivers (1 1/2 cups)

1. In a small bowl, whisk together the orange juice, soy sauce, oyster-flavored sauce, vinegar, chile-garlic sauce (or hot sauce) and cornstarch; set aside.

2. Heat 1 teaspoon oil in a large nonstick skillet or stir-fry pan over high heat. Add half of the steak and cook, without stirring or turning, until browned on the underside, about 1 minute. Stir and turn the slices, then cook just until browned on the other side, about 30 seconds. Transfer to a plate. Add another 1 teaspoon oil, repeat with the remaining steak, and transfer to the plate.

3. Add the remaining 1 teaspoon oil to the skillet, then add the ginger, orange zest, and garlic and stir-fry until fragrant, 10 to 20 seconds. Add the onion and stir-fry for 1 minute. Add the broccoli and bell pepper and stir-fry for 30 seconds. Add 1/4 cup water, cover, and cook just until crisp-tender, about 1 1/2 minutes. Push the vegetables to the outside of the pan. Stir the reserved sauce, pour into the center of the pan, and cook, stirring, until glossy and thickened, about 1 minute. Stir the vegetables into the sauce, return the steak to the skillet, and turn to coat. One serving is 1 1/2 cups.

Per serving: 247 calories, 25 g protein, 17 g carbohydrates, 3 g fiber, 9 g total fat, 3 g saturated fat, 34 mg cholesterol, 655 mg sodium.

Tip: A zester is the easiest way to remove zest from oranges and lemons. If you don't have one, use a vegetable peeler and mince the peels. Or cover a grater with plastic wrap and use the side made for grating hard cheese.

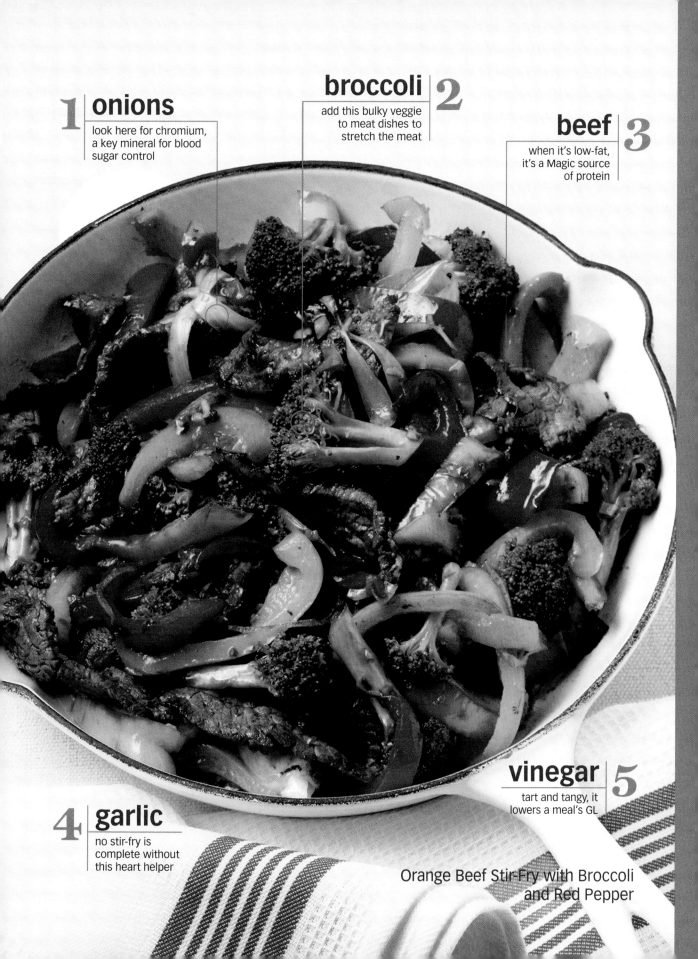

1 onions
look here for chromium, a key mineral for blood sugar control

broccoli 2
add this bulky veggie to meat dishes to stretch the meat

beef 3
when it's low-fat, it's a Magic source of protein

4 garlic
no stir-fry is complete without this heart helper

vinegar 5
tart and tangy, it lowers a meal's GL

Orange Beef Stir-Fry with Broccoli and Red Pepper

Flank Steak with Balsamic Sauce

6 Serves

| Preparation time: 20 minutes |
| Marinating time: 2 hours |
| Cooking time: 12 to 14 minutes |

One of the leaner beef cuts, flank steak is an excellent choice when you're craving a steak dinner. It is economical, has lots of flavor, and becomes nice and tender when marinated. Since you slice the steak before serving, it's easy to control portion sizes. In this recipe, the zesty marinade is transformed into a rich-tasting sauce. We use a ridged grill pan or skillet, but you can also cook the steak on an outdoor grill or broil it. *See photo on page 245.*

1/3 cup orange juice or port

1/4 cup balsamic **vinegar**

1 teaspoon Worcestershire sauce

1 tablespoon chopped fresh thyme or 1 teaspoon dried thyme

2 **garlic** cloves, minced

1/2 teaspoon salt, or to taste

Freshly ground black pepper to taste

1 1/2 pounds (700 grams) **flank steak,** trimmed

2 tablespoons finely chopped **shallot** (1 large)

1 teaspoon **olive oil**

2 teaspoons unsalted butter

1. In a small bowl, whisk together the orange juice (or port), vinegar, Worcestershire sauce, thyme, garlic, salt, and pepper. Place the steak in a shallow glass dish, pour on the orange juice mixture, and turn to coat. Cover and refrigerate for at least 2 hours or up to 8 hours, turning several times.

2. Remove the steak from the marinade and pour the marinade into a small saucepan. Add the shallots and set aside. Brush a ridged grill pan or heavy skillet with oil and place over medium-high heat. Add the steak to the pan and, depending on thickness, cook for 6 to 7 minutes

per side for medium-rare, or until it reaches the desired doneness. Transfer to a cutting board and let stand for 5 minutes.

3. Meanwhile, bring the marinade to a boil over medium-high heat and cook until reduced to 1/3 cup, 3 to 5 minutes. Remove from the heat, add the butter, and whisk until melted.

4. Slice the steak thinly across the grain. Add any accumulated juices on the cutting board to the sauce and serve the sauce with the steak. One serving is 3 ounces (85 grams) steak and 1 tablespoon sauce. Leftover steak will keep, covered, in the refrigerator for up to 2 days.

Per serving: 196 calories, 25 g protein, 4 g carbohydrates, 0 g fiber, 8 g total fat, 3 g saturated fat, 41 mg cholesterol, 269 mg sodium.

Slow-Cooker Beef and Vegetable Stew

8 Serves

| Preparation time: 30 minutes |
| Cooking time: 15 minutes on the stovetop, then 4 to 4 1/2 hours in the slow cooker on high or 7 to 8 hours on low |

The trick to making a healthful, hearty meat stew is to include lots of vegetables and make a generous amount of full-bodied, low-fat gravy. You can't whip up this stew on a busy evening, so plan to make it on the weekend. It keeps well and tastes even better the next day.

1 1/2 pounds (700 grams) cubed boneless **beef** chuck (1 1/2-inch/4-centimeter cubes), trimmed

1/2 teaspoon freshly ground black pepper

1/4 teaspoon salt, or to taste

1 tablespoon **olive oil**

1 medium **onion,** chopped (1 cup)

2 tablespoons all-purpose flour

4 **garlic** cloves, minced

1 cup dry red wine

1 can (14 1/2 ounces/398 milliliters) diced **tomatoes,** undrained

3/4 cup reduced-sodium chicken broth

1 teaspoon Worcestershire sauce

1 1/2 teaspoons dried thyme

2 bay leaves

2 cups peeled baby **carrots**
(10 ounces/280 grams), rinsed

2 medium white turnips, peeled and cut into
bite-size chunks (2 cups)

1 1/2 cups frozen pearl **onions** (6 ounces/170 grams)

1/4 cup chopped fresh parsley

1. Pat the beef dry with paper towels and sprinkle with the pepper and salt. Heat 2 teaspoons oil in a large nonstick skillet over medium-high heat. Add half of the beef and cook, turning with tongs occasionally, until browned, 3 to 5 minutes, then transfer to a plate. Repeat with the remaining beef and transfer to the plate.

2. Add the remaining 1 teaspoon oil to the skillet. Add the chopped onion and cook, stirring frequently, until softened and lightly browned, 1 to 2 minutes. Add the flour and garlic and cook, stirring, for 30 seconds to 1 minute. Add the wine and bring to a boil, stirring to scrape up any browned bits from the skillet. Add the tomatoes and mash with a potato masher. Stir in the broth, Worcestershire sauce, thyme, and bay leaves and bring to a simmer.

3. Place the beef in 4-quart (4-liter) slow cooker and spoon on half of the tomato mixture. Place the carrots and turnips on top of the sauce, then top with the remaining tomato mixture. Cover and cook until the beef and vegetables are very tender, 4 to 4 1/2 hours on high or 7 to 8 hours on low.

4. Shortly before the stew is ready, cook the pearl onions according to package directions, then add to the stew. Discard the bay leaves and sprinkle with the parsley. One serving is 1 cup.

Per serving: 235 calories, 21 g protein, 14 g carbohydrates, 3 g fiber, 8 g total fat, 3 g saturated fat, 42 mg cholesterol, 371 mg sodium.

Lamb Stew with Spring Vegetables

In Step 1, substitute 1 1/2 pounds (700 grams) cubed boneless lamb leg meat, trimmed, for the beef. In Step 2, substitute 1 cup dry white wine for the red wine and 2 tablespoons chopped fresh rosemary for the thyme. In Step 3, omit the turnips. In Step 4, cook 1 1/2 cups frozen pearl onions and 1 1/2 cups frozen peas separately according to package directions, then add to the stew.

Pork Stew with Latin Flavors

In Step 1, substitute 1 1/2 pounds (700 grams) cubed boneless pork (choose a leg cut, also called fresh ham, rather than shoulder, which is higher in fat), trimmed, for the beef. In Step 2, substitute 1 cup lager beer for the wine and 1 can (14 1/2 ounces/398 milliliters) mild green chile–seasoned tomatoes for the diced tomatoes. Substitute 1 1/2 teaspoons ground cumin and 3/4 teaspoon dried oregano for the thyme and bay leaves. In Step 3, omit the carrots and turnips; instead use 1 medium sweet potato, peeled and cut into 1- by 3/4-inch (2.5- by 2-centimeter) chunks. In Step 4, cook 1 1/2 cups frozen pearl onions and 1 1/2 cups frozen corn niblets according to package directions, then add to the stew. Substitute 1/4 cup chopped fresh cilantro for the parsley. Serve with lime wedges and hot sauce.

Beef and Veggie Meat Loaf

8 Serves

Preparation time: 20 minutes

Baking time: 1 hour, 5 minutes to 1 hour, 20 minutes

An old-fashioned favorite gets a new lease on life with this Magic meat loaf makeover. We stretched the ground beef with grated carrots and zucchini, reducing the saturated fat, boosting the vegetable quota, and adding moisture. Whole grain rolled oats play the role of filler and help keep the meat loaf tender. If you're running late and can't wait for the meat loaf to bake, divide the meat mixture among 8 muffin cups coated with cooking spray and bake for about 30 minutes.

1 pound (450 grams) 93–95% extra-lean ground **beef** (ground round)

3/4 cup old-fashioned rolled **oats**

1 cup chopped **onion** (1 medium)

1 cup shredded **carrots** (2–4 medium)

1 cup shredded **zucchini** (1 small)

1 large **egg,** lightly beaten

2 large **egg** whites, lightly beaten

2 tablespoons ketchup

1 tablespoon Worcestershire sauce

2 teaspoons Dijon mustard

1 teaspoon dried thyme

3/4 teaspoon salt

1/2 teaspoon freshly ground black pepper

1. Preheat the oven to 350°F (180°C). Line an 8 x 4- or 9 x 5-inch (20 x 10- or 23 x 12-centimeter) loaf pan with foil, leaving a 1-inch (2.5-centimeter) overhang along the two long sides. Coat the foil with cooking spray.

2. In a large bowl, combine the beef, oats, onion, carrots, zucchini, egg, egg whites, 1 tablespoon ketchup, Worcestershire sauce, mustard, thyme, salt, and pepper and mix well. Transfer to the pan and press into a loaf. Spread the remaining 1 tablespoon ketchup over the top.

3. Place the pan on a baking sheet and bake for 1 hour. Drain off the fat, then bake until firm and an instant-read thermometer inserted in the center registers 165°F (75°C), 5 to 20 minutes, depending on the depth of the pan you're using. Drain off the fat and let the meat loaf stand for 5 minutes. Use the foil overhang to lift it out and transfer to a cutting board, then slice. One serving is 4 ounces (125 grams). Leftover meat loaf will keep, covered, in the refrigerator for up to 2 days.

Per serving: 165 calories, 19 g protein, 11 g carbohydrates, 2 g fiber, 5 g total fat, 2 g saturated fat, 68 mg cholesterol, 380 mg sodium.

Greek Pasta and Beef Casserole

8 Serves

Preparation time: 50 minutes

Baking time: 40 to 50 minutes

Known as pastitsio, this hearty Greek casserole serves up layers of creamy noodles separated by cinnamon-scented meat sauce. Like its Italian cousin, lasagna, it's an ideal make-ahead meal (assemble it through Step 5, then cover and refrigerate for up to 2 days). While there are several parts to this lightened version, none is difficult to make, and you can break up the workload by preparing the meat sauce a day ahead (it's also delicious on its own, tossed with whole wheat pasta).

MEAT SAUCE

12 ounces (340 grams) 93–95% lean ground **beef** (ground round)

2 teaspoons **olive oil**

2 cups chopped **onion** (1 large)

3 **garlic** cloves, minced

1 1/2 teaspoons dried oregano

1 teaspoon ground **cinnamon**

1/2 teaspoon sugar

1/4 teaspoon salt, or to taste

1/2 cup dry white wine or reduced-sodium chicken broth

1 can (14 1/2 ounces/398 milliliters) no-salt-added diced **tomatoes,** with liquid

1/4 cup **tomato** paste

1/4 cup chopped fresh parsley

Freshly ground black pepper to taste

MACARONI AND CHEESE SAUCE

2 1/2 cups 1% **milk**

1/3 cup all-purpose flour

1 large **egg**

2 large **egg** whites

1 cup fat-free cottage **cheese**

1 cup grated Swiss **cheese** (3 ounces/85 grams)

1/4 teaspoon ground nutmeg

1/4 teaspoon salt, or to taste

Freshly ground black pepper to taste

8 ounces (250 grams) **whole wheat elbow macaroni** (2 cups) (see Ingredient Note)

1/4 cup grated Parmesan **cheese** (1/2 ounce/15 grams)

1. Preheat the oven to 400°F (200°C). Coat a 9 x 13-inch (23 x 35-centimeter) baking dish with cooking spray. Bring a large pot of water to a boil.

2. **To make the meat sauce:** Cook the beef in a medium nonstick skillet over medium-high heat, crumbling with a wooden spoon, until browned, 3 to 4 minutes. Drain in a colander set over a bowl.

3. Heat the oil in a Dutch oven over medium heat. Add the onion and cook, stirring frequently, until softened, 3 to 4 minutes. Add the garlic, oregano, cinnamon, sugar, and salt and cook, stirring, for 30 seconds. Add the wine (or broth) and bring to a simmer. Add the tomatoes and

mash with a potato masher. Return to a simmer and stir in the tomato paste and beef. Reduce the heat to medium-low, partially cover, and simmer, stirring occasionally, for 20 minutes. Stir in the parsley and pepper.

4. **To make the macaroni and cheese sauce:** In a small bowl, whisk 1/2 cup milk and the flour until smooth. Heat the remaining 2 cups milk in a medium saucepan over medium heat until steaming. Add the flour mixture and cook, whisking constantly, until the sauce bubbles and thickens, 3 to 4 minutes. Remove from the heat. In a small bowl, blend the egg and egg whites with a fork, then gradually whisk into the sauce. Stir in the cottage cheese, Swiss cheese, nutmeg, salt, and pepper.

5. Add the macaroni to the boiling water and cook for 4 1/2 minutes, then drain and rinse under cold running water (the macaroni will continue to cook during baking). Transfer to a large bowl, add the cheese sauce, and toss to coat. Spread half of the pasta mixture in the baking dish, then spread the meat sauce on top. Top with the remaining pasta mixture and sprinkle with the cheese.

6. Bake, uncovered, until the top is golden and the casserole is bubbling, 40 to 50 minutes. Let stand for 5 minutes before serving. One serving is 1/8 of the casserole (about 1 1/4 cups). Leftovers will keep, covered, in the refrigerator for up to 2 days.

Per serving: 390 calories, 31 g protein, 40 g carbohydrates, 4 g fiber, 11 g total fat, 5 g saturated fat, 85 mg cholesterol, 440 mg sodium.

Ingredient Note: Look for Barilla Plus elbow macaroni, which is higher in fiber, protein, and omega-3 fatty acids than regular pasta.

Mustard-Crusted Lamb Chops

4
Serves

Preparation time: 15 minutes	
Marinating time: 30 minutes	
Cooking time: 10 minutes	

A full-flavored marinade of grainy mustard, rosemary, and garlic brings out the best in delicate lamb chops and forms an appealing crust during grilling. You can also use the marinade for lamb kebabs or increase the proportions for a grilled or roasted leg of lamb.

3 tablespoons coarse-grain mustard

2 tablespoons chopped fresh rosemary

2 tablespoons red-wine **vinegar**

1 tablespoon extra-virgin **olive oil**

1/2 teaspoon Worcestershire sauce

4 **garlic** cloves, minced

1/4 teaspoon salt

Freshly ground black pepper to taste

8 loin **lamb** chops (3 ounces/85 grams each), trimmed

1. In a shallow glass dish, whisk the mustard, rosemary, vinegar, oil, Worcestershire sauce, garlic, salt, and pepper until blended. Add the lamb chops and turn to coat well. Cover and refrigerate for at least 30 minutes or up to 4 hours.

2. Preheat the grill or broiler.

3. Lightly oil the grill or broiler rack by rubbing a piece of oil-soaked paper towel over the surface. Grill or broil the lamb chops for 4 to 5 minutes per side for medium-rare, or until they reach the desired doneness. One serving is 2 chops (about 3 ounces/85 grams boneless meat total).

Per serving: 247 calories, 19 g protein, 1 g carbohydrates, 0 g fiber, 18 g total fat, 7 g saturated fat, 70 mg cholesterol, 355 mg sodium.

Pork Chop and Cabbage Skillet Dinner

4
Serves

Preparation time: 20 minutes	
Cooking time: 20 minutes	

A pork chop dinner usually involves an oversize portion of fatty meat. But if you use thin-cut boneless chops (about 1/2 inch/1 centimeter thick), you can ensure an appropriate portion size and get the protein benefits of lean meat. Teamed with low-calorie cabbage, the chops make a hearty dinner in just minutes. To trim the preparation time, use the food processor slicing disk to slice the onion, carrot, and cabbage or substitute 5 1/2 cups prepared coleslaw mix for the cabbage and carrots. *See photo on page 245.*

1 teaspoon dried thyme

1/4 teaspoon salt

1/4 teaspoon freshly ground black pepper, plus more to taste

1 pound (450 grams) thin-cut boneless **pork** chops, trimmed

1 tablespoon canola oil

1 cup sliced **onion** (1 medium)

5 cups shredded green **cabbage** (1/2 medium head)

1/2 cup sliced **carrots** (2 medium)

1 can (14 ounces/284 milliliters) reduced-sodium chicken broth (1 3/4 cups)

2 teaspoons coarse-grain mustard

1 teaspoon apple cider **vinegar**

1. In a small bowl, combine the thyme, salt, and pepper. Rub the mixture over the pork chops. Heat 2 teaspoons oil in a large nonstick skillet over medium heat. Add the chops and cook until browned and just cooked through, 2 to 3 minutes per side. Transfer to a plate, cover loosely with foil, and keep warm.

2. Add the remaining 1 teaspoon oil to the skillet. Add the onion and cook over medium heat, stirring frequently, until softened, 1 to 2 minutes. Add the cabbage and carrots and cook, stirring, until the cabbage is wilted, about 2 minutes. Add the broth and 3/4 cup water and bring to a simmer. Cover and cook until the cabbage is tender, 10 to 15 minutes. Stir in the mustard and vinegar and season with pepper. Serve the pork chops over the cabbage mixture. One serving is 3 ounces (85 grams) pork and 3/4 cup vegetables.

Per serving: 224 calories, 24 g protein, 9 g carbohydrates, 3 g fiber, 10 g total fat, 2 g saturated fat, 57 mg cholesterol, 564 mg sodium.

Spice-Crusted Pork Tenderloin with Peach Salsa

4
Serves

Preparation time: 35 minutes

Cooking time: 20–25 minutes

Peaches, one of the sweet Magic foods, are not just for desserts. Try them in this lively salsa, which sets off lean pork tenderloin beautifully. If you prefer to roast the pork, brown the tenderloin in 1 teaspoon vegetable oil in a skillet for 2 to 4 minutes, then transfer to a baking sheet and roast in a 400°F (200°C) oven for 15 to 20 minutes.

SALSA

1 cup diced peeled peach (1 large) (see Tip on page 234)

1/2 cup diced red bell pepper (1/2 small)

1/4 cup chopped scallions (2 medium)

2 tablespoons minced seeded jalapeño chile pepper (1 medium)

2 tablespoons lime juice

1 tablespoon chopped fresh cilantro

Pinch of salt

PORK

2 teaspoons ground cumin

1 teaspoon brown sugar

1 teaspoon paprika

1/2 teaspoon ground cinnamon

1/2 teaspoon ground ginger

1/2 teaspoon salt, or to taste

1/4 teaspoon freshly ground black pepper

1 teaspoon canola oil

1 pound (450 grams) pork tenderloin, trimmed

1. Preheat the grill.

2. To make the salsa: In a medium bowl, combine the peach, bell pepper, scallions, jalapeño pepper, lime juice, cilantro, and salt and toss to mix well.

3. To make the pork: In a small bowl, combine the cumin, brown sugar, paprika, cinnamon, ginger, salt, and pepper. Add the oil and mix well. Rub the spice paste over the pork.

4. Lightly oil the grill rack by rubbing it with a piece of oil-soaked paper towel. Grill the pork, covered, over medium heat, turning occasionally, until it reaches an internal temperature of 155°F (65°C), 20 to 25 minutes. Transfer to a cutting board and let stand for 5 minutes. Cut into slices 1/2 inch (1 centimeter) thick. One serving is 3 ounces (85 grams) pork (about 4 slices) and 1/3 cup salsa.

Per serving: 178 calories, 25 g protein, 7 g carbohydrates, 2 g fiber, 6 g total fat, 1 g saturated fat, 74 mg cholesterol, 388 mg sodium.

Ingredient Note: When working with chile peppers, wear rubber or latex gloves to protect your hands from the irritating oils. Keep your hands away from your eyes.

POULTRY

Chicken Breasts with Peaches and Ginger

4
Serves

| Preparation time: 25 minutes |
| Cooking time: 10 to 12 minutes |

Squeezing more fruit into your diet has never been simpler or more delicious. Here, sweet peaches, accented with fresh ginger, dress up a simple chicken sauté. The vinegar in the sauce balances the flavors and helps lower your blood sugar response to the meal. In winter, you can substitute 1 cup frozen peaches for the fresh peach. *See photo on page 244.*

1 bunch **scallions,** trimmed

1 pound (450 grams) boneless skinless **chicken** breast halves, trimmed

1/4 teaspoon salt, or to taste

Freshly ground black pepper to taste

2 teaspoons canola oil

3 tablespoons apple cider **vinegar**

2 tablespoons sugar

1/2 cup no-sugar-added peach juice or nectar, or apple juice

2 tablespoons grated fresh ginger

1 1/4 cups reduced-sodium chicken broth

1 large **peach,** peeled (see Tip) and sliced (1/2-inch/1-centimeter wedges)

2 teaspoons cornstarch

2 teaspoons water

1. Chop the scallions, reserving all of the white portions and 1/4 cup of the green portions separately.

2. If the chicken pieces are large, cut them in half lengthwise so that you have at least 4 pieces. Place the chicken between 2 pieces of plastic wrap and pound with a rolling pin or meat mallet into a 1/2-inch (1-centimeter) thickness. Season with the salt and pepper.

3. Heat the oil in a large nonstick skillet over medium-high heat. Add the chicken and cook until browned and no longer pink in the center, 3 to 3 1/2 minutes per side. Transfer to a plate.

4. Add the vinegar and sugar to the skillet. Stir to dissolve the sugar. Cook, swirling the skillet, until the syrup turns dark amber, 30 to 60 seconds. Add the scallion whites, peach juice, and ginger. Bring to a boil, stirring to scrape up any caramelized bits in the skillet. Cook for 1 minute. Add the broth and peaches. Return to a boil. Cook, turning the peaches from time to time, until tender, 2 to 4 minutes. Mix the cornstarch and water. Add to sauce. Cook, stirring, until slightly thickened, about 30 seconds. Reduce the heat to low and return the chicken and any accumulated juices to the skillet. Simmer gently until the chicken is heated through, about 1 minute. Garnish with the reserved scallion greens.

Per serving: 223 calories, 28 g protein, 17 g carbohydrates, 1 g fiber, 4 g total fat, 1 g saturated fat, 67 mg cholesterol, 275 mg sodium.

Tips:
• To peel peaches, dip them in boiling water for 20 to 30 seconds to loosen skins. Remove with a slotted spoon and let cool slightly. Slip off skins with a paring knife.

• Pounding the chicken breasts to make them thinner ensures quick, even cooking. And, by cutting super-size chicken breasts in half and then pounding them, you can ensure appropriate portion sizes. If you purchase thin-cut chicken breasts, you can skip this step.

VARIATION

Substitute 1 large nectarine or 2 plums for the peach. There's no need to peel either of these fruits.

Chicken Sauté with Apple

4
Serves

Preparation time: 20 minutes

Cooking time: 15 minutes

This simple chicken sauté features delectable morsels of boneless chicken and a generous amount of luxurious sauce that tastes deceptively rich, thanks to tart, fresh apples and a small amount of reduced-fat sour cream.

1 pound (450 grams) **chicken** tenders, trimmed, or 1 pound (450 grams) boneless skinless chicken breasts, trimmed and cut into 1/2-inch (1-centimeter)-thick slices

1/8 teaspoon salt, or to taste

Freshly ground pepper to taste

1 teaspoon **olive oil**

1 medium **apple,** peeled, cored, and sliced (prepare just before cooking)

1/4 cup finely chopped **shallot** (1 large)

3/4 teaspoon dried thyme

1/2 cup apple cider or apple juice

1 1/4 cups reduced-sodium chicken broth

1 1/2 teaspoons cornstarch

2 teaspoons water

1/4 cup reduced-fat sour cream

2 teaspoons coarse-grain mustard

1 tablespoon chopped fresh parsley or chives

1. Season the chicken with salt and pepper. Heat 2 teaspoons of the oil in a large nonstick skillet over medium-high heat. Add the chicken and cook, turning from time to time, until browned and no longer pink in the center, 5 to 6 minutes. Transfer to a plate, cover loosely with foil, and keep warm. (Do not wash the skillet.)

2. Add the remaining 1 teaspoon of oil to the skillet. Add the apple, shallot, and thyme. Cook, stirring often, until apple is lightly browned, 2 to 3 minutes. Add the apple cider (or apple juice) and bring to a boil, stirring to scrape up any browned bits. Cook for 1 1/2 minutes. Add the broth and return to a boil. Cook for 3 minutes.

3. Mix the cornstarch and water in a small bowl. Add to the sauce and cook, stirring, until slightly thickened. Reduce heat to low. Add the sour cream and mustard. Whisk until smooth. Return the chicken and any accumulated juices to the skillet and simmer just until heated through, about 1 minute. Garnish with parsley (or chives). One serving is 1 cup.

Per serving: 322 calories, 20 g protein, 31 g carbohydrates, 2 g fiber, 13 g total fat, 4 g saturated fat, 52 mg cholesterol, 706 mg sodium.

All-New Chicken Cordon Bleu

4
Serves

Preparation time: 25 minutes

Cooking time: 22 minutes

Crispy chicken breasts with a surprise nugget of cheesy filling are a family favorite. This version trims fat and calories by avoiding deep-frying. Instead, the chicken is browned on one side in a skillet and then finished in a hot oven, producing a crisp crust, without all the fat and fuss. If you would like to get things ready ahead of time, prepare the recipe through Step 4. Cover and refrigerate for up to 8 hours.

1/4 cup shredded Swiss, Monterey Jack, or part-skim mozzarella **cheese**

2 tablespoons chopped boiled or baked lean deli ham

1 tablespoon low-fat mayonnaise

2 teaspoons Dijon mustard

1/8 teaspoon freshly ground pepper

4 boneless skinless **chicken** breast halves (1 to 1 1/2 pounds/450 to 700 grams total), trimmed

1/2 cup Italian-style dry bread crumbs

1 large **egg** white

2 teaspoons **olive oil**

1. Preheat the oven to 400°F (200°C). Coat a baking sheet with nonstick spray.

2. Mix the cheese, ham, mayonnaise, mustard, and pepper in a small bowl.

3. Using a small sharp knife, make a horizontal slit along the thinner, long edge of a chicken breast half, cutting nearly through to the opposite side. Open up the breast and place about 1 tablespoon of the cheese mixture in the center. Close the breast over the filling and press the edges firmly together to seal. Repeat with the remaining chicken breast halves and cheese mixture.

4. Place the bread crumbs in a shallow glass dish. Lightly beat the egg white with a fork in a medium bowl. Holding each stuffed chicken breast together, dip them in the egg white, then dredge in the bread crumbs. (Discard any leftover bread crumbs.)

5. Heat the oil in a large nonstick skillet over medium-high heat. Add the chicken breasts and cook until browned on one side, about 2 minutes. Using tongs, place chicken breasts, browned side up, on the baking sheet.

6. Bake the chicken until no longer pink in the center, about 20 minutes. An instant-read thermometer inserted in the center should register 170°F (75°C). One serving is 1 stuffed chicken breast half.

Per serving: 260 calories, 32 g protein, 11 g carbohydrates, 1 g fiber, 9 g total fat, 3 g saturated fat, 76 mg cholesterol, 607 mg sodium.

VARIATION Chicken Breasts Stuffed with Pesto

In Step 2, substitute 2 tablespoons reduced-fat cream cheese and 1 tablespoon prepared basil pesto for the Swiss cheese, ham, mayonnaise, and mustard. Blend the cream cheese, pesto, and pepper together in a small bowl with a fork.

Chicken Pot Pie with a Whole Grain Biscuit Crust

5
Serves

Preparation time: 1 hour

Baking time: 30 to 40 minutes

Everyone loves chicken pot pie, but it's a killer when it comes to calories. We've topped ours with a tender, low-fat crust and included a generous serving of vegetables bathed in a light but still-creamy sauce. Bake this whenever you have cooked poultry or a store-bought rotisserie chicken on hand. If you are cooking for a crowd, double the recipe and use a 9 x 13-inch (23 x 33-centimeter) baking dish. To trim preparation time, purchase cleaned, sliced mushrooms and sliced carrots (fresh or frozen).

FILLING

2 teaspoons canola oil

3 cups sliced white mushrooms (8 ounces/250 grams)

1 1/4 cups sliced **carrots**

1/4 cup all-purpose flour

2 1/4 cups reduced-sodium chicken broth or turkey broth, divided

1/4 cup reduced-fat sour cream

1 1/2 teaspoons freshly grated lemon zest

1/8 teaspoon salt, or to taste

1/8 teaspoon freshly ground pepper

2 cups diced, cooked skinless **chicken** (11 ounces/325 grams)

1 1/4 cups frozen green **peas,** rinsed under cold water to thaw

CRUST

1 cup **whole wheat pastry flour** (see Ingredient Note)

1 teaspoon sugar

3/4 teaspoon baking powder

1/4 teaspoon baking soda

1/8 teaspoon salt

4 tablespoons (2 ounces/60 grams) cold, reduced-fat cream **cheese** (Neufchâtel), cut into small pieces

1 tablespoon cold unsalted butter, cut into small pieces

1 tablespoon canola oil

About 1/3 cup low-fat buttermilk

1 teaspoon low-fat (1%) **milk** for brushing

1. Preheat the oven to 400°F (200°C). Coat an 8-inch (20-centimeter) square (or similar 2-quart/2-liter) baking dish with cooking spray.

2. **To make the filling:** Heat the oil in a large nonstick skillet over medium-high heat. Add the mushrooms and cook, stirring or shaking the skillet from time to time, until browned and tender, 5 to 7 minutes. Steam the carrots until just tender, 3 to 5 minutes. Rinse with cold running water.

3. Whisk the all-purpose flour with 1/2 cup cold broth in a small bowl until smooth. Bring the remaining 1 3/4 cups broth to a simmer in a medium saucepan over medium-high heat. Gradually whisk in the flour mixture. Cook, whisking, until the sauce boils and thickens. Reduce the heat to low and simmer for 1 minute. Remove from the heat and whisk in the sour cream, lemon zest, salt, and pepper. Stir in the chicken, peas, mushrooms, and carrots. Scrape into the baking dish, spreading evenly.

4. **To make the crust:** Whisk the flour, sugar, baking powder, baking soda, and salt in a large bowl until blended. Using a pastry blender or 2 knives, cut in the cream cheese and butter until the mixture resembles coarse crumbs. Add the oil and toss with a fork to blend. With a fork, stir in just enough of the buttermilk until a soft, slightly sticky dough forms. Turn out onto a lightly floured surface and knead several times, just until smooth. Pat or roll the dough into a rough 9 x 7-inch (23 x 18-centimeter) rectangle, about 1/2 inch (1 centimeter) thick. With a sharp knife, cut the dough in half lengthwise, then cut

each half into 5 triangles, trimming as needed. Arrange the biscuit triangles over the filling. Brush the tops with milk.

5. Bake the pie until the filling is bubbly and the biscuits are golden and firm, 30 to 40 minutes. One serving equals 1 cup filling and 2 biscuit triangles. You can prepare the filling ahead through Step 3. (Chill the sauce before mixing with the vegetables and chicken.) Cover and refrigerate for up to 1 day.

Per serving: 390 calories, 28 g protein, 43 g carbohydrates, 8 g fiber, 12 g total fat, 4 g saturated fat, 58 mg cholesterol, 706 mg sodium.

Tip: Cutting the biscuit dough into triangles, rather than the traditional circles, allows you to cover a square baking dish efficiently, minimizing waste.

Ingredient Note: Whole wheat pastry flour is lower in protein than regular whole wheat flour. Since it has less gluten-forming potential, it is an excellent choice for tender baked goods. You can find it in large supermarkets and natural foods stores.

VARIATION Turkey Pot Pie with a Whole Grain Biscuit Crust

In Step 3, substitute diced skinless turkey breast for the chicken.

Oven-Fried Chicken

4 Serves

| Preparation time: 20 minutes |
| Marinating time: 30 minutes |
| Baking time: 40 to 50 minutes |

This simple chicken recipe, loaded with Magic extras like mustard (it contains vinegar, a Magic food) and sesame seeds, makes a great family meal. Marinating the chicken in buttermilk keeps it moist and succulent, and a light coating of whole wheat flour, sesame seeds, and spices replaces the fatty chicken skin and forms an appealing crust during baking.

1/2 cup buttermilk

1 tablespoon Dijon mustard

2 garlic cloves, minced

1 teaspoon hot red pepper sauce, such as Tabasco

2 1/2 –3 pounds (1.25 to 1.5 kilograms) bone-in chicken legs, skin removed, fat trimmed, thighs and drumsticks separated at the joint

1/2 cup whole wheat flour

2 tablespoons sesame seeds

1 1/2 teaspoons baking powder

1 1/2 teaspoons paprika

1 teaspoon dried thyme

Pinch of salt

Freshly ground pepper to taste

1. Whisk the buttermilk, mustard, garlic, and hot sauce in a shallow glass dish until well blended. Add the chicken and turn to coat. Cover and marinate in the refrigerator for at least 30 minutes or up to 8 hours.

2. Preheat the oven to 425°F (220°C). Line a baking sheet with aluminum foil. Set a wire rack on the baking sheet and coat it with non-stick spray.

3. Whisk the flour, sesame seeds, baking powder, paprika, thyme, salt, and pepper in a small bowl. Place the flour mixture in a paper bag or large plastic food bag. One at a time, place the chicken pieces in the bag and shake to coat. Shake off excess flour and place the chicken on the rack. (Discard any leftover flour mixture and marinade.) Spray the chicken pieces lightly with nonstick spray.

4. Bake the chicken until golden brown and no longer pink in the center, 40 to 50 minutes. An instant-read thermometer inserted in the center should register 180°F (85°C). One serving is 1 drumstick and 1 thigh.

Per serving: 227 calories, 34 g protein, 5 g carbohydrates, 1 g fiber, 7 g total fat, 2 g saturated fat, 130 mg cholesterol, 262 mg sodium.

Roasted Moroccan Chicken Thighs with Squash and Pearl Onions

4 Serves

| Preparation time: 25 minutes |
| Cooking time: 40 to 45 minutes |

Try this dinner from a roasting pan for a special meal that's easy to make and serve. Boneless skinless chicken thighs, which cook in the same time as the vegetables, are a convenient option for roasting. A flavorful spice rub gives them a faux skin, sealing in the juices and reducing the fat significantly.

1 pound (450 grams) peeled, seeded butternut squash, cut into 3/4-inch (2-centimeter) cubes (3 cups)

2 cups frozen pearl onions, rinsed in cold water to thaw

4 teaspoons olive oil, divided

1/2 teaspoon salt, divided

Freshly ground pepper to taste

2 teaspoons honey

2 teaspoons plus 1 tablespoon lemon juice, divided

2 teaspoons paprika

1/2 teaspoon ground cumin

1 pound (450 grams) boneless skinless **chicken** thighs, trimmed

12 fresh cilantro sprigs, plus 1/4 cup coarsely chopped cilantro

1 cup reduced-sodium chicken broth

1. Preheat the oven to 450°F (230°C). Coat a large roasting pan with nonstick spray.

2. Combine the squash, onions, 2 teaspoons oil, 1/4 teaspoon salt, and pepper in a large bowl. Toss to coat. Set aside.

3. Mix the remaining 2 teaspoons oil, the honey, and 2 teaspoons lemon juice in a small bowl until smooth. Add the paprika, cumin, remaining 1/4 teaspoon salt, and pepper. Rub this mixture over the chicken thighs.

4. Place the cilantro sprigs in the center of the roasting pan. Set the chicken thighs over the cilantro sprigs. Surround the chicken with the squash and onions. Bake, uncovered, until chicken is cooked through (an instant-read thermometer inserted in the center should register 180°F (85°C) and vegetables are tender, turning vegetables twice, 40 to 45 minutes. Transfer the chicken and vegetables to a platter or individual plates (leave cilantro sprigs in the roasting pan).

5. Add the chicken broth and remaining 1 tablespoon lemon juice to roasting pan and place over high heat. Bring to a simmer, stirring to scrape up any browned bits. Simmer for 1 minute. Strain the broth through a sieve into a medium bowl. Spoon pan sauce over chicken and vegetables. Sprinkle with chopped cilantro. One serving is 2 chicken thighs, 1 cup vegetables, and a few tablespoons pan sauce.

Per serving: 304 calories, 28 g protein, 27 g carbohydrates, 4 g fiber, 10 g total fat, 2 g saturated fat, 107 mg cholesterol, 447 mg sodium.

Turkey-Noodle Casserole with Spinach

8 Serves

| Preparation time: 40 minutes |
| Cooking/baking time: 50 to 60 minutes |

Leftover turkey begs to be made into a creamy casserole. Ours is made with whole wheat pasta, a light, lemony sauce, and extra vegetables. This is an ideal dish to make ahead. Prepare the casserole through Step 3, cover and refrigerate for up to 2 days or freeze for up to 3 months (thaw before baking).

2 tablespoons plus 1 teaspoon **olive oil,** divided

1 medium **onion,** chopped

1/2 cup all-purpose flour

4 cups reduced-sodium chicken broth, heated

1/2 cup reduced-fat sour cream

2 teaspoons freshly grated lemon zest

1 tablespoon **lemon** juice

1/4 teaspoon salt, or to taste

Freshly ground pepper to taste

8 ounces (250 grams) whole wheat **pasta,** such as rotini or fusilli

2 cups sliced **carrots** (4 medium)

1 bag (12 ounces/300 grams) baby **spinach,** rinsed

3 cups diced cooked skinless **turkey** or **chicken** (12 ounces/340 grams)

1/2 cup grated Parmesan **cheese**

1/4 cup fine dry plain bread crumbs

1. Bring a large pot of lightly salted water to a boil. Preheat the oven to 400°F (200°C). Coat a 9 x 13-inch (23 x 33-centimeter) baking dish with nonstick spray.

2. Heat 2 tablespoons of the oil in a large saucepan over medium heat. Add the onion and cook, stirring often, until softened, 2 to 3 minutes. Add the flour and cook, stirring, for 30 to 60 seconds. Remove from the heat. Add the hot broth and whisk to blend. Place the saucepan

over medium-high heat and bring the sauce to a simmer, whisking constantly. Reduce the heat to low and simmer, whisking occasionally, until slightly thickened, about 5 minutes. Remove from the heat and whisk in the sour cream, lemon zest, lemon juice, salt, and pepper.

3. Add the pasta and carrots to the boiling water and cook for 5 minutes. Add the spinach and stir until wilted, 30 to 60 seconds. Drain the pasta and vegetables. Refresh under cold running water. (The pasta will seem quite firm but will continue to cook during baking.) Transfer the pasta mixture to a large bowl. Add the sauce and turkey. Toss to coat well. Scrape the mixture into the prepared baking dish, spreading evenly. Sprinkle with the Parmesan. Mix the bread crumbs and remaining 1 teaspoon oil in a small bowl and sprinkle over the casserole.

4. Bake the casserole, uncovered, until it is bubbly and the topping is lightly browned, 35 to 45 minutes. One serving is 1 1/3 cups.

Per serving: 333 calories, 23 g protein, 32 g carbohydrates, 6 g fiber, 9 g total fat, 3 g saturated fat, 42 mg cholesterol, 378 mg sodium.

Honey-Mustard Turkey Burgers

4 Serves | **Preparation time: 20 minutes**
| **Cooking time: 10 to 12 minutes**

Next time you're hankering for a burger, try this turkey burger. A little low-fat mayonnaise helps keep the patties moist, while mustard and honey perk up the flavor. When shopping for ground turkey, check labels. Regular ground turkey, made from breast and leg meat (and often skin), is almost as high in calories and fat as extra-lean ground beef. Ground turkey breast, on the other hand, is truly lean.

1/4 cup coarse-grain mustard

2 tablespoons honey

1 1/2 teaspoons Worcestershire sauce

1 pound (450 grams) lean ground **turkey** breast

1 tablespoon low-fat mayonnaise

1 **garlic** clove, minced

1/2 teaspoon salt, or to taste

1/4 teaspoon freshly ground pepper

4 **whole wheat hamburger rolls**, split

Optional garnishes: lettuce leaves, sliced tomato, sliced red or sweet onion, ketchup, reduced-fat mayonnaise

1. Stir the mustard, honey, and Worcestershire sauce together in a medium bowl. Reserve 2 tablespoons of this mixture to use as glaze. Add the ground turkey, mayonnaise, garlic, salt, and pepper to the mustard mixture remaining in the bowl. Mix with a potato masher. Divide the mixture into 4 portions, then form each one into a 1/2-inch (1-centimeter)-thick patty.

2. Preheat the grill to medium-high.

3. Lightly oil the grill rack by rubbing the surface with a piece of oil-soaked paper towel. Grill the patties for 4 minutes. Turn the patties over and brush the cooked sides with the reserved glaze. Cook for 4 minutes. Turn the patties over and brush again with the glaze. Cook until the juices run clear and an instant-read thermometer inserted in the center registers 165°F (70°C), 2 to 4 minutes longer. Just before the patties are cooked, place the rolls, cut side down, on the grill until lightly toasted, 30 to 60 seconds. Place a patty on each roll and garnish as desired. One serving is 1 patty and 1 roll.

Per serving (without garnishes): 331 calories, 28 g protein, 33 g carbohydrates, 2 g fiber, 11 g total fat, 3 g saturated fat, 65 mg cholesterol, 952 mg sodium.

Turkey Shepherd's Pie with Sweet Potato Topping

6
Serves

Preparation time: 45 minutes

Baking time: 35 to 40 minutes

A Magic version of an old-fashioned favorite, this shepherd's pie uses lean ground turkey instead of ground beef and sweet potatoes in place of white potatoes in the topping. The taste is reminiscent of a Thanksgiving dinner, but you can enjoy this easy-to-make pie throughout the year. To make it ahead, prepare through Step 4, cover and refrigerate for up to 2 days, then continue with the recipe.

FILLING

1 1/4 pounds (600 grams) lean ground **turkey** breast

2 teaspoons **olive oil** or canola oil

1 cup chopped **onion** (1 medium)

1 cup chopped **carrots** (2–4 medium)

2 **garlic** cloves, minced

1 teaspoon dried thyme

1/3 cup all-purpose flour

2 1/4 cups reduced-sodium chicken broth

1 teaspoon Worcestershire sauce

1 cup frozen green **peas,** rinsed under cold water to thaw

Freshly ground pepper to taste

TOPPING

2 medium-large **sweet potatoes,** peeled and cut into chunks

1/2 cup low-fat (1%) **milk**

1/2 teaspoon freshly grated lemon zest

3/4 teaspoon salt, or to taste

Freshly ground pepper to taste

$1.$ Preheat the oven to 400°F (200°C). Coat an 11 x 7-inch (28 x 18-centimeter) or 9 x 13-inch (23 x 33-centimeter) baking dish with cooking spray.

$2.$ **To make the filling:** Cook the turkey in a large nonstick skillet over medium-high heat, crumbling with a wooden spoon, until no longer pink, 4 to 5 minutes. Transfer to a plate.

$3.$ Add 2 teaspoons oil to the skillet. Add the onion and carrots; cook over medium-high heat, stirring often, until softened, 2 to 4 minutes. Add the garlic and thyme; cook, stirring, for 30 seconds. Sprinkle in the flour and stir to coat well. Gradually stir in the broth and bring to a simmer, stirring. Return the turkey to the skillet and reduce the heat to medium. Partially cover and simmer, stirring occasionally, until the carrots are tender, about 10 minutes. Stir in the peas and Worcestershire sauce. Season with pepper. Transfer the turkey mixture to the baking dish.

$4.$ **To prepare the topping:** Place the sweet potatoes in a large saucepan. Add enough lightly salted water to cover and bring to a simmer. Reduce the heat to medium, cover, and simmer until the sweet potatoes are tender, 10 to 15 minutes. Drain and return the sweet potatoes to the saucepan. Mash with a potato masher or portable electric mixer. Gradually stir or beat in the milk. Season with lemon zest, salt, and pepper. Spoon the sweet potato mixture over the turkey filling. Use the back of a spoon to cover the filling and make decorative swirls.

$5.$ Bake the pie, uncovered, until the filling is bubbling and the topping is heated through, 35 to 40 minutes. One serving is 3/4 cup filling and 1/2 cup topping.

Per serving: 317 calories, 31 g protein, 43 g carbohydrates, 7 g fiber, 3 g total fat, 0 g saturated fat, 39 mg cholesterol, 656 mg sodium.

Turkey Meatballs

8 Serves

Preparation time: 40 minutes

Cooking time: 40 to 50 minutes

Made with lean ground turkey breast, these tender meatballs provide protein without the baggage of saturated fat. The Magic cinnamon seasoning in the meatballs adds a delightful accent to the tomato sauce. Spaghetti and meatballs is a crowd-pleaser, ideal for serving a hungry crowd. But even if you are cooking for one or two, make a batch of meatballs and sauce and freeze it in portion-size containers. Serve over whole wheat spaghetti, allowing 2 ounces (60 grams) uncooked pasta per person, or use in sandwiches.

SAUCE

2 teaspoons olive oil

4 garlic cloves, cut into thin slivers

1/2 teaspoon dried oregano

1/8 teaspoon crushed red pepper

3 cans (14 ounces/398 milliliters each) diced tomatoes

2 cans (8 ounces/213 milliliters each) no-salt-added tomato sauce

MEATBALLS

1 pound (450 grams) lean ground turkey breast

1 cup fresh whole wheat bread crumbs (see Tip)

1 cup finely chopped onion (1 medium)

1 large egg, lightly beaten

1/3 cup grated Parmesan cheese

3/4 teaspoon salt, or to taste

1/2 teaspoon cinnamon

1/4 teaspoon freshly ground pepper

2 teaspoons olive oil, divided

2 tablespoons chopped fresh parsley

1. **To make the sauce:** Heat the oil in a Dutch oven over medium-low heat. Add the garlic, oregano, and red pepper. Cook, stirring, until softened but not browned, 1 to 2 minutes. Add the diced tomatoes and mash with a potato masher. Add the tomato sauce and bring to a simmer over medium-high heat. Reduce heat to medium-low, cover, and simmer while you prepare the meatballs.

2. **To make the meatballs:** Mix the ground turkey, bread crumbs, onion, egg, cheese, salt, cinnamon, and pepper thoroughly in a large bowl. Form into 1/2-inch (1-centimeter) meatballs.

3. Heat 1 teaspoon of the oil in a large nonstick skillet over medium-high heat. Add half of the meatballs and cook, turning occasionally, until browned on all sides. Transfer to a plate. Repeat with the remaining 1 teaspoon oil and meatballs. Add the browned meatballs to the simmering tomato sauce and simmer, covered, for 20 minutes. Uncover and simmer, stirring occasionally, until the meatballs are cooked through and the sauce has thickened slightly, 20 to 40 minutes longer. Sprinkle with parsley. One serving is 3 or 4 meatballs and 1 cup sauce. The meatballs and sauce will keep, covered, in the refrigerator for up to 2 days or in the freezer in an airtight container for up to 3 months (thaw in the refrigerator). Reheat on the stovetop or in the microwave.

Per serving: 184 calories, 19 g protein, 15 g carbohydrates, 3 g fiber, 5 g total fat, 1 g saturated fat, 52 mg cholesterol, 703 mg sodium.

Tip: To make fresh bread crumbs, tear fresh bread into pieces and place in a food processor or blender. Pulse until broken down into fine crumbs. Two slices of bread make 1 cup of crumbs.

Turkey and Bean Chili with Avocado Salsa

8 Serves

Preparation time: 35 minutes

Cooking time: 1 hour, 10 minutes

Beans, with their wallop of sugar-lowering soluble fiber, should be on your menu weekly, and this full-flavored chili's a great way to enjoy them. We lightened up the typical chili by using turkey instead of beef and gave it a Magic boost with avocado salsa, full of good fat. Offer a selection of garnishes, such as chopped scallions, lime wedges, hot sauce, reduced-fat sour cream, and grated low-fat cheese, so your family and guests can personalize their chili bowls. *See photo on page 244.*

CHILI

12 ounces (340 grams) lean ground turkey breast

1/4 cup chili powder

1 tablespoon ground cumin

1 1/2 teaspoons dried oregano

2 teaspoons canola oil

2 cups chopped onion (1 large)

4 garlic cloves, minced

2 cans (4 1/2 ounces/127 milliliters each) chopped green chiles

1 can (28 ounces/796 milliliters) diced tomatoes (undrained)

1 can (14 ounces/398 milliliters) reduced-sodium chicken broth

1 can (19 ounces/540 milliliters) black beans, drained and rinsed

1 can (19 ounces/540 milliliters) red kidney beans, drained and rinsed

AVOCADO SALSA

2 medium Hass avocados, diced

2/3 cup diced, seeded fresh tomato (1 medium plum tomato)

1/4 cup finely diced white or red onion

2 tablespoons minced seeded jalapeño pepper (1 small)

2 tablespoons chopped fresh cilantro

2 tablespoons lime juice

1/4 teaspoon salt, or to taste

1. Cook the ground turkey with the chili powder, cumin, and oregano in a large nonstick skillet over medium-high heat, breaking up the meat and mixing in spices with a wooden spoon, until browned, 4 to 5 minutes. Remove from the heat and set aside.

2. Heat the oil in a Dutch oven over medium heat. Add the onion and cook, stirring often, until softened, 3 to 5 minutes. Add the garlic and green chiles. Cook, stirring, until fragrant, 1 to 2 minutes. Add the tomatoes, broth, and browned ground turkey. Bring to a simmer. Reduce heat to low. Cover and simmer, stirring occasionally, for 45 minutes.

3. Stir in the black beans and kidney beans. Return to a simmer. Cover and simmer over low heat until flavors have blended, 15 to 20 minutes.

4. **To make the Avocado Salsa:** combine the avocado, tomato, onion, jalapeño, cilantro, lime juice, and salt in a medium bowl. Toss gently to mix.

5. Spoon 2 tablespoons of salsa on each serving of chili. One serving of chili is 1 1/4 cups chili and 2 tablespoons salsa. The chili will keep, covered, in the refrigerator for up to 2 days or in the freezer in an airtight container for up to 3 months.

Per serving: 327 calories, 23 g protein, 38 g carbohydrates, 12 g fiber, 11 g total fat, 1 g saturated fat, 17 mg cholesterol, 748 mg sodium.

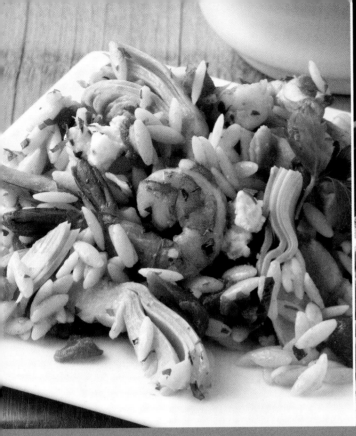
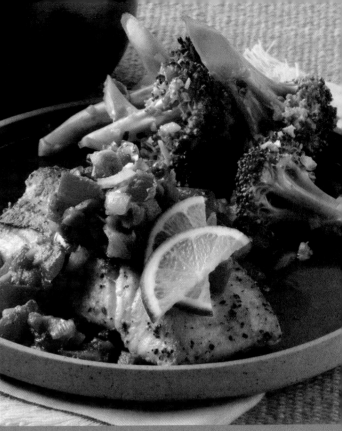

Shrimp and Orzo Casserole *page 251*
olive oil • garlic • tomato • pasta • shrimp • cheese

Seared Fish Steaks with Tomato-Olive Sauce *page 246*
Broccoli with Lemon Vinaigrette page 272
lime • olive oil • halibut • onion • garlic • tomato • olives

Turkey and Bean Chili with Avocado Salsa *page 243*
turkey • onion • garlic • tomato • beans • avocado • lime

Chicken Breasts with Peaches and Ginger *page 234*
Brown Rice Pilaf with Toasted Flaxseeds page 265
scallion •chicken • vinegar • peach

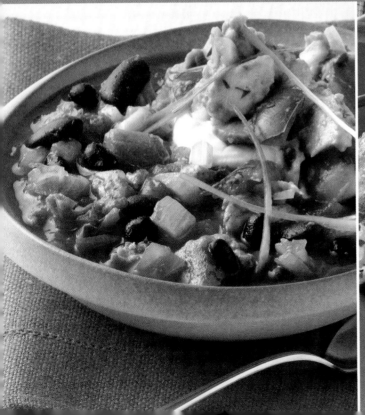
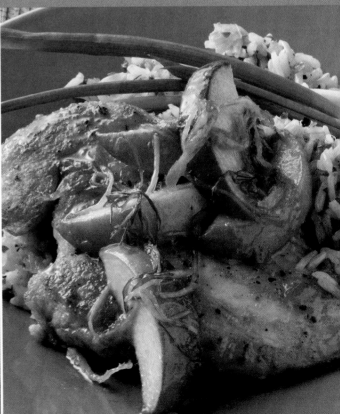

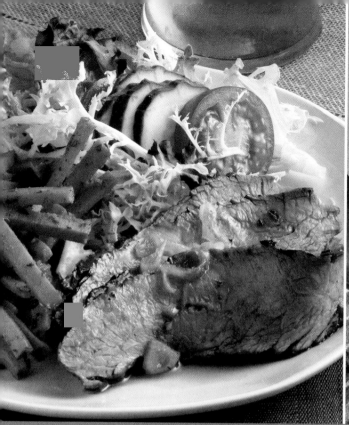

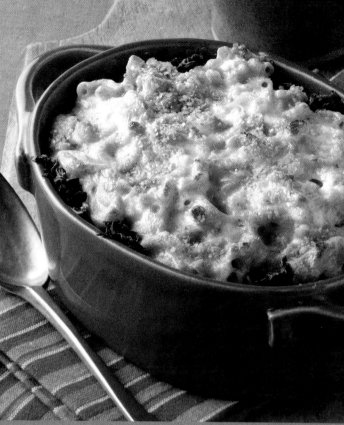

Flank Steak with Balsamic Sauce *page 228*
Moroccan Spiced Carrots page 274
vinegar • garlic • steak • shallot • olive oil

Macaroni and Cheese with Spinach *page 255*
milk • cheese • spinach • pasta • wheat germ

Pork Chop and Cabbage Skillet Dinner *page 232*
pork • onion • cabbage • carrot • vinegar

Mushroom and Herb Pizza *page 258*
whole wheat flour • olive oil • garlic • cheese • onion • tomato

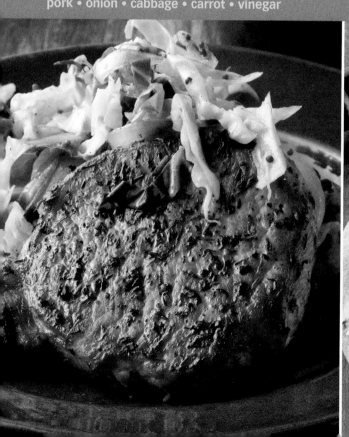

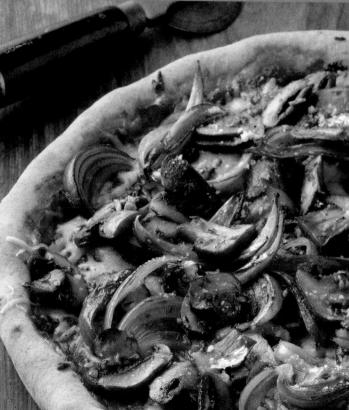

FISH AND SEAFOOD

Seared Fish Steaks with Tomato-Olive Sauce

4
Serves

Preparation time: 25 minutes	
Marinating time: 10 to 20 minutes	
Cooking/baking time: 10 to 12 minutes	

Firm fish like swordfish and halibut benefit from this easy two-step technique of first browning the steaks on one side and then finishing cooking in the oven (cooking the fish entirely in the skillet can make the outside tough and requires more fat). The spicy tomato sauce sets off the succulent fish steaks beautifully. *See photo on page 244.*

1 tablespoon lime juice

4 teaspoons olive oil, divided

1/8 teaspoon salt, or to taste

Freshly ground pepper to taste

4 1-inch (2.5-centimeter) thick halibut steaks (4 ounces/125 grams each) or swordfish steaks (6 ounces/170 grams each)

1/2 cup chopped onion

1 garlic clove, minced

1/2 teaspoon ground cumin

Pinch of crushed red pepper

1 can (10 ounces/398 milliliters) diced tomatoes with green chiles

1/3 cup water

1 tablespoon chopped pitted green olives

2 teaspoons drained capers, rinsed

Lime wedges

1. Preheat the oven to 425°F (220°C). Coat a baking sheet with nonstick spray.

2. Mix the lime juice, 1 teaspoon oil, salt, and pepper in a shallow glass dish. Add the fish steaks and turn to coat. Cover and marinate in the refrigerator for 10 to 20 minutes.

3. Meanwhile, heat 2 teaspoons oil in a medium saucepan over medium heat. Add the onion and cook, stirring often, until softened, 3 to 4 minutes. Add the garlic, cumin, and red pepper. Cook, stirring, for 30 seconds. Add the tomatoes and water. Bring to a simmer. Cook over medium heat, stirring occasionally, until thickened, about 10 minutes.

4. While sauce is simmering, cook the fish. Heat the remaining 1 teaspoon oil in a large nonstick skillet over medium-high heat. Add the fish and cook until browned on one side, 2 to 3 minutes. Transfer the fish to the baking sheet, browned side up. Bake until the fish is opaque in the center, 8 to 10 minutes.

5. Stir the olives and capers into the tomato sauce. Season with black pepper. Top each fish steak with sauce and serve with lime wedges. One serving is 1 fish steak and 1/4 cup sauce.

Per serving: 198 calories, 22 g protein, 6 g carbohydrates, 1 g fiber, 10 g total fat, 2 g saturated fat, 41 mg cholesterol, 551 mg sodium.

Tip: The tomato-olive sauce (Steps 2 and 5) is also delicious over grilled boneless skinless chicken breasts.

Sole Florentine

4	Preparation time: 30 minutes
Serves	Cooking/baking time: 40 to 45 minutes

The term Florentine simply means "with spinach"—the perfect partner for a delicate fish like sole or haddock. The cheesy sauce in this recipe not only enhances the fish and spinach, it also provides calcium, vitamin D, and extra protein.

1 teaspoon freshly grated lemon zest

1 3/4 cups low-fat (1%) milk, divided

3 tablespoons all-purpose flour

1/2 cup grated Parmesan cheese, divided

1/4 teaspoon salt, or to taste

Freshly ground pepper to taste

Pinch of cayenne pepper

1 1/2 packages (10 ounces/300 grams each) frozen spinach

1 pound (450 grams) sole, haddock, flounder, or orange roughy fillets

2 teaspoons lemon juice

3 tablespoons Italian-style bread crumbs

1 teaspoon olive oil

1. Preheat the oven to 425°F (220°C). Coat an 8 x 11 1/2-inch (20 x 30-centimeter) baking dish (or similar 2-quart/2-liter capacity dish) with nonstick spray. Sprinkle the baking dish with lemon zest.

2. Whisk 1/4 cup of the cold milk and the flour in a small bowl until smooth. Heat the remaining 1 1/2 cups milk in a heavy medium saucepan over medium heat until steaming. Add the flour mixture and cook, whisking constantly, until the sauce bubbles and thickens, 2 to 3 minutes. Remove from the heat. Stir in 1/4 cup Parmesan, salt, pepper, and cayenne.

3. Meanwhile, cook the spinach according to package directions. Drain and refresh under cold running water. Press out excess moisture.

4. Spread the spinach over the bottom of the baking dish. Arrange the fish fillets, slightly overlapping, over the spinach. Sprinkle with the lemon juice. Spoon the cheese sauce evenly over the fish. Sprinkle the remaining 1/4 cup Parmesan over the sauce. Mix the bread crumbs and oil in a small bowl and sprinkle over the sauce.

5. Bake until golden and bubbly and the fish flakes when poked with a small sharp knife, 30 to 35 minutes.

Per serving: 278 calories, 35 g protein, 19 g carbohydrates, 4 g fiber, 8 g total fat, 3 g saturated fat, 70 mg cholesterol, 661 mg sodium.

Mustard-Glazed Salmon with Lentils

4	Preparation time: 10 minutes
Serves	Cooking time: 12 to 15 minutes

It doesn't get much easier than this: canned lentil soup (drained so it has the consistency of braised lentils), topped with roasted salmon. This delightful pairing of two Magic foods is actually a French bistro classic, which translates seamlessly into healthy home cooking.

2 cans (19 ounces/540 milliliters each) lentil soup

1 pound (450 grams) salmon fillet, cut into 4 portions

Freshly ground pepper to taste

3 tablespoons coarse-grain or Dijon mustard

2 teaspoons olive oil

2/3 cup scallions, trimmed and chopped (1 bunch)

1/2 teaspoon dried thyme

1 tablespoon lemon juice

Lemon wedges

1. Preheat the oven to 450°F (230°C). Line a small baking pan with aluminum foil and coat it with nonstick spray.

2. Place the lentil soup in a sieve set over a bowl. Set aside to drain for several minutes.

3. Place the salmon, skin side down, in the baking pan. Season with pepper and spread with the mustard. Bake the salmon until opaque in the center, 12 to 15 minutes.

4. Meanwhile, heat the oil in a medium saucepan over medium heat. Add the scallions and cook, stirring, until softened, 1 to 2 minutes. Add the drained lentil soup and thyme. Heat through. Stir in the lemon juice. Spoon the lentils onto plates and top each serving with a piece of salmon. Garnish with lemon wedges. One serving is 3 ounces (85 grams) salmon and 2/3 cup lentils.

Per serving: 330 calories, 34 g protein, 28 g carbohydrates, 9 g fiber, 10 g total fat, 1 g saturated fat, 59 mg cholesterol, 981 mg sodium.

Tip: To cook salmon in the microwave, place in a microwave-safe dish, cover with wax paper, and microwave on high for 5 to 7 minutes.

Salmon with Lemon and Dill Sauce

4

Serves

Preparation time: 20 minutes

Baking time: 15 to 20 minutes

Salmon is your best source of omega 3 fatty acids, which can actually *improve* insulin sensitivity, benefiting your blood sugar. Here is a foolproof way to prepare it. Baking salmon with a small amount of liquid and shallots produces exceptionally moist and succulent results. The creamy sauce, a lighter, much easier version of Hollandaise, is made with low-fat mayonnaise and brightened with fresh herbs and lemon.

SALMON

1 pound (450 grams) center-cut salmon fillet
(about 1 1/4 inches/3 centimeters thick),
cut into 4 portions

2 tablespoons dry white wine or water

2 tablespoons finely chopped shallots (1 medium)

1/4 teaspoon salt, or to taste

Freshly ground pepper to taste

Lemon wedges

SAUCE

1/4 cup reduced-fat mayonnaise

1/4 cup low-fat (1%) milk

2 tablespoons chopped fresh dill

1 teaspoon freshly grated lemon zest

1 tablespoon lemon juice

2 teaspoons Dijon mustard

1. Preheat the oven to 425°F (220°C). Coat a shallow baking dish, such as a 9-inch (23-centimeter) glass pie plate, with nonstick spray. Place the salmon pieces, skin side down, in the dish. Sprinkle with wine (or water), then sprinkle with shallots and season with salt and pepper. Cover with aluminum foil and bake until the salmon is opaque in center, 15 to 20 minutes.

2. **To make the sauce:** Place the mayonnaise in a small saucepan. Gradually whisk in the milk. Set the saucepan over medium-low heat and cook, whisking constantly, until mixture is smooth and heated through but not bubbling, about 2 minutes. Remove from the heat and stir in dill, lemon zest and juice, mustard, and pepper. Keep warm.

3. Divide the salmon among 4 plates. Pour the liquid remaining in the baking dish into the sauce and stir to mix. Spoon the sauce over the salmon and serve with lemon wedges. One serving is 3 ounces (85 grams) salmon and 2 tablespoons sauce.

Per serving: 250 calories, 23 g protein, 4 g carbohydrates, 0 g fiber, 14 g total fat, 3 g saturated fat, 68 mg cholesterol, 384 mg sodium.

Warm Salmon Salad with Olive Toasts

4 Serves

| Preparation time: 25 minutes |
| Cooking time: 5 minutes |

Chunks of pink salmon contrast beautifully with dark, leafy greens in this satisfying but light main-course salad, perfect for a warm summer evening. The olive oil dressing is sharpened with fresh lemon juice, which gives the salad an appealing kick and also dampens your blood sugar response to the meal. Crisp toasts, spread with appetite-teasing black olive spread, round out the salad. This is an excellent opportunity to enjoy the rye or pumpernickel bread that is recommended for Magic eating.

2 tablespoons plus 2 teaspoons extra-virgin olive oil

1 tablespoon plus 1/4 cup lemon juice

1/2 teaspoon Dijon mustard

1 garlic clove, minced

1/4 teaspoon salt, divided

Freshly ground pepper to taste

8 cups (5 ounces/140 grams) mesclun salad mix, rinsed and dried

4 slices rye or pumpernickel bread

1 pound (450 grams) salmon fillet, skin removed, cut into 1 1/4-inch (3-centimeter) chunks

1/2 cup finely chopped red onion

4 teaspoons drained capers, rinsed

2 tablespoons black olive spread (*olivada*) or tapenade or finely chopped pitted kalamata olives

1. Combine 2 tablespoons of the oil, 1 tablespoon lemon juice, mustard, garlic, 1/8 teaspoon salt, and pepper in a small bowl or jar with a tight-fitting lid. Whisk or shake to blend. Place the salad mix in a large bowl. Drizzle with the lemon dressing and toss to coat well. Divide the salad among 4 plates. Toast the bread slices.

2. Season the salmon with the remaining 1/8 teaspoon salt and pepper. Heat 2 teaspoons of the oil in a large nonstick skillet over medium-high heat. Add the salmon and cook, turning several times, until browned, 3 to 4 minutes. Add the remaining 1/4 cup lemon juice, onion, and capers. Cook, shaking the skillet, until salmon is opaque in the center, 30 to 60 seconds. Spoon the salmon, onion, capers, and pan juices over the salads. Cut each slice of toast in half and spread with the olive paste (or chopped olives). Garnish each salad with 2 olive toasts. One serving is 2 cups of salad, 3 ounces (85 grams) salmon, and 1 slice of bread.

Per serving: 347 calories, 22 g protein, 9 g carbohydrates, 2 g fiber, 25 g total fat, 5 g saturated fat, 62 mg cholesterol, 399 mg sodium.

VARIATION Warm Tuna Salad with Olive Toasts

In Step 2, substitute fresh tuna for the salmon.

Shrimp and Scallop Stew

4
Serves

Preparation time: 25 minutes
Cooking time: 15 minutes

If you think seafood cookery is all about deep-frying, think again. This simple but elegant stew demonstrates how poaching keeps seafood moist and provides a flavorful base for the sauce. Cooking fish in wine is a method preferred by French chefs, but it is also a good idea for home cooks everywhere because the acids in the wine have blood sugar–control benefits. Although butter is at the top of The Magic Foods Pyramid, just a little goes a long way here in delivering a delicious finish.

2 teaspoons **olive oil**

1 cup sliced **leek** (1 large; white and light green part only)

1/2 cup dry white wine

3/4 cup reduced-sodium chicken broth

8 ounces (250 grams) medium **shrimp** (61/70 count), peeled and deveined

8 ounces (250 grams) **sea scallops,** halved (See Ingredient Note)

4 teaspoons butter, cut into small pieces

2 teaspoons freshly grated lemon zest

1/8 teaspoon salt, or to taste

Freshly ground black pepper to taste

Pinch of cayenne pepper

2 tablespoons coarsely chopped fresh tarragon or snipped fresh chives

1. Heat the oil in a deep sauté pan or Dutch oven over medium-low heat. Add the leek and cook until tender but not browned, 4 to 6 minutes. (Add 1 tablespoon water, if necessary, to prevent scorching.) Add the wine and broth. Bring to a simmer. Add the shrimp and scallops, cover, and simmer over medium-low heat until shrimp are pink and scallops are opaque in the center, 4 to 5 minutes.

2. Transfer the shrimp and scallops to a warm bowl with a slotted spoon. Cover and keep warm. Increase the heat under the pan to medium-high. Boil the cooking liquid for 2 to 3 minutes to intensify flavor. Remove from the heat. Add the butter, whisking until melted and incorporated into the sauce. Whisk in the lemon zest, salt, black pepper, and cayenne. Spoon the sauce over the shrimp and scallops and garnish with the tarragon (or chives). One serving is 1 cup.

Per serving: 205 calories, 23 g protein, 6 g carbohydrates, 1 g fiber, 7 g total fat, 3 g saturated fat, 140 mg cholesterol, 323 mg sodium.

Ingredient Note: Fish counters sell two types of scallops. Sea scallops are the largest and the most commonly available. Bay scallops are considerably smaller—about the diameter of a quarter. For the best quality (you'll need access to a good fishmonger), seek out "dry-pack" scallops. These have not been treated with phosphates, which are often added to improve appearance and extend shelf life, or soaked in water. "Dry-pack" scallops have a better texture and shrink less when they are cooked than "wet-pack" scallops. Scallops should be used within a day or two of purchase.

Shrimp and Orzo Casserole

 6 Serves | **Preparation time: 20 minutes**
Baking time: 20 to 25 minutes

This easy recipe for heart-healthy shrimp is prepared Greek-style, with tomatoes, orzo pasta cooked just until al dente, and tangy reduced-fat feta cheese. Convenient canned artichokes are a surprisingly good source of fiber. *See photo on page 244.*

2 teaspoons **olive oil**

2 **garlic** cloves, minced

1/2 teaspoon dried oregano

Pinch of crushed red pepper

1 can (14 1/2 ounces/398 milliliters) diced **tomatoes** (undrained)

1 can (14 1/2 ounces/398 milliliters) reduced-sodium chicken broth

1 cup (6 ounces/170 grams) orzo **pasta** (See Ingredient Note)

1 can (14 ounces/398 milliliters) artichoke hearts, drained, rinsed, and quartered

1 teaspoon freshly grated lemon zest

Freshly ground pepper to taste

1 pound (450 grams) cooked medium **shrimp,** tails removed (see Tip)

2 tablespoons chopped fresh parsley

1 cup (3 ounces/85 grams) crumbled reduced-fat feta **cheese**

1. Preheat the oven to 425°F (220°C). Coat an 8 x 11 1/2-inch (20 x 30-centimeter) baking dish (2-quart/2-liter capacity) with cooking spray.

2. Heat the oil in a large saucepan over medium heat. Add the garlic, oregano, and red pepper. Cook, stirring, until fragrant but not colored, 30 to 60 seconds. Add the tomatoes and mash with a potato masher. Add the broth and bring to a simmer. Stir in the orzo, artichoke hearts, lemon zest, and pepper. Transfer to the baking dish. Cover tightly with aluminum foil.

3. Bake the casserole for 15 minutes. Stir the ingredients in the casserole, then stir in the shrimp. Sprinkle with the parsley, then the feta. Bake, uncovered, until the orzo is firm-tender and the feta starts to melt, 5 to 10 minutes longer. One serving is 1 cup.

Per serving: 273 calories, 27 g protein, 33 g carbohydrates, 6 g fiber, 4 g total fat, 2 g saturated fat, 154 mg cholesterol, 544 mg sodium.

Tip: To cook shrimp, place in a large saucepan of lightly salted boiling water. Cook until shrimp turn pink, 2 to 3 minutes, then drain. You can also use frozen cooked shrimp. Thaw before using.

Ingredient Note: If possible, use whole wheat orzo for extra fiber and whole grain goodness. It's not yet widely available in stores, but it is available online at sites such as amazon.com.

PASTA AND PIZZA

Penne with Asparagus, Ricotta and Lemon

4 | **Preparation time: 15 minutes**
Serves | **Cooking time: 8 to 10 minutes**

Bulking up a pasta dish with vegetables can be as easy as tossing veggies into the boiling water along with the pasta. Just watch the timing. In most cases, add the vegetables midway through cooking. This super-simple pasta dish, highlighting asparagus, lemon, and herbs and finished with a ricotta sauce, is perfect for a light spring supper.

1/2 cup reduced-fat ricotta **cheese**

1/2 cup freshly grated Parmesan **cheese,** divided

2 tablespoons chopped fresh parsley

2 teaspoons freshly grated lemon zest

2 teaspoons **lemon** juice

1/2 teaspoon salt, or to taste

Freshly ground pepper to taste

2 cups (8 ounces/250 grams) **whole wheat penne**

1 pound (450 grams) asparagus, stem ends snapped off, cut into 1 1/2-inch (4-centimeter) lengths (2 cups)

1. Bring a large pot of lightly salted water to a boil for cooking the penne.

2. Stir the ricotta, 1/4 cup of the Parmesan, parsley, lemon zest, lemon juice, salt, and pepper in small bowl until smooth.

3. Add the penne to the boiling water and cook, stirring occasionally, for 4 minutes. Add the asparagus and cook until the penne is al dente (just tender) and the asparagus is tender, 4 to 6 minutes longer. Reserve 1/3 cup of the pasta cooking water. Drain the pasta and asparagus and place in a large bowl.

4. Add 1/3 cup of the reserved pasta cooking water to the ricotta mixture, whisking until smooth. Toss the pasta with the ricotta sauce. Pass the remaining Parmesan separately. One serving is 1 1/2 cups.

Per serving: 306 calories, 15 g protein, 49 g carbohydrates, 7 g fiber, 6 g total fat, 2 g saturated fat, 16 mg cholesterol, 482 mg sodium.

VARIATION Penne with Spinach, Ricotta, and Lemon

In Step 3, omit the asparagus; cook the penne for 8 to 12 minutes. While the penne is cooking, cook one 10-ounce (300-gram) package frozen spinach according to package directions. In Step 4, toss the penne with the ricotta sauce and spinach.

Quick Spinach and Sausage Lasagna

6 Serves

Preparation time: 30 minutes

Cooking/baking time: 1 hour

You can't beat lasagna for crowd-pleasing appeal and make-ahead convenience. We've given our favorite lasagna a healthier spin by lightening up the meat and cheese layers and bulking up the spinach layer. Oven-ready noodles speed up preparation time. You can assemble the recipe in advance through Step 4, cover, and refrigerate for up to 2 days or freeze for up to 3 months (thaw in the refrigerator before baking).

1 link (4 ounces/125 grams) hot Italian turkey sausage, casing removed

1 jar (26 ounces/700 milliliters) **marinara sauce** (3 cups)

1 teaspoon dried oregano

1/4 teaspoon crushed red pepper

1 1/2 packages (10 ounces/300 grams each) frozen **spinach**

1 large **egg**

1 container (15 ounces/475 grams) reduced-fat ricotta **cheese**

1/2 cup grated Parmesan **cheese,** divided

1/8 teaspoon ground nutmeg

Freshly ground pepper to taste

12 oven-ready lasagna noodles (see Tip)

1 1/3 cups shredded part-skim mozzarella **cheese**

1. Preheat the oven to 400°F (200°C). Coat a 9 x 13-inch (23 x 33-centimeter) baking dish with nonstick spray.

2. Cook the sausage in a small nonstick skillet over medium heat, crumbling with a wooden spoon, until browned, 2 to 4 minutes. Blot the sausage with paper towel. Transfer to a medium bowl. Stir in the marinara sauce, oregano, and red pepper.

3. Cook the spinach according to package directions. Drain and refresh under cold running water. Drain the spinach well and press out moisture. Whisk the egg and ricotta in a medium bowl until smooth. Add the spinach, 1/4 cup of the Parmesan, the nutmeg, and the black pepper. Mix well.

4. Place 3 of the lasagna noodles in a deep dish or bowl and cover with warm water. Let soak while you assemble the lasagna. Spread about 3/4 cup of the marinara sauce mixture in the baking dish. Place 3 of the remaining unsoaked noodles crosswise over the sauce. Spread about 1 1/3 cups of the spinach mixture over the noodles. Spoon 1/2 cup marinara sauce over the spinach mixture. Sprinkle with 1/3 cup mozzarella. Add another layer of unsoaked noodles and repeat layering with spinach mixture and marinara sauce and mozzarella 2 more times. Lift the soaked noodles from the water, shake off excess, and arrange over lasagna. Spread the remaining marinara sauce evenly over the final layer of noodles.

5. Cover the lasagna with aluminum foil and bake for 35 minutes. Sprinkle with the remaining 1/4 cup Parmesan and 1/3 cup mozzarella. Bake, uncovered, until noodles are tender and lasagna is bubbly, about 15 minutes longer. Let stand for 5 minutes before serving. One serving is one 4 1/2 x 3 1/2-inch (11 x 9-centimeter) piece.

Per serving: 400 calories, 24 g protein, 34 g carbohydrates, 5 g fiber, 19 g total fat, 8 g saturated fat, 82 mg cholesterol, 986 mg sodium.

Tip: Oven-ready lasagna noodles eliminate the step of boiling the noodles. However, even when the top layer of oven-ready noodles is thoroughly covered with sauce, it never seems to tenderize properly. To remedy this problem, soak the 3 noodles for the top layer in warm water before assembling the lasagna.

Whole Wheat Pasta with Sausage, Beans and Greens

6 Serves

Preparation time: 25 minutes

Cooking time: 20 to 25minutes

A small amount of lean turkey sausage goes a long way in imparting a full flavor to this quick pasta sauce. We've boosted the fiber with cannellini beans and the vegetable content with vibrant Swiss chard, which cooks conveniently in the pasta water.

1 link (4 ounces/125 grams) hot Italian turkey sausage, casing removed

1 teaspoon **olive oil**

3/4 cup chopped **onion** (1 small)

3 **garlic** cloves, minced

1 can (15 ounces/398 milliliters) no-salt-added diced **tomatoes**

1 can (8 ounces/213 milliliters) no-salt-added tomato sauce

1 can (19 or 15 ounces/540 or 398 milliliters) cannellini **beans,** drained and rinsed

1/4 cup water

Freshly ground pepper to taste

4 cups (12 ounces/340 grams) whole wheat **pasta,** fusilli, penne, or rigatoni

1 bunch (1 pound/450 grams) **Swiss chard,** stems trimmed (see Tip), leaves washed, and torn into bite-size pieces

6 tablespoons grated Parmesan **cheese**

1. Bring a large pot of lightly salted water to a boil for cooking pasta. Cook the sausage in a large nonstick skillet over medium heat, crumbling the sausage with a wooden spoon, until browned, 3 to 5 minutes. Transfer the sausage to a paper towel–lined plate to drain.

2. Add the oil to the skillet. Add the onion and cook over medium heat, stirring often, until softened, 1 to 2 minutes. Add the garlic and cook, stirring, for 10 to 20 seconds. Add the diced tomatoes and mash with a wooden spoon. Add the tomato sauce, beans, water, and browned sausage. Bring to a simmer. Cook, uncovered, at a lively simmer over medium-low heat, stirring occasionally, until flavors have blended, 10 to 15 minutes. Season with pepper.

3. Meanwhile, add the pasta to the boiling water and cook for 5 minutes. Add the Swiss chard and stir to immerse. Cook until the pasta is just tender and the chard has wilted, 3 to 5 minutes longer. Drain well and transfer to a large bowl. Toss with the tomato sauce. Sprinkle each serving with Parmesan cheese. One serving is 1 1/3 cups pasta and sauce and 1 tablespoon cheese.

Per serving: 390 calories, 19 g protein, 65 g carbohydrates, 11 g fiber, 6 g total fat, 1 g saturated fat, 22 mg cholesterol, 409 mg sodium.

Tips

• The celery-like stems of Swiss chard are edible and have a pleasant, mild taste. Cut them into bite-size pieces and steam or boil until tender, 6 to 8 minutes.

• Leftovers? Transform them into a pasta gratin. Spread the leftovers in a shallow baking dish coated with cooking spray. Moisten with a little water and top with grated Parmesan and bread crumbs. Bake, uncovered, at 425°F (220°C) until the top is golden and crusty, 25 to 30 minutes.

Macaroni and Cheese with Spinach

6
Serves

Preparation time: 15 minutes

Cooking/baking time: 45 to 55 minutes

A crusty casserole of mac and cheese is pure comfort food—and it can be a Magic food as well. We've improved the dish with your blood sugar in mind by using whole wheat pasta, a lightened cheese sauce, a surprise layer of spinach, and a topping of wheat germ. You can assemble the recipe through Step 5 in advance, cover, and refrigerate for up to 2 days or freeze for up to 3 months (thaw in the refrigerator before baking). *See photo on page 245.*

1 3/4 cups low-fat (1%) milk, divided

3 tablespoons all-purpose flour

2 cups (6 ounces/170 grams) grated extra-sharp cheddar cheese

1 cup 1% low-fat cottage cheese

1/8 teaspoon ground nutmeg

1/2 teaspoon salt, or to taste

Freshly ground pepper to taste

1 package (10 ounces/300 grams) frozen spinach or 4 cups individually quick-frozen spinach

2 cups (8 ounces/250 grams) whole wheat macaroni

1/4 cup toasted wheat germ

1. Preheat the oven to 400°F (200°C). Coat an 8-inch (20-centimeter) square baking dish (2-quart/2-liter capacity) with nonstick spray. Bring a large pot of lightly salted water to a boil for cooking the macaroni.

2. Whisk 1/4 cup of the cold milk with the flour in a small bowl until smooth. Set aside. Heat the remaining 1 1/2 cups milk in a heavy medium saucepan over medium heat until steaming. Add the flour mixture and cook, whisking constantly, until the sauce boils and thickens, 2 to 3 minutes. Remove from the heat. Add the cheddar cheese,

stirring until melted. Stir in the cottage cheese, nutmeg, salt, and pepper.

3. Cook the spinach according to package directions. Drain, refresh under cold water, and press out excess moisture.

4. Cook the macaroni, stirring often, in the boiling water until not quite tender, 4 to 5 minutes. (The macaroni will continue to cook during baking.) Drain, rinse with cold running water, then drain again.

5. Mix the macaroni with the cheese sauce in a large bowl. Spread half of the macaroni mixture in the baking dish. Spoon the spinach on top. Spread the remaining macaroni mixture over the spinach layer. Sprinkle with wheat germ.

6. Bake the casserole until bubbly and golden, 35 to 45 minutes. One serving is 1 1/3 cups.

Per serving: 357 calories, 22 g protein, 40 g carbohydrates, 6 g fiber, 12 g total fat, 7 g saturated fat, 35 mg cholesterol, 606 mg sodium.

VARIATION Southwestern Macaroni and Cheese and Peppers

In Step 1, substitute a mixture of 1 cup shredded pepper Jack cheese and 1 cup shredded extra-sharp cheddar cheese for the 2 cups cheddar. Omit the nutmeg. Add 4 1/2 ounces (125 milliliters) canned chopped mild green chiles, 1/3 cup chopped fresh cilantro, and a dash of cayenne pepper to the cheese sauce. In Step 3, omit the spinach. Instead, sauté 2 cups frozen pepper stir-fry vegetables in 1 teaspoon olive oil until tender, 3 to 4 minutes. In Step 5, spread the pepper mixture over bottom macaroni layer.

Penne with Tomato and Eggplant Sauce

6
Serves

Preparation time: 20 minutes

Cooking time: 25 minutes

Whole wheat pasta has come a long way in recent years. Supermarkets now stock a wide array of shapes. The nutty taste of the whole wheat pasta pairs well with assertive flavors like this full-flavored tomato sauce, which has a rich, meaty taste thanks to the Magic eggplant, an excellent meat substitute.

4 teaspoons **olive oil,** divided

1 large (8 ounces/250 grams) baby **eggplant,** cut into 3/4-inch (2-centimeter) cubes (3 cups)

1 cup chopped **onion** (1 medium)

4 **garlic** cloves, minced

1/8 teaspoon crushed red pepper

1 can (28 ounces/796 milliliters) diced **tomatoes**

3 tablespoons chopped fresh parsley or basil, divided

1/8 teaspoon salt, or to taste

Freshly ground pepper to taste

4 cups (12 ounces/340 grams) whole wheat **pasta,** such as penne or rigatoni (see Tip)

3/4 cup crumbled reduced-fat feta **cheese**

6 tablespoons pine **nuts,** toasted (see Tip)

1. Bring a large pot of lightly salted water to a boil for cooking the pasta.

2. Heat 2 teaspoons of the oil in a large non-stick skillet over medium-high heat. Add the eggplant and cook, turning from time to time, until browned and tender, 5 to 7 minutes. Transfer to a plate.

3. Reduce the heat to medium and add the remaining 2 teaspoons oil to the skillet. Add onion and cook, stirring often, until softened,

2 to 3 minutes. Add the garlic and red pepper. Cook, stirring, until fragrant, about 30 seconds. Add the tomatoes and mash with a potato masher. Bring to a simmer. Add the eggplant. Simmer, uncovered, over medium-low heat until the flavors have developed and the sauce has thickened, 15 to 20 minutes. (Add a little water if the sauce thickens too quickly.) Stir in 2 tablespoons of the parsley. Season with salt and pepper.

4. Meanwhile, cook the pasta in the boiling water until al dente (just tender), 8 to 10 minutes, or according to package directions. Drain and add to the sauce in the skillet. Toss to coat well. Sprinkle each serving with feta, pine nuts, and some of the remaining parsley (or basil). One serving is 1 1/3 cups pasta and sauce, 2 tablespoons feta, and 1 tablespoon pine nuts.

Per serving: 390 calories, 15 g protein, 57 g carbohydrates, 8 g fiber, 13 g total fat, 2 g saturated fat, 8 mg cholesterol, 556 mg sodium.

Tips

• Toast the pine nuts in a small dry skillet over medium-low heat, stirring constantly, until golden and fragrant, 1 to 3 minutes.

• Test the pasta often toward the end of cooking, so you will be sure to catch it when it has just become tender or "al dente." When pasta is overcooked, not only does it lose its appeal, it has a higher GL.

2 tomato
their lycopene may have special power against diabetes

3 pine nuts
their "good" fats help slow the digestion of your dinner

pasta 4
whole wheat has three times the fiber per serving

1 cheese
reduced-fat feta provides calcium, which may help boost your sensitivity to insulin

olive oil 8
this liquid gold helps "spike-proof" your meals

eggplant 7
adding bulky veggies like eggplant to pasta lowers the GL of the dish

onions 6
indispensable onions may lower high blood sugar

5 garlic
it helps keep blood clots and cholesterol in check

Penne with Tomato and Eggplant Sauce

Quick Whole Wheat Pizza Dough

1 pizza

Preparation time: 10 minutes

Rising time: 10 to 20 minutes

Makes 12 ounces (340 grams) pizza dough, enough for one 12-inch (30-centimeter) pizza

A food processor mixes and kneads this "better blood sugar" pizza dough in just minutes. You can also make this dough in a bread machine; use bread-machine yeast and room temperature water. Place the ingredients in your bread machine in the order recommended by the manufacturer and select the manual setting.

3/4 cup **whole wheat flour**

3/4 cup all-purpose flour

2 teaspoons quick-rising yeast (see Ingredient Note)

3/4 teaspoon salt

1/4 teaspoon sugar

1/2–2/3 cup hot water (120–130°F/50–55°C)

2 teaspoons **olive oil**

1. Combine the whole wheat flour, all-purpose flour, yeast, salt, and sugar in a food processor. Pulse to mix. Combine the hot water and oil in a measuring cup. With the motor running, gradually pour the hot liquid through food processor feed tube. Process until dough forms a ball, then process 1 minute to knead. The dough should be quite soft. If it seems dry, add 1 to 2 tablespoons warm water. If too sticky, add 1 to 2 tablespoons flour.

2. Transfer the dough to a lightly floured surface. Spray a sheet of plastic wrap with nonstick spray and place it, sprayed side down, over the dough. Let the dough rest for 10 to 20 minutes before rolling.

Ingredient Note: Quick-rising yeast is a special variety of yeast that can be mixed directly with dry ingredients, works with hotter liquids than regular yeast, and requires only a 10-minute rest rather than the standard 1 1/2-hour rising time. Fleischmann's RapidRise yeast is the most common brand. You can find it in the refrigerated dairy case.

Mushroom and Herb Pizza

4 Serves

Preparation time: 30 minutes

Cooking/baking time: 20 minutes

Yes, pizza, can be part of your Magic Foods eating plan, especially when you make your own with a thin whole grain crust, topped with lots of vegetables and a moderate amount of cheese. Using our Quick Whole Wheat Pizza Dough, you can bake your own wholesome pizza in about the same time it takes for delivery pizza to arrive at your door. We offer two toppings, one with meaty-tasting mushrooms and a variation with broccoli and olives. *See photo on page 245.*

12 ounces (340 grams) Quick Whole Wheat Pizza Dough or purchased whole wheat pizza dough

Cornmeal for dusting

1 tablespoon **olive oil,** divided

3 cups (8 ounces/250 grams) baby bella or cremini mushrooms, stem ends trimmed, wiped clean, and sliced

2 **garlic** cloves, minced

Pinch of salt

Freshly ground pepper to taste

2 tablespoons chopped fresh parsley

2/3 cup prepared **marinara sauce**

2 tablespoons chopped fresh marjoram or oregano

1/8 teaspoon crushed red pepper

1 cup shredded part-skim mozzarella **cheese**

1/2 cup diced red **onion**

1/4 cup grated Parmesan **cheese**

1. Prepare the Quick Whole Wheat Pizza Dough, if using.

2. Place a baking stone or inverted baking sheet on lowest rack of oven. Preheat the oven to 500°F (260°C) or highest setting. Coat a 12 1/2-inch (32-centimeter) pizza pan with nonstick spray. Dust with the cornmeal.

3. Heat 2 teaspoons of the oil in a large non-stick skillet over medium-high heat. Add the mushrooms and cook, stirring or shaking the skillet from time to time, until tender and lightly browned, 3 to 4 minutes. Add the garlic and cook, stirring, for 30 seconds longer. Remove from the heat and stir in parsley, salt, and pepper.

4. Mix the marinara sauce, marjoram (or oregano), and red pepper in a small bowl.

5. On a lightly floured surface, roll the dough into a 13-inch (33-centimeter) circle. Transfer to the pizza pan. Turn the edges under to make a slight rim around the outside edge. Brush the remaining 1 teaspoon oil over the rim. Spread the marinara sauce over the crust, leaving a 1/2-inch (1-centimeter) border. Sprinkle the mozzarella over the sauce. Scatter the mushrooms over the mozzarella. Sprinkle with the onion. Top with the Parmesan cheese.

6. Place the pizza pan on heated baking stone (or baking sheet) and bake until the bottom crust is crisp and golden, 10 to 14 minutes. One serving is 1/4 of a 12-inch (30-centimeter) pizza.

Per serving: 368 calories, 18 g protein, 45 g carbohydrates, 6 g fiber, 14 g total fat, 5 g saturated fat, 22 mg cholesterol, 916 mg sodium.

VARIATION Whole Wheat Pizza with Broccoli and Olives

In Step 3, steam 2 cups broccoli florets (3/4-inch/2-centimeter pieces) until crisp-tender, 2 to 3 minutes. In Step 4, mix 2/3 cup prepared marinara sauce with 1 teaspoon dried oregano and 1/8 teaspoon crushed red pepper. In Step 5, spread the marinara sauce over the crust. Sprinkle 1 cup shredded part-skim mozzarella cheese over the sauce. Scatter the broccoli, 1/2 cup diced red onion, and 1/4 cup coarsely chopped, pitted kalamata olives over top. Spritz the top lightly with olive oil nonstick spray. Bake the pizza as directed in Step 6.

MEATLESS MAIN DISHES

Spring Vegetable Stir-Fry with Tofu

4 Serves

Preparation time: 25 minutes	
Marinating time: 10 minutes	
Cooking time: 10 minutes	

This colorful stir-fry celebrates spring with seasonal asparagus and sweet onions. It is a protein-rich vegetarian dish, thanks to the tofu. And with its zesty sauce, it will appeal even to resolute meat lovers. You can vary the recipe by using snow peas instead of asparagus and red bell pepper rather than carrots. Substitute sliced boneless chicken breast for the tofu, if you like—just be sure that it is cooked through when you brown it in Step 2.

1 package (14 to16 ounces/400 to 425 grams) extra-firm water-packed **tofu,** drained

1/2 cup orange juice

2 tablespoons reduced-sodium soy sauce

1 tablespoon oyster-flavored sauce (see Ingredient Note)

1 tablespoon medium-dry sherry, rice wine, or nonalcoholic white wine

1 1/2 teaspoons chile-garlic sauce (see Ingredient Note)

1 teaspoon sugar

1 1/2 teaspoons cornstarch

1 tablespoon vegetable oil, divided

1 tablespoon grated fresh ginger

2 teaspoons freshly grated orange zest

3 **garlic** cloves, minced

1 cup thinly sliced sweet **onion,** such as Vidalia or Walla Walla (1 small)

1 pound (450 grams) asparagus, stem ends snapped off, cut into 1 1/4-inch (3-centimeter) lengths (2 cups)

1 cup baby **carrots,** quartered lengthwise

1/4 cup water

1. Pat the tofu dry and cut into 3/4-inch (2-centimeter) pieces. Whisk the orange juice, soy sauce, oyster-flavored sauce, sherry (or wine), chile-garlic sauce, and sugar in a medium bowl. Add the tofu and toss gently to coat. Marinate for about 10 minutes, turning from time to time, while you prepare the vegetables.

2. When you are ready to cook, drain the tofu, reserving the marinade in a medium bowl. Add the cornstarch to the reserved marinade and whisk until smooth. Reserve for the sauce. Heat 2 teaspoons of the oil in nonstick skillet or stir-fry pan over high heat. Add the tofu and cook, turning from time to time, until browned and crusty, 3 to 5 minutes. Transfer to a plate.

3. Add the remaining 1 teaspoon oil to the skillet. Add the ginger, orange zest, and garlic. Stir-fry until fragrant, 10 to 20 seconds. Add the onion and stir-fry for 1 minute. Add the asparagus and carrots. Stir-fry for 30 seconds. Add the water, cover, and cook just until vegetables are crisp-tender, about 2 minutes. Push vegetables to the outside perimeter of the skillet. Stir the reserved sauce and add it to the center of the skillet. Cook, stirring the sauce, until it becomes glossy and thickens, about 1 minute. Stir the vegetables into the sauce and return the tofu to the skillet. Stir to coat. One serving is 1 1/3 cups.

Per serving: 263 calories, 19 g protein, 23 g carbohydrates, 6 g fiber, 12 g total fat, 2 g saturated fat, 0 mg cholesterol, 454 mg sodium.

Ingredient Note: Oyster-flavored sauce and chile-garlic sauce can be found in the Asian foods section of large supermarkets.

Dahl with Spinach

6 Serves

| Preparation time: 20 minutes |
| Cooking time: 45 to 50 minutes |

Dahl turns up frequently in Indian cooking and it is one of those confusing terms that refer to both a preparation and an ingredient. As an ingredient, dahl encompasses a wide variety of dried pulses (legumes), including lentils and split peas, all of which are valuable sources of soluble fiber and vegetable protein. The preparation is a dish like this one, made with seasoned stewed pulses. We've squeezed three Magic seasonings—turmeric, fenugreek, and garlic—into this spicy stew.

DAHL

1 cup yellow split peas or chana dahl (see Ingredient Note), sorted and rinsed

3 cups water

1/2 teaspoon turmeric

1 tablespoon canola oil

1 teaspoon cumin seeds

1 cup chopped onion (1 medium)

1 tablespoon grated fresh ginger or 1/2 teaspoon ground ginger

3 garlic cloves, minced

1 teaspoon ground fenugreek (optional)

1/4 teaspoon cayenne pepper

1 can (14 1/2 ounces/398 milliliters) diced tomatoes (undrained)

1 package (10 ounces/300 grams) frozen cut-leaf spinach

1/2 teaspoon salt, or to taste

RAITA

1 cup low-fat plain yogurt

4 teaspoons lime juice

1 teaspoon ground cumin

1/8 teaspoon salt, or to taste

1. **To make the dahl:** Combine the split peas (or chana dahl), water, and turmeric in a large saucepan. Bring to a simmer. Partially cover, reduce heat to medium-low, and cook until the split peas are tender, 40 to 45 minutes.

2. Meanwhile, heat the oil in a large nonstick skillet over medium heat. Add the cumin seeds and cook, stirring, until fragrant, 10 to 20 seconds. Add the onion and cook, stirring often, until softened, 2 to 3 minutes. Add the ginger, garlic, fenugreek, if using, and cayenne. Cook, stirring, until fragrant, 20 to 30 seconds. Add the tomatoes and cook until most of the liquid has evaporated, 5 to 10 minutes.

3. Cook the spinach according to package directions. Drain, pressing out excess moisture.

4. When the split peas are tender, stir them (and any remaining cooking liquid) into the tomato mixture, along with the spinach. Cook for 2 to 3 minutes to blend the flavors. Season with salt.

5. **To make the raita:** Mix all the raita ingredients in a small bowl. Serve the dahl with raita. One serving is 3/4 cup dahl and 2 1/2 tablespoons raita. Leftover dahl will keep, covered, in the refrigerator for up to 2 days. Reheat on the stovetop or in the microwave, adding a little additional water, if necessary.

Per serving: 199 calories, 12 g protein, 33 g carbohydrates, 12 g fiber, 4 g total fat, 0 g saturated fat, 0 mg cholesterol, 412 mg sodium.

Ingredient Note: Chana dahl are split chickpeas. You can find them in Indian markets and some supermarkets.

Barley Risotto with Asparagus and Lemon

4 Serves | **Preparation time: 20 minutes**
Cooking time: 20 minutes

A creamy risotto is traditionally made with arborio rice, which falls in the top (undesirable) tier of the Magic Foods Carb Pyramid (see page 43). We've created this blood sugar-friendly version, which swaps nutty tasting whole grain barley for the white rice. Since risotto requires almost constant stirring, quick-cooking barley is a more practical choice then pearl barley.

2 cans (14 1/2 ounces/284 milliliters) vegetable broth or reduced-sodium chicken broth (3 1/2 cups)

3/4 cup water

1 pound (450 grams) asparagus, stem ends snapped off, cut into 1-inch (2.5-centimeter) lengths (2 cups)

1 tablespoon **olive oil**

1/2 cup chopped **scallions**

1 cup quick-cooking **barley**

1/2 cup grated Parmesan **cheese**

1/4 cup chopped fresh parsley or snipped chives

2 teaspoons freshly grated lemon zest

1 tablespoon **lemon** juice

Pinch of salt

Freshly ground pepper to taste

1. Combine the broth and water in a medium saucepan. Bring to a simmer over medium heat. Drop in the asparagus and cook, uncovered, until crisp-tender, 2 to 4 minutes. Transfer the asparagus to a plate with a slotted spoon and set aside. Reduce the heat to low and keep the broth at a bare simmer.

2. Heat the oil in a Dutch oven over medium heat. Add the scallions and cook, stirring, until softened, about 1 minute. Add the barley and cook, stirring, for 30 seconds. Add about 1 cup of the hot broth and cook, stirring, until most of the liquid has been absorbed, 1 to 1 1/2 minutes.

Continue to simmer and stir almost constantly, adding broth about 1/2 cup at a time and waiting until most of it has been absorbed before adding more, until barley is tender and risotto has creamy consistency, about 15 minutes.

3. Add the reserved asparagus and stir until heated through, about 1 minute. Remove the risotto from the heat. Stir in the Parmesan, parsley, lemon zest, lemon juice, salt, and pepper. One serving is 1 cup.

Per serving: 221 calories, 9 g protein, 7 g carbohydrates, 3 g fiber, 7 g total fat, 3 g saturated fat, 13 mg cholesterol, 319 mg sodium.

Lentil and Bean Chili

8 Serves | **Preparation time: 20 minutes**
Cooking time: 50 minutes

Nothing takes the chill out of a winter evening like a bowl of steaming, spicy chili. The combination of lentils and beans produces a vegetarian version that is rich in soluble fiber and protein, both strong allies in the battle against blood sugar spikes. Garnish the chili with diced avocado, grated pepper Jack or cheddar cheese, chopped fresh cilantro, chopped scallions, and reduced-fat sour cream.

2 teaspoons **olive oil**

1 cup chopped **onion** (1 medium)

1 cup diced **carrots** (2–4 medium)

3 **garlic** cloves, minced

5 teaspoons chili powder

4 teaspoons ground cumin

1 teaspoon dried oregano

4 cups vegetable broth or reduced-sodium chicken broth

3/4 cup brown **lentils,** sorted and rinsed

2 cans (10 ounces/398 milliliters each) diced **tomatoes** with green chiles

2 cans (15 or 19 ounces/398 or 540 milliliters each) dark red kidney **beans,** drained and rinsed

Freshly ground pepper to taste

1. Heat the oil in a Dutch oven over medium heat. Add the onion and carrots. Cook, stirring often, until softened, 3 to 5 minutes. Add the garlic, chili powder, cumin, and oregano. Cook, stirring, until fragrant, 30 to 60 seconds. Add the broth and lentils. Bring to a simmer. Reduce the heat to medium-low, cover, and simmer for 25 minutes.

2. Add the tomatoes, beans, and pepper. Return to a simmer. Cook, covered, over medium-low heat until lentils are tender, 15 to 20 minutes longer. One serving is 1 cup. Leftovers will keep, covered, in the refrigerator for up to 2 days. Reheat on the stovetop or in the microwave.

Per serving: 199 calories, 12 g protein, 36 g carbohydrates, 12 g fiber, 3 g total fat, 0 g saturated fat, 0 mg cholesterol, 691 mg sodium.

Black Bean and Sweet Potato Burritos

8
Serves

| Preparation time: 25 minutes |
| Cooking time: 20 minutes |

Sweet potatoes and fiber-rich beans are a Magic marriage in this flavor-packed vegetarian entrée. If you are cooking for just one or two, make up the sweet potato–bean filling (through Step 2) and store, covered, in the refrigerator for up to 2 days. For a quick pick up meal, just heat leftover filling and individual tortillas in the microwave (see Tip).

2 teaspoons canola oil

1 cup chopped onion (1 medium)

2 garlic cloves, minced

4 teaspoons ground cumin

1/2 teaspoon dried oregano

3/4 cup vegetable broth or reduced-sodium chicken broth

1 medium sweet potato, peeled and diced (3 cups)

1 can (14 1/2 ounces/398 milliliters) mild green chile-seasoned diced tomatoes (undrained)

1 can (15 1/2 ounces/398 milliliters) black beans, drained and rinsed

3/4 cup frozen corn

1/4 cup chopped fresh cilantro

1 tablespoon fresh lime juice

1/8 teaspoon freshly ground pepper

8 (8-inch/20-centimeter) whole wheat wraps or tortillas

1 cup shredded pepper Jack or Monterey Jack cheese

1/2 cup reduced-fat sour cream

1. Preheat the oven to 325°F (160°C).

2. Heat the oil in a large nonstick skillet over medium heat. Add the onion and cook, stirring often, until softened, 2 to 3 minutes. Add the garlic, cumin, and oregano. Cook, stirring, until fragrant, 10 to 20 seconds. Add the broth and sweet potato. Bring to a simmer. Cover and cook for 5 minutes. Add the tomatoes, beans, and corn. Return to a simmer. Cover and cook until the sweet potato is tender, 5 to 10 minutes longer. Mash about 1/4 of the vegetable mixture with a potato masher. Stir the mashed and unmashed portions together. Stir in the lime juice, cilantro, and pepper.

3. Meanwhile, enclose the wraps (or tortillas) in aluminum foil and heat in oven for 10 to 15 minutes.

4. To serve, spoon about 2/3 cup of the sweet potato filling down center of each tortilla. Sprinkle with about 2 tablespoons cheese. Fold in edges of wrap, then fold 1 side over filling and wrap up the burrito. Serve with sour cream for dipping. One serving is 1 wrap, 2/3 cup filling, 2 tablespoons shredded cheese, and 1 tablespoon sour cream.

Per serving: 262 calories, 14 g protein, 35 g carbohydrates, 15 g fiber, 10 g total fat, 4 g saturated fat, 21 g cholesterol, 784 mg sodium.

Tip: To heat individual wraps or flour tortillas in the microwave, place 1 wrap between 2 paper towels and microwave on high for 10 to 12 seconds.

SIDE DISHES

Bulgur with Ginger and Orange

4
Serves

| Preparation time: 15 minutes |
| Cooking time: 25 minutes |

Instead of cooking a side of rice or potatoes (both high-GL foods) to go with your next chicken, beef, or pork dinner, reach for the bag of bulgur instead. Bulgur cooks in about the same time as white rice but offers the blood sugar benefits of a whole grain rich in soluble fiber.

2 **oranges,** scrubbed

2 teaspoons canola oil

2 tablespoons minced fresh ginger

2 **garlic** cloves minced

1 cup **bulgur,** rinsed

2 teaspoons firmly packed brown sugar

1/4 teaspoon salt, or to taste

2/3 cup chopped **scallions**

1 tablespoon reduced-sodium soy sauce

1/3 cup slivered **almonds,** toasted (see Tip)

1. Grate the orange peels to make 1 tablespoon zest. Juice the oranges and add enough water to measure 1 1/2 cups.

2. Heat the oil in a large, heavy saucepan over medium-high heat. Add the ginger and garlic. Cook, stirring, until fragrant, about 30 seconds. Add the bulgur and stir to coat. Add the diluted orange juice, sugar, and salt. Bring to a simmer. Reduce heat to low, cover, and simmer until the bulgur is tender and most of the liquid has been absorbed, 15 to 20 minutes.

3. Add scallions, soy sauce, and the reserved orange zest to the bulgur. Mix gently and fluff with a fork. Sprinkle with almonds. One serving is 3/4 cup. Leftovers will keep, covered, in the refrigerator for up to 2 days. Reheat in the microwave.

Per serving: 234 calories, 7 g protein, 38 g carbohydrates, 8 g fiber, 7 g total fat, 1 g saturated fat, 0 mg cholesterol, 295 mg sodium.

Tip: Toast almonds in a small dry skillet over medium-low heat, stirring constantly, until light golden and fragrant, 2 to 3 minutes. Transfer to a plate and let cool.

VARIATION Bulgur with Carrot Juice and Sesame Seeds

Substitute carrot juice for the orange juice and toasted sesame seeds for almonds.

Mushroom-Barley Pilaf

6
Serves

| Preparation time: 15 minutes |
| Cooking time: 10 to 15 minutes |

Taking its inspiration from the classic barley-mushroom soup, this easy pilaf is an ideal side dish to accompany beef, pork, or chicken entrées. Finishing the pilaf with a splash of vinegar heightens the flavors while dampening the blood-sugar effects of your whole meal.

4 teaspoons **olive oil,** divided

1 cup chopped **onion** (1 medium)

1 cup quick-cooking **barley**

1 can (14 ounces/284 milliliters) reduced-sodium chicken broth or vegetable broth (1 3/4 cups)

8 ounces (250 grams) mushrooms, stem ends trimmed, caps wiped clean, sliced (3 cups)

1 medium red bell pepper, seeded and diced

1 **garlic** clove, minced

1/4 cup chopped fresh dill

1 tablespoon balsamic **vinegar** or **lemon** juice

Freshly ground pepper to taste

1. Heat 2 teaspoons of the oil in a large sauce-pan over medium heat. Add the onion and cook, stirring often, until softened, 2 to 3 minutes. Add the barley and cook, stirring, for 1 minute. Add the broth and bring to a simmer. Reduce the heat to low, cover, and simmer until the barley is tender and the liquid has been absorbed, 10 to 15 minutes.

2. Meanwhile, heat the remaining 2 teaspoons oil in a large nonstick skillet over medium-high heat. Add the mushrooms, bell pepper, and garlic. Cook, stirring often, until tender, 3 to 5 minutes. Add to the barley, along with dill, vinegar, and pepper. Stir gently to mix. One serving is 2/3 cup. The pilaf will keep, covered, in the refrigerator for up to 2 days. Reheat in the microwave.

Per serving: 128 calories, 5 g protein, 21 g carbohydrates, 3 g fiber, 4 g total fat, 1 g saturated fat, 1 mg cholesterol, 45 mg sodium.

Brown Rice Pilaf with Toasted Flaxseeds

6
Serves

| Preparation time: 10 minutes |
| Cooking time: 45 to 55 minutes |

Nutty flaxseeds give a simple rice pilaf a soluble-fiber boost to help lower blood sugar. If you don't have time to cook brown rice, substitute parboiled (converted) white rice; use 1/4 cup water and cook the pilaf for about 20 minutes. With its fresh lemon and parsley accent, this pilaf makes an excellent accompaniment to fish or chicken entrées.

2 teaspoons olive oil

1 cup chopped onion (1 medium)

1 cup long-grain brown rice

1 can (14 ounces/284 milliliters) reduced-sodium chicken broth or vegetable broth (1 3/4 cups)

3/4 cup water

1/4 cup whole flaxseeds

2 teaspoons freshly grated lemon zest

1 tablespoon lemon juice

1/4 cup chopped fresh parsley

Freshly ground pepper to taste

1. Heat the oil in a large, heavy saucepan over medium heat. Add the onion and cook, stirring often, until softened, 2 to 3 minutes. Add the rice and stir for 30 seconds. Add the broth and water and bring to a simmer. Reduce heat to low, cover, and simmer until the rice is tender and the liquid has been absorbed, 45 to 55 minutes.

2. Meanwhile, toast the flaxseeds in a small dry skillet over medium-low heat, stirring constantly, until fragrant and starting to pop, 2 to 3 minutes. Transfer to a small bowl and let cool. Place the flaxseeds in a spice grinder or blender and pulse several times until broken down but not ground.

3. When rice is ready, add the flaxseeds, lemon zest, lemon juice, parsley, and pepper. Fluff and mix gently with a fork. One serving is 1/2 cup. Leftovers will keep, covered, in the refrigerator for up to 2 days. Reheat in the microwave.

Per serving: 166 calories, 4 g protein, 27 g carbohydrates, 3 g fiber, 5 g total fat, 0 g saturated fat, 0 mg cholesterol, 166 mg sodium.

> **VARIATION** Brown Rice Pilaf with Flaxseeds, Lime, and Cilantro
>
> Substitute 1 teaspoon lime zest for 2 teaspoons lemon zest, lime juice for lemon juice, and cilantro for parsley.

Wheatberry Salad with Dried Apricots and Mint

6
Serves

Preparation time: 25 minutes

Cooking time: 1 1/2 to1 3/4 hours

You may have to plan ahead to purchase and cook the wheatberries, but you'll be rewarded with a great-tasting, whole grain salad that's truly blood sugar–friendly. Look for wheatberries in the bulk bins of natural foods markets and allow enough time to cook them—plan on about 1 1/2 hours for unsoaked berries. These chewy, nutty berries are lovely in salads. Here they are complemented by a spiced citrus vinaigrette, dried fruit, and nuts. Serve as a side dish with lamb or poultry.

3/4 cup hard **wheatberries** or spelt berries, rinsed (see Tip)

1/2 cup dried apricots, diced

1/4 cup extra-virgin **olive oil**

3 tablespoons orange juice

2 tablespoons **lemon** juice

1/2 teaspoon honey

1/2 teaspoon **cinnamon**

1 **garlic** clove, minced

1/2 teaspoon salt, or to taste

Freshly ground pepper to taste

1/2 cup chopped **scallions**

1/3 cup chopped fresh mint

1/3 cup slivered **almonds** or chopped peeled pistachios, toasted (see Tip)

1. Place the wheatberries in a large saucepan and cover generously with water. Bring to a simmer over medium-high heat. Reduce heat to medium-low, partially cover, and cook until the wheatberries are tender, 1 1/2 to 1 3/4 hours. (Add more water, if necessary.) Drain and rinse with cold running water.

2. Meanwhile, place the apricots in a small bowl. Cover with boiling water and let soak for 5 to 10 minutes. Drain.

3. Combine the oil, orange juice, lemon juice, honey, cinnamon, garlic, salt, and pepper in a medium bowl or a jar with a tight-fitting lid. Whisk or shake to blend.

4. Combine the cooked wheatberries, soaked dried apricots, scallions, and mint in a large bowl. Add the orange juice dressing and toss to coat well. Just before serving, sprinkle with nuts. One serving is 2/3 cup. The salad will keep, covered, in the refrigerator for up to 2 days.

Per serving: 262 calories, 6 g protein, 32 g carbohydrates, 5 g fiber, 13 g total fat, 2 g saturated fat, 0 mg cholesterol, 200 mg sodium.

Tip: If you soak the wheatberries for at least 8 hours or overnight in a large bowl of water, you can reduce cooking time to about 1 hour (cook the wheatberries in fresh water).

Quinoa with Chiles and Cilantro

6
Serves

Preparation time: 15 minutes

Cooking time: 30 minutes

Quinoa, a delicately flavored whole grain that originated in South America, is higher in protein than any other grain. You can find it in natural foods stores or in the natural foods section of large supermarkets. The good news for busy cooks is that it takes no longer to cook than white rice. Accented with Latin flavors, this versatile side pairs well with seafood, poultry, or pork. *See photo on page 271.*

1 cup **quinoa**

2 teaspoons canola oil

1 cup chopped **onion** (1 medium)

1 can (4 ounces) chopped green chiles

2 **garlic** cloves, minced

1 3/4 cups reduced-sodium chicken broth or vegetable broth

3/4 cup coarsely chopped fresh cilantro

1/2 cup chopped **scallions**

1/4 cup **pepitas** (pumpkin seeds), toasted (see (Tip)

2 tablespoons **lime** juice

1/4 teaspoon salt, or to taste

1. Toast the quinoa in a large dry skillet over medium heat, stirring often, until it crackles and becomes aromatic, 3 to 5 minutes. Transfer to a fine sieve and rinse thoroughly.

2. Heat the oil in a large saucepan over medium heat. Add the onion and cook, stirring often, until softened, 2 to 3 minutes. Add the chiles and garlic. Cook, stirring, for 30 seconds. Add the broth and quinoa and bring to a simmer. Reduce the heat to low, cover, and cook until the quinoa is tender and most of the liquid has been absorbed, 20 to 25 minutes.

3. Add the cilantro, scallions, pepitas, lime juice, and salt to the quinoa. Mix gently and fluff with a fork. One serving is 2/3 cup.

Per serving: 182 calories, 7 g protein, 27 g carbohydrates, 4 g fiber, 6 g total fat, 1 g saturated fat, 0 mg cholesterol, 145 mg sodium.

Tip: Toast the pepitas in a small dry skillet over medium-low heat, stirring constantly, until fragrant, 3 to 5 minutes.

Mashed Sweet Potatoes with Ginger and Orange

6 Serves	Preparation time: 20 minutes
	Cooking time: 12 to 15 minutes

Like French fries, mashed potatoes are blood sugar nightmares—but not if they're made from sweet potatoes, one of our favorite Magic foods. In this dish, fresh citrus and ginger provide delicious accents. Reducing the orange juice enhances its natural sweetness, while just a touch of butter provides exceptional enrichment with a minimum of saturated fat. This puree makes a superb holiday side dish, but it is also easy enough for simple weeknight suppers. Try it with chicken, turkey, or pork tenderloin.

1 1/2 pounds (700 grams) **sweet potatoes** (2 medium-large), peeled and cut into 1 1/2- to 2-inch (4- to 5-centimeter) chunks

1 1/4 cups fresh orange juice (4 oranges)

1 tablespoon grated fresh ginger

1 **garlic** clove, minced

2 teaspoons unsalted butter

1/4 teaspoon salt, or to taste

Freshly ground pepper to taste

1. Place the sweet potatoes in a large saucepan, add enough water to cover, and bring to a boil. Reduce heat to medium, cover, and simmer until the sweet potatoes are tender, 10 to 12 minutes.

2. Meanwhile, combine the orange juice, ginger, and garlic in a small saucepan and bring to a boil. Reduce the heat to medium and simmer, uncovered, until the juice is reduced to 3/4 cup, 5 to 8 minutes. Remove from the heat, add the butter, and stir until melted.

3. When the sweet potatoes are tender, drain them and return to the saucepan. Mash with a potato masher or portable electric mixer. Gradually add the reduced orange juice mixture,

stirring with wooden spoon or beating at low speed with the electric mixer. Season with the salt and pepper. One serving is 1/2 cup. Leftovers will keep, covered, in the refrigerator for up to 2 days. Reheat in the microwave.

Per serving: 116 calories, 2 g protein, 24 g carbohydrates, 3 g fiber, 2 g total fat, 1 g saturated fat, 3 mg cholesterol, 130 mg sodium.

Sweet Potato Oven Fries

4 Serves | **Preparation time: 10 minutes**
| **Cooking time: 25 to 30 minutes**

French fries are one of the top 10 worst foods for blood sugar. But these fries, made in the oven with sweet potatoes, have a dramatically lower GL and more nutrition to boot. They're so tasty you might even prefer them to French fries. *See photo on page 271.*

2 medium **sweet potatoes**
  (12–16 ounces/340–450 grams), peeled

2 teaspoons **olive oil**

1/2 teaspoon paprika

1/4 teaspoon salt, or to taste

1/8 teaspoon freshly ground pepper

1. Preheat the oven to 450°F (230°C). Coat a baking sheet that has a rim or a large roasting pan with cooking spray.

2. Cut the sweet potatoes in half crosswise, then lengthwise into 1/2-inch (1-centimeter)-wide wedges. Place on the baking sheet. Toss with the oil, paprika, salt, and pepper.

3. Bake the sweet potatoes, turning wedges over several times, until golden brown and tender, 25 to 30 minutes. One serving is 1 cup.

Per serving: 100 calories, 2 g protein, 19 g carbohydrates, 3 g fiber, 2 g total fat, 0 g saturated fat, 0 mg cholesterol, 177 mg sodium.

Jerusalem Artichoke Pancakes

4 Serves | **Preparation time: 20 minutes**
| **Cooking/baking time: 25 minutes**

Believe it or not, you can enjoy delicious "potato" pancakes without the potatoes! Here we've used Jerusalem artichokes, also called sunchokes. Not to be confused with leafy globe artichokes, these low-GL tubers are plenty starchy, slightly sweet, and perfect for these pancakes.

1 pound (450 grams) **Jerusalem artichokes** (sunchokes), peeled

1 medium **onion,** halved and peeled

1 large **egg**

3 tablespoons all-purpose flour

1/2 teaspoon salt, or to taste

Freshly ground pepper to taste

4 teaspoons vegetable oil, divided

1/2 cup low-fat plain **yogurt**

1. Preheat the oven to 425°F (220°C). Coat a large baking sheet with nonstick spray.

2. Grate the artichokes and onion in a food processor fitted with a grating disk or on a box grater. (You should have about 2 1/2 cups grated vegetables.)

3. Whisk the egg in a large bowl. Add the grated artichoke mixture, flour, salt, and pepper, and mix well with a fork.

4. Brush 2 teaspoons of the oil over a large non-stick skillet; heat over medium-high heat. Allowing a heaping tablespoon of the artichoke mixture per pancake, drop 4 pancakes into the skillet, spacing evenly. Flatten each pancake with the back of a spatula. Cook until golden, 1 1/2 to 2 1/2 minutes per side. Transfer the pancakes to the prepared baking sheet. Repeat 2 more times

with the remaining artichoke mixture and oil, using 1 teaspoon oil for each successive batch.

5. Place the baking sheet in the oven and bake until crisp and heated through, about 10 minutes. Serve with yogurt. One serving is 3 pancakes and 2 tablespoons yogurt.

Per serving: 167 calories, 5 g protein, 23 g carbohydrates, 2 g fiber, 6 g total fat, 1 g saturated fat, 55 mg cholesterol, 328 mg sodium.

Tip: Once grated, Jerusalem artichokes discolor quickly. Make up the batter and cook the pancakes right away.

Ingredient Note: Jerusalem artichokes are gnarly and look similar to ginger root. Choose smooth, unblemished tubers that are firm, not soft.

Curried Butternut Squash Puree

4
Serves

| Preparation time: 10 minutes |
| Cooking time: 30 to 35 minutes |

A departure from traditional sweet winter squash preparations, this recipe has an exotic flavor thanks to a simple seasoning of fenugreek seeds and turmeric, two Magic spices. Fenugreek seeds have a distinctive aroma reminiscent of curry.

1 tablespoon vegetable oil

2 medium onions, chopped (2 cups)

2 teaspoons ground fenugreek seeds (see Ingredient Note)

1/2 teaspoon turmeric

Pinch of cayenne pepper

4 cups cubed (1 1/2-inch/4-centimeter chunks) peeled butternut squash (20 ounces/575 grams) (see Ingredient Note)

1 cup water

1/2 teaspoon salt, or to taste

2 teaspoons lemon juice

1. Heat the oil in a Dutch oven over medium heat. Add the onions and cook, stirring often, until softened but not colored, 2 to 3 minutes. Add the fenugreek seeds, turmeric, and cayenne. Stir for a few seconds until fragrant. Add the squash, water, and salt. Stir to coat. Return to a simmer, then cook, covered, over medium-low heat until the squash is very tender, 25 to 30 minutes. (Add a little additional water, if necessary.)

2. Mash the squash coarsely with a potato masher. Stir in the lemon juice. One serving is 2/3 cup. Leftovers will keep, covered, in the refrigerator for up to 2 days. Reheat in the microwave.

Per serving: 129 calories, 2 g protein, 25 g carbohydrates, 4 g fiber, 4 g total fat, 1 g saturated fat, 0 mg cholesterol, 299 mg sodium.

Ingredient Note: Fenugreek can be found in the bulk bins of natural foods stores, at Indian grocers, and at Web sites, such as www.kalustyans.com or www.namaste.com. If using whole fenugreek seeds, grind them in a spice mill (a coffee grinder reserved for spices works well).

Cauliflower and Spinach Casserole

6 | Preparation time: 20 minutes
Serves | Cooking/baking time: 50 minutes

This crispy-topped casserole will win over even fussy eaters who claim they don't like vegetables. It's great for special occasions and potlucks because it can be prepared in advance and baked just before serving. (Prepare through Step 4. Cover and refrigerate for up to 2 days.) Frozen vegetables can also be used. Substitute 1 1/2 packages (16 ounces/450 grams) frozen cauliflower and 1 package (10 ounces/300 grams) frozen spinach for fresh. *See photo on opposite page.*

3 tablespoons plain dry bread crumbs

1 teaspoon **olive oil**

1/4 teaspoon paprika

1 medium **cauliflower**
(about 2 1/2 pounds/1.25 kilograms),
cored and cut into 1 1/2-inch (4-centimeter)
florets (about 7 cups)

1 package (10 ounces/300 grams) fresh **spinach**
(12 cups), stems trimmed, washed

1 3/4 cups low-fat (1%) **milk,** divided

3 tablespoons all-purpose flour

1 1/3 cups grated extra-sharp cheddar **cheese**

1 1/2 teaspoons dry mustard

1/2 teaspoon salt, or to taste

Freshly ground pepper to taste

1. Preheat the oven to 425°F (220°C). Coat a 12 x 8-inch (30 x 20-centimeter) shallow baking dish (2 1/2-quart/2 1/2-liter capacity) with non-stick spray.

2. Mix the bread crumbs, oil, and paprika in a small bowl.

3. Cook the cauliflower, uncovered, in a large pot of lightly salted boiling water until tender, about 6 minutes. Stir in the spinach. Cook until the spinach has wilted, about 1 minute longer. Drain cauliflower and spinach. Rinse with cold water to stop further cooking. Drain the vegetables thoroughly and spread in the baking dish.

4. Whisk 1/4 cup of the cold milk with the flour in a small bowl until smooth. Heat the remaining 1 1/2 cups milk in a heavy medium saucepan over medium heat until steaming. Remove from the heat and whisk in the flour mixture. Return to medium heat and cook, whisking constantly, until the sauce bubbles and thickens, 2 to 3 minutes. Remove from the heat. Stir in the cheese, mustard, salt, and pepper. Pour the sauce over the vegetables, spreading evenly. Sprinkle with the reserved bread crumb mixture.

5. Bake the casserole, uncovered, until golden and bubbly, 30 to 35 minutes. One serving is 1 cup.

Per serving: 175 calories, 13 g protein, 14 g carbohydrates, 10 g fiber, 9 g total fat, 5 g saturated fat, 23 mg cholesterol, 519 mg sodium.

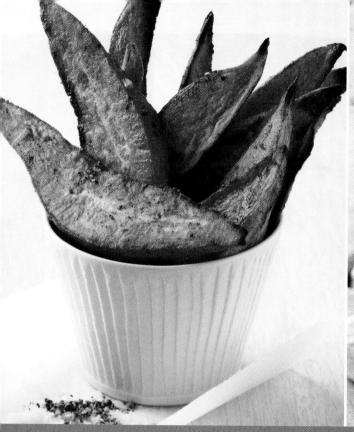

Sweet Potato Oven Fries *page 268*
sweet potato • olive oil

Caulilflower and Spinach Casserole *page 270*
olive oil • cauliflower • cheese

Sautéed Brussels Sprouts with Red Pepper
and Caraway Seeds *page 273*
Brussels sprouts • onion • seeds • vinegar

Quinoa with Chiles and Cilantro *page 266*
quinoa • onion • garlic • scallion • seeds • lime

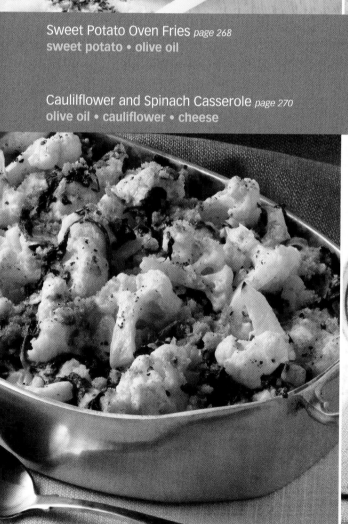

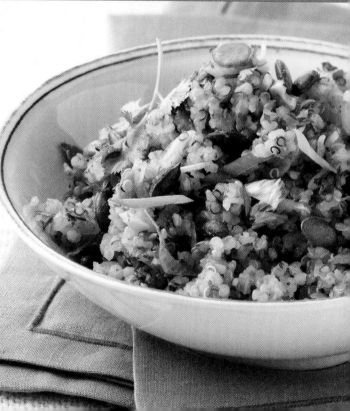

Spiced Cauliflower with Peas

6 | Preparation time: 25 minutes
Serves | Cooking time: 15 minutes

This vegetable braise from India gets its golden hue from the spice turmeric, which boasts anti-inflammatory properties and is believed to have positive affects on blood sugar. The aromatic spice mixture transforms plain old cauliflower and peas into a star-attraction side dish to accompany chicken or dahl (stewed lentils). Since the complex flavors of the spice blend develop as the dish sits, it is a good candidate for making ahead.

1 tablespoon canola oil

1 teaspoon cumin seeds

2 medium **onions,** thinly sliced (2 cups)

2 jalapeño peppers, seeded, deveined, and minced

4 **garlic** cloves, minced

1 tablespoon grated fresh ginger

1 tablespoon ground coriander

1 teaspoon ground cumin

1/2 teaspoon **turmeric**

1 cup water

1 medium head **cauliflower,** cut into florets (7–8 cups)

3/4 teaspoon salt, or to taste

1 medium **tomato,** diced (1 cup)

1 cup frozen green **peas,** rinsed under cold water to thaw

1/3 cup chopped fresh cilantro

Lime wedges

1. Heat the oil in a Dutch oven over medium-high heat. Add the cumin seeds and cook, stirring, until they sizzle, 10 to 20 seconds. Add the onions, jalapeños, garlic, and ginger. Cook, stirring often, until softened, 2 to 3 minutes.

Add the coriander, ground cumin, and turmeric. Stir until fragrant, 10 to 20 seconds. Add the water, cauliflower, and salt. Stir to coat well. Cover and cook until the cauliflower is almost tender, about 8 minutes.

2. Stir in the tomato and peas. Cover and cook until the cauliflower is tender and the peas are heated through, 2 to 3 minutes. Sprinkle with the cilantro and serve with the lime wedges. One serving is 1 cup. Leftovers will keep, covered, in the refrigerator for up to 2 days. Reheat in the microwave.

Per serving: 85 calories, 4 g protein, 13 g carbohydrates, 4 g fiber, 3 g total fat, 0 g saturated fat, 0 mg cholesterol, 349 mg sodium.

Broccoli with Lemon Vinaigrette

4 | Preparation time: 10 minutes
Serves | Cooking time: 5 to 8 minutes

Heaping your plate with a generous portion of broccoli is an excellent strategy for Magic eating—but not if you drown it in butter or cheese sauce. Follow the example in this recipe and use a flavorful olive oil–lemon dressing to moisten steamed broccoli. For convenience, you can substitute one 16-ounce (450-gram) package frozen broccoli florets for fresh; cook according to the package directions.

1 teaspoon freshly grated **lemon** zest

2 tablespoons **lemon** juice

1 tablespoon extra-virgin **olive oil**

2 **garlic** cloves, minced

1/4 teaspoon salt, or to taste

1/8 teaspoon crushed red pepper

Freshly ground pepper to taste

1 large bunch (1 1/2 pounds/700 grams) **broccoli**

1. Whisk the lemon zest, lemon juice, oil, garlic, salt, red pepper, and black pepper in a large bowl.

2. Separate the broccoli florets and cut into 1-inch (2.5-centimeter) pieces. Trim about 3 inches (7.5 centimeters) from stems. Peel remaining portions of stems with a paring knife and cut into 1/2-inch (1-centimeter)-thick slices. Rinse the broccoli. Place in steamer basket over boiling water. Cover and steam until crisp-tender, 5 to 8 minutes. Add to the bowl with the lemon dressing and toss to coat well. (Serve right away. The lemon juice will cause the broccoli to discolor.) One serving is 1 cup.

Per serving: 85 calories, 5 g protein, 10 g carbohydrates, 5 g fiber, 4 g total fat, 1 g saturated fat, 0 mg cholesterol, 192 mg sodium.

Sautéed Brussels Sprouts with Red Pepper and Caraway Seeds

4 Serves | **Preparation time: 15 minutes**
| **Cooking time: 12 minutes**

Brussels sprouts are often enjoyed as part of a Thanksgiving feast but ignored during the rest of the year. That's a shame, because this hardy vegetable is loaded with Magic benefits. Sautéed with colorful red pepper, they make a superb side dish to accompany lean meat or poultry for a simple weeknight dinner. *See photo on page 271.*

3 cups (10 ounces/280 grams) Brussels sprouts, trimmed and cored

2 teaspoons canola oil

1 cup sliced onion (1 medium)

1 medium red bell pepper, cored, seeded, and cut into 2-inch (5-centimeter)-long slivers

1 1/2 teaspoons caraway seeds

1/2 cup reduced-sodium chicken broth or vegetable broth

3 tablespoons cider vinegar

1/4 teaspoon salt, or to taste

Freshly ground pepper to taste

1. Quarter Brussels sprouts with a sharp knife or shred in a food processor fitted with a slicing disk.

2. Heat the oil in a large nonstick skillet over medium-high heat. Add the onion and bell pepper. Cook, stirring often, until softened, 3 to 4 minutes. Add the caraway seeds and cook, stirring, for 30 seconds. Add the Brussels sprouts and cook, stirring, for 2 minutes. Add the broth, cover, and cook until the sprouts are crisp-tender, about 2 or 3 minutes. Stir in the vinegar, salt, and pepper. One serving is 3/4 cup.

Per serving: 75 calories, 3 g protein, 11 g carbohydrates, 4 g fiber, 3 g total fat, 0 g saturated fat, 0 mg cholesterol, 233 mg sodium.

Moroccan Spiced Carrots

4
Serves

Preparation time: 10 minutes

Cooking time: 8 minutes

It is hard to believe that humble carrots can be transformed into such a rich-tasting yet low-calorie dish. The secret is the Moroccan spice blend, which includes a subtle hint of Magic cinnamon. And of course, we've used olive oil instead of butter.

1 1/2 pounds (700 grams) carrots (8–10 medium), peeled and cut into 2 1/2 x 1/2-inch (6 x 1-centimeter) sticks (4 cups)

1 tablespoon extra-virgin olive oil

1 garlic clove, minced

3/4 teaspoon paprika

1/2 teaspoon ground cumin

1/8 teaspoon cinnamon

Pinch of cayenne pepper

3 tablespoons lemon juice

2 tablespoons chopped fresh parsley or cilantro

1/4 teaspoon salt, or to taste

1. Steam the carrots until crisp-tender, 4 to 6 minutes.

2. Heat the oil in a large nonstick skillet over medium-low heat. Add the garlic, paprika, cumin, cinnamon, and cayenne. Cook, stirring, until fragrant, 1 to 2 minutes. Add the carrots, lemon juice, parsley (or cilantro), and salt. Stir to coat the carrots with the spice mixture. One serving is 3/4 cup.

Per serving: 107 calories, 2 g protein, 18 g carbohydrates, 5 g fiber, 4 g total fat, 1 g saturated fat, 0 mg cholesterol, 265 mg sodium.

Spinach with Pine Nuts and Currants

4
Serves

Preparation time: 10 minutes

Cooking time: 10 minutes

Even if you haven't had time to shop for fresh produce or are too busy to rinse fresh greens, there is no excuse for not including a side of Magic spinach on your menu. Frozen spinach works beautifully in this adaptation of a traditional Spanish recipe. Note: Use the frozen cut-leaf spinach that is packed loose in a poly bag (rather than frozen in a block and packed in a box). It is easier to sauté and tastes more like fresh spinach.

1/3 cup dried currants or coarsely chopped dark raisins

Boiling water

2 teaspoons extra-virgin olive oil

1/4 cup pine nuts

1 cup finely chopped onion (1 medium)

1 garlic clove, minced

1 bag (16 ounces/450 grams) frozen cut-leaf spinach

1 tablespoon balsamic vinegar

1/2 teaspoon salt, or to taste

Freshly ground pepper to taste

1. Place the currants in a small bowl and pour in enough boiling water to cover. Let plump for 5 to 10 minutes. Drain, reserving the soaking liquid.

2. Heat the oil in a large nonstick skillet over medium-low heat. Add the pine nuts and cook, stirring, until light golden, 1 to 2 minutes. Transfer pine nuts to a small bowl and set aside. (Do not wash the skillet.)

3. Add the onion and garlic to the skillet. Cook, stirring, until softened and light golden, 2 to 3 minutes. Add the frozen spinach and 2 tablespoons of the reserved soaking liquid. Increase

heat to medium-high and cook, stirring, until heated through and no frozen bits remain, 3 to 5 minutes. Stir in the currants and pine nuts. Season with vinegar, salt, and pepper. One serving is 3/4 cup.

Per serving: 165 calories, 6 g protein, 19 g carbohydrates, 5 g fiber, 9 g total fat, 1 g saturated fat, 0 mg cholesterol, 434 mg sodium.

Sautéed Spinach with Ginger and Soy Sauce

2
Serves

Preparation time: 10 minutes

Cooking time: 5 to 8 minutes

You cannot have enough recipes for simple spinach side dishes in your repertoire. This one has an Asian flair and features aromatic toasted sesame oil, which is low in saturated fat and has an appealing nutty flavor. You can also use frozen spinach for this recipe. In Step 1, substitute one package (10 ounces/300 grams) frozen spinach for fresh; cook according to package directions.

1 package (10 ounces/300 grams) fresh **spinach** (12 cups), stems trimmed, washed

1 tablespoon reduced-sodium soy sauce

2 teaspoons rice **vinegar**

1 teaspoon toasted sesame oil

1/4 teaspoon firmly packed brown sugar

2 teaspoons canola oil

1 **garlic** clove, minced

1 1/2 teaspoons minced fresh ginger

Dash of crushed red pepper

1 tablespoon sesame **seeds,** toasted (see Tip)

1. With just the water clinging to the leaves after washing, cook the spinach in a large, wide pot over medium-high heat just until wilted, 3 to 5 minutes. Drain, refresh under cold running water, and press out excess moisture.

2. Mix the soy sauce, vinegar, sesame oil, and sugar in a small bowl. Heat the oil in a large nonstick skillet over medium-high heat. Add the garlic, ginger, and red pepper. Stir-fry until fragrant but not browned, about 10 seconds. Add the spinach and cook, stirring often, until heated, through 2 to 3 minutes. Stir in the soy sauce mixture and toss to coat well. Sprinkle with the sesame seeds. One serving is 3/4 cup.

Per serving: 119 calories, 4 g protein, 7 g carbohydrates, 3 g fiber, 10 g total fat, 2 g saturated fat, 0 mg cholesterol, 348 mg sodium.

Tip: To toast sesame seeds, heat a small heavy skillet over medium-low heat. Add sesame seeds and stir constantly for 2 to 3 minutes or until light golden and fragrant. Transfer to a small bowl and let cool.

DESSERTS

Cantaloupe and Blueberry Compote with Green Tea and Lime

6 Serves | **Preparation time: 10 minutes**
Cooking time: 0 minutes

Cantaloupe and blueberries are a natural pairing of Magic foods. Here a tart lime seasoning and light green tea syrup give a distinctive and thoroughly refreshing finish to a low-calorie dessert or breakfast compote.

2 green **tea** bags

2/3 cup boiling water

2 tablespoons sugar

1 teaspoon grated lime zest

2 tablespoons **lime** juice

1/2 **cantaloupe,** cut into 1 1/2-inch (4-centimeter) cubes (3 cups)

2 cups **blueberries,** rinsed and dried

1. Place the tea bags in the boiling water and let steep for 3 to 4 minutes. Remove the tea bags. Add the sugar to the tea and stir until dissolved. Stir in the lime zest and lime juice. Let cool to room temperature.

2. Combine the cantaloupe and blueberries in a large bowl. Pour the green tea mixture over the fruit and toss to coat well. One serving is 2/3 cup. The compote will keep, covered, in the refrigerator for up to 2 days.

Per serving: 72 calories, 1 g protein, 18 g carbohydrates, 2 g fiber, 0 g total fat, 0 g saturated fat, 0 mg cholesterol, 13 mg sodium.

Mixed Berry and Stone Fruit Soup

8 Serves | **Preparation time: 20 minutes**
Cooking time: 0 minutes

Don't let the title mislead you—this "soup" is actually a cool, refreshing dessert. Made with some of our favorite Magic berries and stone fruits, it bursts with flavor but contains surprisingly few calories and no fat. Serve this pretty dessert with pride.

1/4 cup orange juice

1 tablespoon **lemon** juice

3 tablespoons sugar

2 medium **nectarines,** pitted and cut into 1 x 1/2-inch (2.5 x 1-centimeter) pieces (1 1/2 cups)

3 medium **plums,** pitted and cut into 1 x 1/2-inch (2.5 x 1-centimeter) pieces (1 1/2 cups)

1 cup fresh **blueberries,** rinsed

1 cup fresh **blackberries,** rinsed

2 tablespoons frozen orange juice concentrate

2 ice cubes, crushed (see Tip)

1/2 cup nonfat vanilla **yogurt**

Mint sprigs for garnish

1. Combine the orange juice, lemon juice, and sugar in a large bowl. Stir to dissolve the sugar. Gently stir in the nectarines, plums, blueberries, and blackberries. Transfer 3/4 cup of the fruit and juices to a blender. Add the frozen orange juice concentrate and ice cubes to the blender and blend until smooth. Scrape the puree into the bowl containing the remaining fruit. Stir gently to combine.

2. To serve, ladle the "soup" into dessert bowls and garnish each serving with a dollop of yogurt and a mint sprig. One serving is 1/2 cup.

Per serving: 88 calories, 2 g protein, 21 g carbohydrates, 2 g fiber, 0 g total fat, 0 g saturated fat, 0 mg cholesterol, 10 mg sodium.

Tips

• This "soup" is best served chilled. The addition of frozen orange juice concentrate and ice cubes cools down the fruit puree base quickly, so you can serve it right away. But if you have time, cover and refrigerate the "soup" for at least 1 hour before serving.

• To crush ice cubes, place them in a resealable plastic bag, seal, and smash with a rolling pin or saucepan.

Pink Grapefruit Brûlée

2 Serves | **Preparation time: 5 minutes** | **Cooking time: 5 to 7 minutes**

Chilled fresh grapefruit is always a refreshing breakfast treat, but when it is caramelized with a cinnamon-scented honey drizzle and warmed, it becomes a simple and satisfying winter dessert or brunch dish.

1 pink **grapefruit**

2 teaspoons honey

Pinch of **cinnamon**

1. Preheat the broiler. Line a small baking sheet with aluminum foil (the caramelized drippings can be hard to clean up). Cut the grapefruit in half crosswise. Use a paring knife or grapefruit knife to separate the flesh from the rind and membrane. Drizzle 1 teaspoon honey over each grapefruit half and spread evenly. Sprinkle with cinnamon. Set the grapefruit halves on the baking sheet and broil until the grapefruit skin is lightly browned in places and the grapefruit is warmed through, 5 to 7 minutes. One serving is 1/2 grapefruit.

Per serving: 59 calories, 1 g protein, 15 g carbohydrates, 1 g fiber, 0 g total fat, 0 g saturated fat, 0 mg cholesterol, 0 mg sodium.

Instant Strawberry Frozen Yogurt

6 Serves | **Preparation time: 5 minutes** | **Cooking time: 0 minutes**

Homemade desserts don't come faster or easier than this one. Even if you don't own an ice cream maker, you can still enjoy frozen yogurt that is better tasting—and better for you—than anything you can buy. Start with unsweetened frozen fruit and use your food processor to whirl in yogurt for a low-calorie frozen treat in just minutes.

16 ounces (450 grams) unsweetened frozen **strawberries** (3 1/2 cups)

1/2 cup sugar

1/2 cup nonfat plain **yogurt**

1 tablespoon orange juice

1. Place the strawberries and sugar in a food processor. Pulse until coarsely chopped. Mix the yogurt and lemon juice in a measuring cup. With the motor running, gradually pour the yogurt mixture through feed tube. Process until smooth and creamy, stopping once or twice to scrape down the side of workbowl. Serve the frozen yogurt directly from the food processor workbowl or place in freezer for 30 minutes to harden before serving. One serving is 1/2 cup.

Per serving: 100 calories, 1 g protein, 25 g carbohydrates, 2 g fiber, 0 g total fat, 0 g saturated fat, 0 mg cholesterol, 13 mg sodium.

VARIATION Instant Peach Frozen Yogurt

Substitute unsweetened frozen peaches for the strawberries.

Orange and Pomegranate Compote

4 Serves | **Preparation time: 15 minutes**
Cooking time: 0 minutes

The best strategy for making Magic desserts is to celebrate the fruits of the season. This simple but elegant compote brightens a winter meal with two seasonal favorites, oranges and pomegranates, and a splash of orange liqueur. Ruby-red pomegranate seeds, renowned for their antioxidant content and high in fiber, lend an exquisite, tart flavor and an appealing crunch.

2 tablespoons orange liqueur, such as Grand Marnier or Cointreau, or orange juice

1 tablespoon sugar

3 medium-large navel **oranges**

1/2 pomegranate

1. Stir the orange liqueur (or orange juice) and sugar together in a medium bowl. Peel the oranges, removing the white pith with a paring knife. Quarter the oranges and slice. Add the orange segments to the bowl with the orange liqueur. Toss to coat.

2. Scoop the seeds from the pomegranate half into a small bowl, discarding the membrane. Sprinkle the pomegranate seeds over the oranges. One serving is 3/4 cup. The compote will keep, covered, in the refrigerator for up to 2 days.

Per serving: 94 calories, 2 g protein, 23 g carbohydrates, 3 g fiber, 0 g total fat, 0 g saturated fat, 0 mg cholesterol, 1 mg sodium.

Pumpkin Custards

6 Serves | **Preparation time: 20 minutes**
Baking time: 50 to 55 minutes

Think of these custards as the best part of a pumpkin pie and enjoy the fact that they are significantly lower in calories and much easier to make. A pumpkin filling is distinguished by its seasoning. This one has a generous amount of cinnamon, which not only makes it taste good, it helps with blood sugar control. Vanilla soy milk makes exceptionally rich-tasting, low-fat custards. If you don't have any on hand, substitute low-fat (1%) milk and increase the vanilla to 1 teaspoon. *See photo on page 281.*

2 large **eggs**

2 large **egg** whites

2/3 cup sugar

3/4 cup canned unseasoned pumpkin puree

1 1/2 teaspoons **cinnamon**

1/2 teaspoon ground nutmeg

1/4 teaspoon salt

1/2 teaspoon vanilla extract

1 1/2 cups vanilla **soy milk**

3 tablespoons whipped cream or low-calorie whipped topping

1. Preheat the oven to 325°F (160°C). Line a roasting pan with a folded kitchen towel (this prevents the custard cups from sliding around). Put a kettle of water on to boil for the water bath.

2. Whisk the eggs, egg whites, and sugar in a large bowl until smooth. Add the pumpkin puree, cinnamon, nutmeg, salt, and vanilla. Whisk until blended. Gently whisk in the soy milk.

3. Divide the mixture among six 6-ounce/ 180-milliliter (3/4-cup) custard cups. Skim foam from the surface of the custards. Set the custard cups on the towel in the roasting pan. Pour enough boiling water into the roasting pan to come halfway up sides of the custard cups. Place the roasting pan in the oven and bake, uncovered, until custards are set, 50 to 55 minutes. Transfer

the custard cups to a rack and let cool. Cover the custards and refrigerate until chilled, at least 1 hour. Just before serving, top each custard with a dollop of whipped cream (or whipped topping). One serving is 1 custard and 1/2 tablespoon whipped cream.

Per serving: 166 calories, 5 g protein, 28 g carbohydrates, 1 g fiber, 4 g total fat, 1 g saturated fat, 75 mg cholesterol, 165 mg sodium.

Lemony Blueberry Cheesecake Bars

24 Bars | **Preparation time:** 25 minutes
Cooking time: 55 to 60 minutes

If you love cheesecake—and who doesn't?—you will certainly enjoy this wholesome bar cookie. We've used naturally sweet blueberries to stretch the creamy filling. We've also swapped out the traditional shortbread crust (made with white flour and a copious amount of butter) for a whole wheat crust, which contains more fiber and a fraction of the saturated fat. *See photo on page 281.*

CRUST

1 1/2 cups **whole wheat pastry flour** (see Ingredient Note, page 280)

1/4 teaspoon baking powder

1/4 teaspoon baking soda

1/4 teaspoon salt

2 tablespoons unsalted butter, softened

2 tablespoons canola oil

1/2 cup sugar

1 large **egg,** lightly beaten

1 teaspoon vanilla extract

CREAM CHEESE FILLING

12 ounces (340 grams) reduced-fat cream **cheese** (Neufchâtel)

1/2 cup sugar

1 tablespoon cornstarch

2 large **eggs,** lightly beaten

4 teaspoon freshly grated lemon zest

1 1/2 teaspoon vanilla extract

3 cups fresh or partially thawed frozen **blueberries**

1. Preheat the oven to 350°F (180°C). Coat a 9 x 13-inch (23 x 33-centimeter) baking dish with nonstick spray.

2. To make the crust: Whisk the flour, baking powder, baking soda, and salt in a medium bowl. Beat the butter, oil, and sugar with an electric mixer in a mixing bowl until smooth. Add the egg and vanilla. Beat until smooth. Add the dry ingredients and mix with a rubber spatula just until the dry ingredients are moistened. Transfer the dough to the prepared baking dish. Use a piece of plastic wrap to press it into an even layer.

3. Bake the crust, uncovered, until puffed and starting to brown around the edges, about 20 minutes.

4. To make the cream cheese filling: Blend the cream cheese, sugar, and cornstarch with an electric mixer or in a food processor until smooth and creamy. Add the eggs, lemon zest, and vanilla. Beat or process until smooth. Spread the blueberries over the crust. Pour the cream cheese batter over the blueberries, spreading evenly.

5. Bake the bars until the filling has set, 35 to 40 minutes. Let cool completely in the pan on a wire rack. Cut into 24 bars with a sharp knife that has been coated with nonstick spray. One serving is 1 bar. The bars will keep, covered, in the refrigerator for up to 4 days or in the freezer for up to 1 month.

Per serving: 140 calories, 3 g protein, 17 g carbohydrates, 1 g fiber, 6 g total fat, 3 g saturated fat, 40 mg cholesterol, 105 mg sodium.

Fudge Brownies

24 Bars

Preparation time: 20 minutes

Baking time: 20 to 25 minutes

Nearly everyone has a craving for a chewy chocolate treat from time to time. Here is a way to indulge yourself with a whole grain brownie that contains much less saturated fat than traditional recipes. We've lowered the GL by replacing some of the flour with oat bran and seasoning the brownies with cinnamon, a delicious complement to the chocolate. *See photo on next page.*

3 ounces/85 grams (3 squares) unsweetened chocolate

2/3 cup whole wheat pastry flour (see Ingredient Note)

1/3 cup oat bran

1/2 teaspoon cinnamon

1/4 teaspoon salt

1/3 cup unsweetened cocoa powder

4 large egg whites (see Tip)

3 large eggs

1 1/3 cups firmly packed light brown sugar

3/4 cup unsweetened applesauce or Lighter Bake (see Ingredient Note)

1/4 cup canola oil

1 teaspoon vanilla extract

1/2 cup bittersweet or semisweet chocolate chips

1/3 cup chopped pecans or walnuts

1. Preheat the oven to 350°F (180°C). Coat a 9 x 13-inch (23 x 33-centimeter) baking dish with nonstick spray.

2. Melt the chocolate in a double boiler over barely simmering water or in the microwave.

3. Combine the flour, oat bran, cinnamon, and salt in a medium bowl. Sift in the cocoa. Whisk to blend the dry ingredients.

4. Beat the egg whites, eggs, and sugar in a large mixing bowl with an electric mixer or a whisk until smooth. Add the applesauce (or Lighter Bake), oil, and vanilla. Beat until blended. Add the melted chocolate and beat until blended. Add the flour mixture and mix at low speed just until dry ingredients are moistened. Stir in the chocolate chips. Scrape the batter into the prepared baking dish, spreading evenly. Sprinkle with the nuts.

5. Bake the brownies until the top springs back when touched lightly, 20 to 25 minutes. Let cool completely on a wire rack. Cut into 24 bars. One serving is one 2 x 2-inch (5 x 5-centimeter) square.

Per serving: 156 calories, 3 g protein, 22 g carbohydrates, 2 g fiber, 8 g total fat, 3 g saturated fat, 26 mg cholesterol, 48 mg sodium.

Tip To avoid wasting the extra egg yolks, use reconstituted dried egg whites, such as Just Whites, which can be found in the baking section of most supermarkets.

Ingredient Notes

• Whole wheat pastry flour is lower in protein than regular whole wheat flour. Since it has less gluten-forming potential, it is an excellent choice for tender baked goods. You can find it in large supermarkets and natural foods stores.

• Lighter Bake is a product produced by Sunsweet Growers. It is made from prunes and apples and designed for use as a fat replacement in baking. You can find it in large supermarkets in the baking section or with the dried fruits.

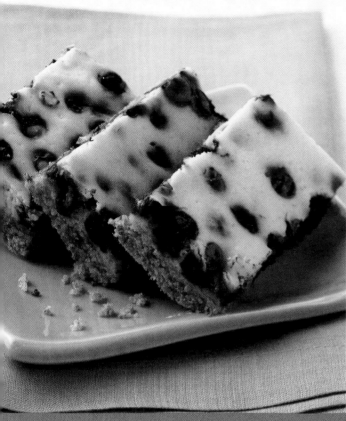

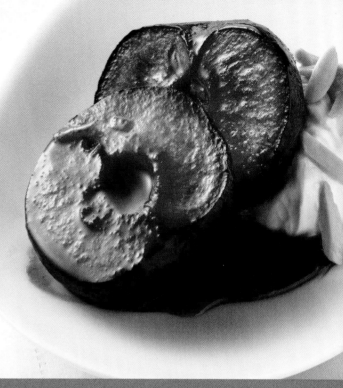

Lemony Blueberry Cheesecake Bars *page 279*
whole wheat flour • egg • cheese • blueberries

Orange-Glazed Roasted Plums *page 282*
plum • almonds • yogurt

Pumpkin Custards *page 278*
egg • cinnamon • soy milk

Fudge Brownies *page 280*
whole wheat flour • oats • cinnamon • egg • pecans

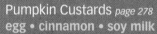

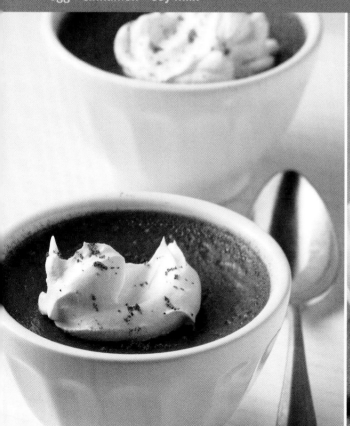

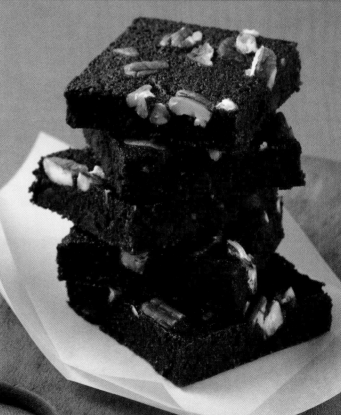

Maple-Walnut Roasted Apples

4 — **Preparation time: 15 minutes**

Serves — **Baking time: 30 to 40 minutes**

Eaten out of hand, crisp raw apples are one of the tastiest, healthiest snacks going, but when cooked they can also be the starting point for an easy low-calorie dessert. Our sophisticated yet simple baked apple features walnuts for a dose of protein and "good" fat and maple syrup instead of brown sugar. If possible, use Red Rome or Cortland apples, considered the best choice for baking because they retain their shape, as well as their tart flavor, during baking.

1/3 cup maple syrup

3 tablespoons apple cider or apple juice

2 teaspoons unsalted butter

2 large **apples,** halved

2 tablespoons chopped **walnuts**

1 cup reduced-fat ice cream or low-fat vanilla
 frozen yogurt

1. Preheat the oven to 400°F (200°C). Coat an 8-inch (20-centimeter) square baking dish with nonstick spray.

2. Combine the maple syrup, apple cider, and butter in a small saucepan. Bring to a simmer, stirring. Remove from the heat.

3. Wash and dry the apple halves (leave the skin on) and remove cores. Place the apples cut side up, in the baking dish. Pour the maple syrup mixture over apples. Cover with aluminum foil and bake for 20 minutes.

4. Baste the apples with the maple syrup mixture. Sprinkle with the walnuts. Return to the oven and bake, uncovered, until the apples are tender and glazed, 10 to 20 minutes, basting once or twice. Let cool slightly. Place an apple half on each dessert dish and drizzle with syrup. Serve with a scoop of vanilla ice cream (or frozen yogurt). One serving is 1 apple half, about 2 table-spoons syrup, and 1/4 cup ice cream.

Per serving: 207 calories, 2 g protein, 38 g carbohydrates, 2 g fiber, 6 g total fat, 2 g saturated fat, 10 mg cholesterol, 29 mg sodium.

Orange-Glazed Roasted Plums

4 — **Preparation time: 15 minutes**

Serves — **Baking time: 30 to 40 minutes**

Roasting brings out the natural sweetness in fruits and is a delicious way to prepare fiber-rich stone fruits. Here, an orange-scented syrup provides a delicate balance to the tart plums. Pluots, which are hybrids of plum and apricot, have become increasingly available and also work well in this recipe. *See photo on page 281.*

1 teaspoon grated orange zest or grated fresh ginger

1/4 cup fresh orange juice (1 orange)

3 tablespoons firmly packed brown sugar

2 teaspoons unsalted butter

4 medium **plums** or pluots (1–1 1/4 pounds/
 450–600 grams), halved and pitted

2 tablespoons slivered **almonds**

1/2 cup fat-free vanilla **yogurt**

1. Preheat the oven to 400°F (200°C). Coat an 8-inch (20-centimeter) square baking dish with nonstick spray.

2. Combine the orange zest (or ginger), orange juice, and brown sugar in a small saucepan. Bring to a simmer, stirring to dissolve the sugar. Remove from the heat, add butter, and stir until melted.

3. Place the plums, cut side up, in the baking dish. Pour the orange juice mixture over the

plums. Cover with aluminum foil and bake until the plums are almost tender, 20 to 25 minutes.

4. Baste the plums with the orange syrup and sprinkle with the almonds. Bake, uncovered, until the plums are tender and glazed, 10 to 15 minutes, basting once or twice. Serve the plums warm or chilled, drizzled with the syrup and accompanied by a dollop of yogurt. One serving is 2 plum halves, about 2 tablespoons syrup, and 2 tablespoons yogurt.

Per serving: 151 calories, 3 g protein, 28 g carbohydrates, 1 g fiber, 4 g total fat, 1 g saturated fat, 6 mg cholesterol, 25 mg sodium.

Cherry Clafouti

8	Preparation time: 25 minutes
Serves	Baking time: 35 to 40 minutes

Cherries are one of our favorite low-GL foods, and it's hard to think of a more delicious way to enjoy them than in a clafouti. This rustic French dessert is a cross between a custard and a baked pancake. It's simple to make and ever-so-comforting. If you're using fresh cherries, use a cherry pitter to speed the pitting process. Or use frozen cherries, which are already pitted.

2 tablespoons plus 1/2 cup sugar, divided

1/2 cup all-purpose flour

2 large eggs

2 large egg whites (see Tip page 280)

1 cup low-fat (1%) milk

1 tablespoon unsalted butter, melted

1 teaspoon vanilla extract

1 pound/450 grams (3 cups) fresh or partially thawed frozen sweet cherries, such as Bing, pitted

Confectioners' sugar for dusting

1. Preheat the oven to 400°F (200°C). Coat a 9- or 9 1/2-inch (23- or 24-centimeter) pie pan with nonstick spray. Sprinkle with 1 tablespoon sugar and tilt to coat.

2. Place 1/2 cup sugar, the flour, eggs, egg whites, milk, butter, and vanilla in a food processor or blender. Process until smooth.

3. Spread the cherries in the pie pan. Pour the egg batter over the cherries. Sprinkle with the remaining 1 tablespoon sugar. Bake the clafouti until light brown and puffed, 35 to 40 minutes. Let cool slightly. (The clafouti will sink as it cools.) Dust with confectioners' sugar and serve warm. (Leftovers are also delicious chilled.)

Per serving: 176 calories, 5 g protein, 33 g carbohydrates, 1 g fiber, 3 g total fat, 2 g saturated fat, 59 mg cholesterol, 48 mg sodium.

VARIATION Pear-Berry Clafouti

In Step 2, add 2 teaspoons grated lemon zest to the custard. In Step 3, substitute 2 sliced, peeled Anjou pears and 1 cup fresh or unsweetened frozen raspberries for the cherries.

Chocolate-Raspberry Cheesecake

12 | Preparation time: 40 minutes
Serves | Baking time: 60 to 70 minutes

This rich-tasting, fudgy cheesecake plays on the delicious contrast of tart raspberries and dark chocolate to make a truly impressive dessert. No one will ever guess that it is relatively low in calories and saturated fat. The secret ingredient is silken tofu. It bakes up into a velvety cheesecake, and the protein it provides helps to offset the carbohydrates in the dessert.

CRUST

1 1/4 cups chocolate wafer cookies
(see Ingredient Note)

1/3 cup **walnuts**

4 teaspoons light brown sugar

1/8 teaspoon **cinnamon**

3 tablespoons canola oil

FILLING

1 package (12 ounces/350 grams) reduced-fat firm silken **tofu**

1 package (8 ounces/250 grams) reduced-fat cream **cheese** (Neufchâtel)

3/4 cup firmly packed light brown sugar

1/2 cup granulated sugar

2/3 cup unsweetened cocoa powder

4 ounces (125 grams) bittersweet (*not* unsweetened) chocolate, melted (see Ingredient Note)

2 tablespoons cornstarch

2 teaspoons vanilla extract

3 large **eggs,** lightly beaten

1 1/2 cups fresh **raspberries**

GARNISH

1 1/4 cups Raspberry Sauce (*recipe follows*)

2 cups fresh **raspberries**

1/4 cup chocolate shavings (see Tip)

Confectioners' sugar for dusting

1. Preheat the oven to 325°F (160°C). Coat a 9-inch (23-centimeter) springform pan with cooking spray. Wrap the outside of pan with a double thickness of foil to keep water out while cheesecake is baking.

2. To make the crust: Put the cookies, walnuts, 4 teaspoons brown sugar, and cinnamon in a food processor. Pulse until fine crumbs form. Add the oil and pulse until the crumbs are moistened. Transfer to the pan and use the bottom of a glass to press the crumb mixture over bottom and 1/2 inch (1 centimeter) up the sides. Bake the crust until firm to the touch, 10 to 15 minutes. Set aside to cool. (Rinse and dry the food processor workbowl.)

3. To make the filling: Put the tofu in a food processor and process until smooth, stopping to scrape down sides of workbowl once or twice. Add the cream cheese, 3/4 cup brown sugar, granulated sugar, cocoa, chocolate, cornstarch, and vanilla. Process until well blended. Add the eggs and pulse just until mixed in.

4. Put a kettle of water on to boil for the waterbath. Rinse the raspberries and pat thoroughly dry. Scatter the raspberries over the bottom of the baked crust. Scrape the chocolate batter into the pan and spread evenly. Place the cheesecake in a shallow roasting pan and pour in enough boiling water to come 1/2 inch (1 centimeter) up sides of springform pan. Bake the cheesecake until set around edges but center still jiggles when pan is tapped, 50 to 55 minutes. Turn off the oven and prop oven door open with a wooden spoon. Let the cheesecake cool in oven for 1 hour.

5. Remove the foil and place the springform pan on a wire rack to cool completely. Cover with plastic wrap and refrigerate until chilled, at least 4 hours or up to 4 days.

6. To prepare the garnish: Make the Raspberry Sauce. Rinse 2 cups raspberries and pat thoroughly dry. Run a small, sharp knife between cheesecake and pan rim to loosen edges, then remove pan rim. Set the cheesecake on a serving platter and arrange raspberries over the top. Sprinkle with chocolate shavings and dust with confectioners' sugar. Serve with Raspberry Sauce. One serving is 1/12th of the cheesecake and 1 1/2 tablespoons Raspberry Sauce.

Per serving: 352 calories, 8 g protein, 52 g carbohydrates, 6 g fiber, 16 g total fat, 6 g saturated fat, 11 mg cholesterol, 138 mg sodium.

Tip: To make chocolate shavings, warm a chunk or piece of bittersweet chocolate at low power in the microwave for a few seconds, just until pliable but not melted. Use a vegetable peeler to shave off curls.

Ingredient Notes:
 • It's worth going to the natural foods section or store to find chocolate wafers for the crust that don't contain hydrogenated oils.

 • Seek out the best dark chocolate, preferably one with 70 percent cocoa content. Not only do these chocolates have the truest chocolate flavor, they are richest in antioxidants.

Raspberry Sauce

12
Serves

| Preparation time: 5 minutes |
| Makes 1 1/4 cups |

This elegant sauce is made by simply pureeing raspberries (frozen berries work just fine). Use it to dress up a compote of strawberries or mixed berries or as a topping for low-fat vanilla ice cream or yogurt. It does contain sugar, so keep your serving sizes small.

1 package (12 ounces/300 grams) frozen unsweetened **raspberries,** thawed

1/3 cup confectioners' sugar

1 tablespoon orange juice

1. Put the raspberries, sugar, and orange juice in a food processor. Process until pureed. Pass the puree through a fine sieve set over a medium bowl. Discard seeds. One serving is a generous 1 1/2 tablespoons.

Per serving: 25 calories, 0 g protein, 6 g carbohydrates, 0 fiber, 0 g total fat, 0 g saturated fat, 0 mg cholesterol, 0 mg sodium.

Apple-Cranberry Crumble

8 | **Preparation time: 20 minutes**
Serves | **Baking time: 40 to 55 minutes**

With its emphasis on whole grains and fruit, this could be the ideal Magic dessert. We've replaced the white flour in the typical recipe with whole wheat to make a 100 percent whole grain topping and substituted fruit juice concentrate and canola oil for much of the butter. This is an extremely versatile concept. The variations at right offer a special dessert for every season. Top off the crumble with a dollop of fat-free vanilla yogurt.

5 cups sliced peeled **apples** (4–5 medium)

1 cup fresh or frozen **cranberries**

1/3 cup granulated sugar

2/3 cup **whole wheat flour**

1/2 cup old-fashioned rolled **oats**

1/2 cup firmly packed light brown sugar

2 teaspoons **cinnamon**

Pinch of salt

1 tablespoon unsalted butter, cut into small pieces

1 tablespoon canola oil

3 tablespoons frozen apple juice concentrate

1 tablespoon chopped **walnuts**

1. Preheat the oven to 375°F (190°C). Coat an 8-inch (20-centimter) square baking dish (2-quart/2-liter capacity) with nonstick spray.

2. Combine the apples, cranberries, and granulated sugar in the baking dish. Toss to mix. Cover with aluminum foil and bake for 20 minutes (25 minutes, if using some frozen fruit).

3. Meanwhile, mix the flour, oats, brown sugar, cinnamon, and salt with a fork in a medium bowl. Add the butter and crumble with a pastry blender or your fingertips until well blended. Add the oil and stir to coat. Add the apple juice concentrate and stir and toss until the dry ingredients are moistened.

4. When the crumble has baked for 20 minutes, sprinkle the flour mixture evenly over the fruit. Sprinkle with the walnuts. Bake, uncovered, until the fruit is bubbly and tender and the topping is lightly browned, 20 to 30 minutes longer. Let cool for at least 10 minutes before serving warm or at room temperature. One serving is 1/2 cup.

Per serving: 241 calories, 3 g protein, 46 g carbohydrates, 4 g fiber, 6 g total fat, 1 g saturated fat, 4 mg cholesterol, 26 mg sodium.

Rhubarb-Blackberry Crumble

8 | **Preparation time: 20 minutes**
Serves | **Baking time: 40 to 55 minutes**

If you enjoy the tart taste of rhubarb, you'll adore this sweet and tangy springtime dessert.

5 cups diced (1/2-inch/1-centimeter pieces) rhubarb (1 1/2 pounds/700 grams before trimming)

1 cup **blackberries**

1/2 cup granulated sugar

1 tablespoon cornstarch

2/3 cup **whole wheat flour**

1/2 cup old-fashioned rolled **oats**

1/2 cup firmly packed light brown sugar

1 teaspoon **cinnamon**

Pinch of salt

1 tablespoon unsalted butter, cut into small pieces

1 tablespoon canola oil

3 tablespoons frozen orange juice concentrate

1 tablespoon chopped slivered **almonds**

1. Preheat the oven to 375°F (190°C). Coat an 8-inch (20-centimter) square baking dish (2-quart/2-liter capacity) with nonstick spray.

2. Combine the rhubarb, blackberries, granulated sugar and cornstarch in the baking dish. Toss to mix. Cover with aluminum foil and bake for 20 minutes.

3. Meanwhile, mix the flour, oats, brown sugar, cinnamon, and salt with a fork in a medium bowl. Add the butter and crumble with a pastry blender or your fingertips until well blended. Add the oil and stir to coat. Add the orange juice concentrate and stir and toss until the dry ingredients are moistened.

4. When the crumble has baked for 20 minutes, sprinkle the flour mixture evenly over the fruit. Sprinkle with the walnuts. Bake, uncovered, until the fruit is bubbly and tender and the topping is lightly browned, 20 to 30 minutes longer. Let cool for at least 10 minutes before serving warm or at room temperature. One serving is 1/2 cup.

Per serving: 227 calories, 4 g protein, 45 g carbohydrates, 4 g fiber, 4 g total fat, 1 g saturated fat, 4 mg cholesterol, 28 mg sodium.

Peach-Raspberry Crumble

In Step 2, combine 5 cups sliced peeled peaches (2 pounds/1 kilogram), 1 cup raspberries, 2 tablespoons sugar, and 1 tablespoon lemon juice in the baking dish. Toss to mix.

In Step 3, reduce cinnamon to 1 teaspoon and substitute frozen orange juice concentrate for the apple juice concentrate.

In Step 4, substitute chopped slivered almonds for the walnuts.

Cherry-Raspberry Crumble

In Step 2, combine 5 cups pitted sweet cherries, such as Bing, (1 1/2 pounds/ 700 grams), 1 cup raspberries, 1/3 cup sugar, 1 tablespoon cornstarch, and 1 tablespoon lemon juice in the baking dish. Toss to mix.

In Step 2, reduce the cinnamon to 1 teaspoon and substitute frozen orange juice concentrate for the apple juice concentrate. In Step 3, substitute chopped slivered almonds for the walnuts.

Plum-Walnut Crumble

In Step 2, combine 6 cups sliced plums (2 pounds/1 kilogram), 1/3 cup sugar, 2 teaspoons freshly grated orange zest, and 1 tablespoon orange juice in the baking dish. Toss to mix.

In Step 3, reduce the cinnamon to 1 teaspoon.

Cherry-Almond Gratin

6 Serves

Preparation time: 30 minutes

Baking time: 30 to 40 minutes

Fruit baked in a rich-tasting almond cream makes a homey yet special dessert. Tofu may seem like a surprising ingredient, but it makes a very successful and healthful substitute for butter in this almond cream.

1/3 cup slivered **almonds**

1/3 cup sugar

1 tablespoon all-purpose flour

Pinch of salt

1 large **egg**

1 large **egg** white

1/2 cup reduced-fat firm silken **tofu**

1 tablespoon unsalted butter, softened

1/4 teaspoon almond extract

3 cups fresh or partially thawed frozen sweet **cherries**, such as Bing, pitted

Confectioners' sugar for dusting

1. Preheat the oven to 375°F (190°C). Coat a 9 1/2-inch (24-centimeter) pie pan with nonstick spray.

2. Spread the almonds in a small baking dish. Toast in the oven until light golden and fragrant, 4 to 6 minutes. Let cool.

3. Combine the almonds, sugar, flour, and salt in a food processor. Process until the almonds are ground. Add the egg, egg white, tofu, butter, and almond extract. Process until smooth.

4. Spread the cherries in the pie pan. Scrape the tofu mixture evenly over the cherries. Bake the gratin until light golden and firm to the touch, 30 to 40 minutes. Let cool slightly. Dust with confectioners' sugar. Serve warm or at room temperature.

Per serving: 168 calories, 5 g protein, 26 g carbohydrates, 2 g fiber, 6 g total fat, 2 g saturated fat, 40 mg cholesterol, 28 g sodium.

VARIATIONS

Mixed Berry-Almond Gratin

In Step 4, substitute 3 cups mixed berries, such as raspberries, blackberries, and blueberries (fresh or frozen and partially thawed) for the cherries.

Pear and Dried Cranberry Gratin

In Step 4, substitute 3 sliced peeled firm pears, such as Anjou or Bosc, and 1/2 cup plumped dried cranberries (microwave with 2 tablespoons water on high for 1 minute) for the cherries.

7 day MEAL PLANS

Incorporating a few Magic foods into your diet is easy as pie. But what does a whole day of Magic eating look like? How do you know if you're eating too many carbohydrates—or not enough? How do you know if you're eating too much *food?*

To help you put the *Magic Foods* approach to work on your plate, we designed week-long meal plans based on three different calorie goals. Each meal, snack, and dessert incorporates the Seven Secrets of Magic Eating, and each day features at least a dozen different Magic foods.

You'll see for yourself not only how much food you should be eating but also what a good breakdown of carbohydrates, protein, and fat looks like; what three daily servings of whole grains look like; and what five or more daily servings of fruits and vegetables look like.

How do you know which calorie target is right for you? (Remember, controlling portion sizes and calories is key to controlling your blood sugar.) If you're trying to lose some weight, simply multiply your current weight in pounds by 10 to get the number of calories you should be eating. For instance, if you currently weigh 180 pounds and want to shed some of them, 1,800 calories a day would be about right for you. (To convert kilograms to pounds, multiply by 2.2. To convert pounds back to kilograms, multiply by 0.453.)

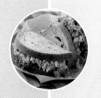

Otherwise, consider the 1,400-calorie target appropriate for most smaller women or women trying to lose weight; the 1,800-calorie target for most larger women, average-size men, and larger men who want to lose weight; and the 2,200-calorie target for larger or highly active men.

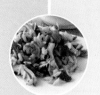

We don't necessarily expect you to follow every day's meal plan to the letter (although if you want to, terrific!), but do try one or two days' worth to see what the *Magic Foods* approach is like—and how good it makes you feel.

1400 calorie MEAL PLAN

	monday	tuesday	wednesday
breakfast	2/3 cup Oatmeal with Apples and Flaxseeds *page 193* Coffee or tea	1 orange 1 cup low-fat fruit yogurt Coffee or tea	3/4 cup Raisin Bran cereal with 1/2 cup sliced strawberries and 1/2 cup fat-free milk Coffee or tea
lunch	1 cup Turkey and Bean Chili with Avocado Salsa *page 243* 1 sliced pear with 1/2 ounce (15 grams) sliced low-fat Swiss cheese Unsweetened iced tea or mineral water	Turkey sandwich on whole grain bread with 3 slices turkey, 1 slice avocado, lettuce, tomato, and mustard 2 celery sticks (5 inches/13 centimeters) with 1 tablespoon peanut butter 1/2 apple Water	2 cups Grilled Chicken Salad with Oranges *page 210* 2-inch (5-centimeter) pumpernickel dinner roll Water or mineral water
snack	6 red bell pepper rings 2 tablespoons Asian Peanut Dip *page 204* Water	2 tablespoons White Bean Spread with Italian Flavors *page 205* 4 Whole Wheat Pita Crisps *page 207*	2 tablespoons Mediterranean Split Pea Spread *page 205* 3 small melba toast crackers
dinner	3/4 cup Chicken Sauté with Apple *page 235* 1/2 cup Mushroom-Barley Pilaf *page 264* 1 cup steamed green beans Water with lemon	1 2/3 cups Greek Pasta and Beef Casserole *page 230* 1 cup Broccoli with Lemon Vinaigrette *page 272* Unsweetened iced tea or mineral water	1 serving Mustard-Glazed Salmon with Lentils *page 247* 1/2 cup Brown Rice Pilaf with Toasted Flaxseeds *page 265* 6 steamed asparagus spears Water or mineral water
dessert			1 serving Pumpkin Custard *page 278*
NUTRITIONAL INFORMATION	Calories: 1402; Protein: 82 g; Carbohydrate: 185 g; Fat: 42 g; Fiber: 33 g Percentage of calories from carbs: 53; protein: 23; fat: 27	Calories: 1445; Protein: 88 g; Carbohydrate: 197 g; Fat: 43 g; Fiber: 27 g Percentage of calories from carbs: 54; protein: 24; fat: 28	Calories: 1429; Protein: 90 g; Carbohydrate: 180 g; Fat: 44 g; Fiber: 30 g Percentage of calories from carbs: 50; protein: 25; fat: 28

thursday	friday	saturday	sunday
3/4 cup Kashi GoLean cereal with 1/2 cup fat-free milk 1 nectarine 1/2 cup orange juice	3/4 cup hot oat bran with 1/2 cup blueberries and 1/2 cup fat-free milk Coffee or tea	2 Multi-Grain Pancakes with syrup and strawberries *page 192* 1/2 cup fat-free milk	Spinach and Goat Cheese Omelet *page 194* 2 cantaloupe wedges Coffee or tea
Tuna and Carrot Sandwich on Rye *page 222* 8 Spiced Almonds *page 203* 1 peach Unsweetened iced tea	Whole wheat wrap with 3 slices lean ham, 1 slice low-fat Muenster cheese, lettuce, and tomato 3/4 cup grapes 1 container (4 ounces/ 125 milliliters) low-fat fruit yogurt Water with lemon	1 1/2 cups Curried Red Lentil Soup *page 224* 1 tablespoon hummus 8 baby carrots Water	1 1/4 cups Whole Wheat Chicken and Noodles with Peanut Sauce *page 214* 2 fresh pineapple slices Water with lemon
1 Oatmeal–Peanut Butter Trail Bar *page 207*	1 1/2 cups popcorn mixed with 7 peanuts and 1/2 tablespoon Smart Balance or Becel (in Canada) spread	1 1/2 ounces (45 grams) semisoft goat cheese drizzled with lemon juice 1 Wasa Crispbread rye cracker	4 whole wheat pretzel sticks 1 stick reduced-fat string cheese
5 ounces (140 grams) Flank Steak with Balsamic Sauce *page 228* 3/4 cup brown rice 2 cups romaine lettuce salad with cherry tomatoes, cucumber, 1/4 cup chickpeas, and 1 tablespoon each olive oil and balsamic vinegar Water	1 1/2 cups Shrimp and Orzo Casserole *page 251* 1 cup green beans 2 cups baby spinach salad with tomato and cucumber and 1 tablespoon each olive oil and balsamic vinegar Unsweetened iced tea or mineral water	1 1/2 cups Slow-Cooker Beef and Vegetable Stew *page 228* 1/2 slice Whole Wheat Flaxseed Bread *page 196* 1 1/4 cups romaine lettuce salad with cherry tomatoes, cucumber, and 1/2 tablespoon each olive oil and vinegar Water with lemon	1 3/4 cups Spring Vegetable Stir-Fry with Tofu *page 260* 1/2 cup brown rice Green tea
		3/4 cup Orange and Pomegranate Compote *page 278*	1/2 cup Instant Strawberry Frozen Yogurt *page 277*
Calories: 1417; Protein: 83 g; Carbohydrate: 175 g; Fat: 50 g; Fiber: 28 g Percentage of calories from carbs: 49; protein: 24; fat: 31	Calories: 1399; Protein: 84 g; Carbohydrate: 172 g; Fat: 42 g; Fiber: 26 g Percentage of calories from carbs: 49; protein: 24; fat: 27	Calories: 1444; Protein: 81 g; Carbohydrate: 186 g; Fat: 41 g; Fiber: 35 g Percentage of calories from carbs: 52; protein: 22; fat: 26	Calories: 1401; Protein: 82 g; Carbohydrate: 169 g; Fat: 49 g; Fiber: 25 g Percentage of calories from carbs: 48; protein: 23; fat: 32

1800
calorie MEAL PLAN

	monday	tuesday	wednesday
breakfast	3/4 cup Oatmeal with Apples and Flaxseeds *page 193* with 4 slivered almonds 1/2 cup unsweetened grapefruit juice	1 Blueberry Oatmeal Muffin *page 198* 1 orange 1/2 cup low-fat fruit yogurt Coffee or tea	3/4 cup Raisin Bran cereal with 1/2 cup sliced strawberries, 5 walnuts (chopped), and 1/2 cup fat-free milk Coffee or tea
lunch	1 1/4 cups Turkey and Bean Chili with Avocado Salsa *page 243* 1 sliced pear with 1/2 ounce (15 grams) sliced low-fat Swiss cheese Unsweetened iced tea	Turkey sandwich on whole grain bread with 3 slices turkey, 1 slice avocado, lettuce, tomato, and mustard 2 celery sticks (5 inches/13 centimeters) with 2 tablespoons peanut butter 1 apple Water	2 1/2 cups Grilled Chicken Salad with Oranges *page 210* 2-inch (5-centimeter) pumpernickel dinner roll Water
snack	6 red bell pepper rings 3 tablespoons Asian Peanut Dip *page 204* Water	3 tablespoons White Bean Spread with Italian Flavors *page 205* 8 Whole Wheat Pita Crisps *page 207*	2 tablespoons Mediterranean Split Pea Spread *page 205* 5 small melba toast crackers
dinner	1 1/4 cups Chicken Sauté with Apple *page 235* 1/2 cup Mushroom-Barley Pilaf *page 264* 1 cup steamed green beans Water with lemon	2 cups Greek Pasta and Beef Casserole *page 230* 1 cup Broccoli with Lemon Vinaigrette *page 272* Unsweetened iced tea	1 1/2 servings Mustard-Glazed Salmon with Lentils (use 6 ounces/170 grams fish) *page 247* 1/2 cup Brown Rice Pilaf with Toasted Flaxseeds *page 265* 6 steamed asparagus spears Water
dessert			1 serving Pumpkin Custard *page 278*
NUTRITIONAL INFORMATION	Calories: 1814; Protein: 102 g; Carbohydrate: 233 g; Fat: 59 g; Fiber: 39 g Percentage of calories from carbs: 51; protein: 23; fat: 29	Calories: 1781; Protein: 103 g; Carbohydrate: 229 g; Fat: 60 g; Fiber: 34 g Percentage of calories from carbs: 51; protein: 23; fat: 30	Calories: 1804; Protein: 118 g; Carbohydrate: 209 g; Fat: 63 g; Fiber: 38 g Percentage of calories from carbs: 46; protein: 26; fat: 31

thursday	friday	saturday	sunday
1 cup Kashi GoLean cereal with 1/2 cup fat-free milk 1 nectarine 1/2 cup orange juice	3/4 cup hot oat bran with 1/2 cup blueberries, 4 pecans (chopped), and 1/2 cup fat-free milk Coffee or tea	2 Multi-Grain Pancakes with syrup and strawberries *page 192* 1/2 tablespoon Smart Balance or Becel (in Canada) spread 1/2 cup fat-free milk	1 Spinach and Goat Cheese Omelet *page 194* 1/2 whole wheat English muffin 1/2 tablespoon Smart Balance or Becel (in Canada) spread 2 cantaloupe wedges Coffee or tea
Tuna and Carrot Sandwich on Rye *page 222* 15 Spiced Almonds *page 203* 1 peach Unsweetened iced tea	Whole wheat wrap with 3 slices lean ham, 1 slice low-fat Muenster cheese, lettuce, tomato, and mustard 1 cup grapes 1/2 cup low-fat fruit yogurt with 2 tablespoons ground flaxseeds Water with lemon	2 cups Curried Red Lentil Soup *page 224* 2 tablespoons hummus 8 baby carrots Water	1 2/3 cups Whole Wheat Chicken and Noodles with Peanut Sauce *page 214* 2 slices fresh pineapple Water with lemon
1 Oatmeal–Peanut Butter Trail Bar *page 207*	2 cups popcorn mixed with 7 peanuts and 1 tablespoon Smart Balance or Becel (in Canada) spread	1 1/2 ounces (45 grams) semisoft goat cheese drizzled with lemon juice 2 Wasa Crispbread rye crackers	6 whole wheat pretzel sticks 2 ounces (60 grams) low-fat Colby cheese (2 1-inch/2.5-centimeter squares)
6 ounces (170 grams) Flank Steak with Balsamic Sauce *page 228* 1 cup brown rice 2 cups romaine lettuce salad with cherry tomatoes, cucumber, 3/4 cup chickpeas, and 1 tablespoon each olive oil and vinegar Water	2 cups Shrimp and Orzo Casserole *page 251* 1 cup steamed green beans 2 cups baby spinach salad with tomato, cucumber, and 1 tablespoon each olive oil and balsamic vinegar Unsweetened iced tea	2 cups Slow-Cooker Beef and Vegetable Stew *page 228* 1 slice Whole Wheat Flaxseed Bread *page 196* 1 1/4 cups romaine lettuce salad with cherry tomatoes, cucumber, and 1/2 tablespoon each olive oil and vinegar Water with lemon	2 1/4 cups Spring Vegetable Stir-Fry with Tofu *page 260* 3/4 cup brown rice Green tea
		3/4 cup Orange and Pomegranate Compote *page 278*	1/2 cup Instant Strawberry Frozen Yogurt *page 277*
Calories: 1813; Protein: 101 g; Carbohydrate: 1237 g; Fat: 59 g; Fiber: 37 g Percentage of calories from carbs: 52; protein: 22; fat: 29	Calories: 1797; Protein: 103 g; Carbohydrate: 204 g; Fat: 65 g; Fiber: 36 g Percentage of calories from carbs: 45; protein: 23; fat: 32	Calories: 1828; Protein: 108 g; Carbohydrate: 222 g; Fat: 64 g; Fiber: 35 g Percentage of calories from carbs: 48; protein: 24; fat: 31	Calories: 1836; Protein: 103 g; Carbohydrate: 231 g; Fat: 55 g; Fiber: 47 g Percentage of calories from carbs: 50; protein: 23; fat: 27

2200 calorie MEAL PLAN

	monday	tuesday	wednesday
breakfast	3/4 cup Oatmeal with Apples and Flaxseeds *page 193* with 4 slivered almonds 1/2 cup unsweetened grapefruit juice Coffee or tea	1 Blueberry Oatmeal Muffin *page 198* 1 orange 1 cup low-fat fruit yogurt Coffee or tea	1 cup Raisin Bran cereal with 3/4 cup sliced strawberries, 7 walnuts (chopped), and 3/4 cup fat-free milk Coffee or tea
lunch	2 cups Turkey and Bean Chili with Avocado Salsa *page 243* 1 sliced pear with 4 (1/2 ounce/15 grams) slices low-fat Swiss cheese Unsweetened iced tea	Turkey sandwich on whole grain bread with 3 slices turkey, 1 slice provolone cheese, 1 slice avocado, lettuce, tomato, and mustard 4 celery sticks (5 inches/13 centimeters) with 2 tablespoons peanut butter 1 apple Water	3 cups Grilled Chicken Salad with Oranges *page 210* 2-inch (5-centimeter) pumpernickel dinner roll Water
snack	6 red bell pepper rings 3 tablespoons Asian Peanut Dip *page 204* Water	4 tablespoons White Bean Spread with Italian Flavors *page 205* 8 Whole Wheat Pita Crisps *page 207* 1/4 cucumber, sliced	3 tablespoons Mediterranean Split Pea Spread *page 205* 5 small melba toast crackers
dinner	2 cups Chicken Sauté with Apple *page 235* 1/2 cup Mushroom-Barley Pilaf *page 264* 1 cup steamed green beans Water with lemon	2 1/2 cups Greek Pasta and Beef Casserole *page 230* 1 cup Broccoli with Lemon Vinaigrette *page 272* Unsweetened iced tea	8 ounces (250 grams) Mustard-Glazed Salmon with Lentils *page 247* 3/4 cup Brown Rice Pilaf with Toasted Flaxseeds *page 265* 8 steamed asparagus spears Water
dessert			1 serving Pumpkin Custard *page 278*
NUTRITIONAL INFORMATION	Calories: 2202; Protein: 123 g; Carbohydrate: 278 g; Fat: 74 g; Fiber: 47 g Percentage of calories from carbs: 50; protein: 22; fat: 30	Calories: 2196; Protein: 131 g; Carbohydrate: 272 g; Fat: 74 g; Fiber: 37 g Percentage of calories from carbs: 49; protein: 24; fat: 30	Calories: 2196; Protein: 149 g; Carbohydrate: 259 g; Fat: 72 g; Fiber: 47 g Percentage of calories from carbs: 47; protein: 27; fat: 29

thursday	friday	saturday	sunday
1 1/4 cups Kashi GoLean cereal with 1/2 cup low-fat milk 1 nectarine 1/2 cup orange juice	1 1/4 cups hot oat bran with 2/3 cup blueberries and 6 pecans (chopped) 3/4 cup fat-free milk Coffee or tea	2 Multi-Grain Pancakes with syrup and strawberries *page 192* 1 tablespoon Smart Balance or Becel (in Canada) spread 3/4 cup fat-free milk	1 Spinach and Goat Cheese Omelet *page 194* 1/2 whole wheat English muffin 1/2 tablespoon Smart Balance or Becel (in Canada) spread 2 cantaloupe wedges Coffee or tea
2 Tuna and Carrot Sandwiches on Rye *page 222* 15 Spiced Almonds *page 203* 1 peach Unsweetened iced tea	Whole wheat wrap with 3 slices lean ham, 2 slices low-fat Muenster cheese, lettuce, and tomato 1 1/2 cups grapes 1/2 cup low-fat fruit yogurt with 2 tablespoons ground flaxseeds Water with lemon	2 1/2 cups Curried Red Lentil Soup *page 224* 2 tablespoons hummus 8 baby carrots Water	1 2/3 cups Whole Wheat Chicken and Noodles with Peanut Sauce *page 214* 1/4 cup edamame 2 pineapple slices Water with lemon
1 Oatmeal–Peanut Butter Trail Bar *page 207*	2 cups popcorn mixed with 7 peanuts and 1 tablespoon Smart Balance or Becel (in Canada) spread	2 ounces (60 grams) semi-soft goat cheese drizzled with lemon juice 2 Wasa Crispbread rye crackers	4 whole wheat pretzel sticks 1 stick reduced-fat string cheese
6 ounces (170 grams) Flank Steak with Balsamic Sauce *page 228* 1 cup brown rice 2 cups salad with romaine lettuce, cherry tomatoes, cucumber, 1/2 cup chickpeas, and 1 tablespoon each olive oil and vinegar Water	2 1/4 cups Shrimp and Orzo Casserole *page 251* 1 cup steamed green beans 2 cups baby spinach salad with tomato, cucumber, and 1 tablespoon each olive oil and balsamic vinegar Unsweetened iced tea	2 1/2 cups Slow-Cooker Beef and Vegetable Stew *page 228* 1 slice Whole Wheat Flaxseed Bread *page 196* 2 1/2 cups salad with romaine lettuce, cherry tomatoes, cucumber, and 1 tablespoon each olive oil and vinegar Water with lemon	2 3/4 cups Spring Vegetable Stir-Fry with Tofu *page 260* 1 cup brown rice Green tea
		3/4 cup Orange and Pomegranate Compote *page 278*	3/4 cup Instant Strawberry Frozen Yogurt *page 277*
Calories: 2232; Protein: 121 g; Carbohydrate: 272 g; Fat: 73 g; Fiber: 44 g Percentage of calories from carbs: 49; protein: 22; fat: 29	Calories: 2177; Protein: 124 g; Carbohydrate: 248 g; Fat: 77 g; Fiber: 42 g Percentage of calories from carbs: 46; protein: 23; fat: 32	Calories: 2221; Protein: 126 g; Carbohydrate: 256 g; Fat: 75 g; Fiber: 55 g Percentage of calories from carbs: 46; protein: 23; fat: 30	Calories: 2201; Protein: 126 g; Carbohydrate: 275 g; Fat: 76 g; Fiber: 43 g Percentage of calories from carbs: 50; protein: 23; fat: 31

index

Page numbers in *italic* type indicate recipe titles. Page numbers in **bold italic** type indicate recipe photos.